# CURRENT

# PRACTICE IN

# Ophthalmology

**LAWRENCE W. HIRST,** MD
Lions Professor
Department of Ophthalmology
Princess Alexandra Hospital
Brisbane, Australia

**GARY N. HOLLAND,** MD
Associate Professor of Ophthalmology
Director, UCLA Ocular Inflammatory Disease
    Center
Jules Stein Eye Institute
University of California Los Angeles School of
    Medicine
Los Angeles, California

**HENRY D. JAMPEL,** MD
Assistant Professor
The Wilmer Ophthalmological Institute
The Johns Hopkins University School of
    Medicine
Baltimore, Maryland

**CHARLES D. KELMAN,** MD
Clinical Professor
Department of Ophthalmology
New York Medical College
New York, New York

**JAMES E. KEY,** MD
Clinical Associate Professor
Department of Ophthalmology
Baylor College of Medicine
Houston, Texas

**LANNING B. KLINE,** MD
Associate Professor
Departments of Ophthalmology, Neurology,
    and Neurosurgery
University of Alabama School of Medicine
Birmingham, Alabama

**RICHARD L. LINDSTROM,** MD
Clinical Professor
Department of Ophthalmology
University of Minnesota School of Medicine
Minneapolis, Minnesota

**JAN M. McDONNELL,** MD
Departments of Ophthalmology and
    Pathology
Estelle Doheny Eye Institute
University of Southern California School of
    Medicine
Los Angeles, California

**PETER J. McDONNELL,** MD
Associate Professor
Department of Ophthalmology
Estelle Doheny Eye Institute
University of Southern California School of
    Medicine
Los Angeles, California

**RONALD G. MICHELS,** MD
Deceased

**CARLOS AUGUSTO MOREIRA, Jr.,** MD
Prof de Oftalmologia da Fac. Evangelica de
    Medicina
Curitiba, Brasil

**G. EDWARD MORGAN,** MD
Vice Chairman and Assistant Professor of
    Anesthesiology
Department of Anesthesiology
University of Southern California School of
    Medicine
Los Angeles, California

**J. DANIEL NELSON,** MD
Associate Professor
Department of Ophthalmology
University of Minnesota
Minneapolis, Minnesota

**ROBERT B. NUSSENBLATT,** MD
Director, Clinical Branch
National Eye Institute
Laboratory of Immunology
Bethesda, Maryland

**TERRENCE P. O'BRIEN,** MD
Assistant Professor
The Wilmer Ophthalmological Institute
The Johns Hopkins University School of
    Medicine
Baltimore, Maryland

**PAUL PALMBERG,** MD, PhD
Associate Professor
Department of Ophthalmology
Bascom Palmer Eye Institute
University of Miami School of Medicine
Miami, Florida

**ARNALL PATZ,** MD
Professor
The Wilmer Ophthalmological Institute
The Johns Hopkins University School of
    Medicine
Baltimore, Maryland

**IRVIN P. POLLACK,** MD
Director, Kreiger Eye Institute
Sinai Hospital
Baltimore, Maryland

**MICHAEL J. POTTER,** MD
The Wilmer Ophthalmological Institute
The Johns Hopkins University School of
    Medicine
Baltimore, Maryland

**PETER A. RAPOZA,** MD
Assistant Professor
Department of Ophthalmology
University of Wisconsin Medical School
Madison, Wisconsin

**VIVIAN RISMONDO,** MD
Departments of Ophthalmology and
    Neurological Surgery
University of Southern California School of
    Medicine
Los Angeles, California

**ALAN ROBIN,** MD
Associate Professor
The Wilmer Ophthalmological Institute
The Johns Hopkins University School of
    Medicine
Baltimore, Maryland

**BENJAMIN RUBIN,** MD
National Eye Institute
Laboratory of Immunology
Bethesda, Maryland

**GARY S. RUBIN,** MD
Assistant Professor
The Wilmer Ophthalmological Institute
The Johns Hopkins University School of
    Medicine
Baltimore, Maryland

**ALFREDO A. SADUN,** MD
Associate Professor
Departments of Ophthalmology and
    Neurological Surgery
University of Southern California School of
    Medicine
Los Angeles, California

**JAMES SALZ,** MD
Clinical Professor
Department of Ophthalmology
University of Southern California School of
    Medicine
Los Angeles, California

**MARK R. SAWUSCH,** MD
Department of Ophthalmology
Estelle Doheny Eye Institute
University of Southern California School of
    Medicine
Los Angeles, California

**ANDREW P. SCHACHAT,** MD
Associate Professor
The Wilmer Ophthalmological Institute
The Johns Hopkins University School of
    Medicine
Baltimore, Maryland

**ARTHUR L. SCHWARTZ,** MD, FACS
Assistant Clinical Professor
Department of Ophthalmology
Georgetown University School of Medicine
Washington, DC

**DANIEL J. SIGBAND,** MD, FACS
Huntington Beach, California

**LAWRENCE J. SINGERMAN,** MD
Associate Clinical Professor
Case Western Reserve University School of
    Medicine
Cleveland, Ohio

**DAVID B. SOLL,** MD
Clinical Professor of Surgery
University of Medicine and Dentistry of New
 Jersey
Camden, New Jersey

**H. KAZ SOONG,** MD
Associate Professor
Department of Ophthalmology
Kellogg Eye Center
University of Michigan Medical School
Ann Arbor, Michigan

**GISÈLE SOUBRANE,** MD
Assistant Clinical Professor
Department of Ophthalmology
University of Paris
Paris, France

**WALTER J. STARK,** MD
Professor
The Wilmer Ophthalmological Institute
The Johns Hopkins University School of
 Medicine
Baltimore, Maryland

**PAUL STERNBERG, Jr.,** MD
Associate Professor
Department of Ophthalmology
Emory University School of Medicine
Atlanta, Georgia

**MICHAEL E. SULEWSKI,** MD
Scheie Eye Institute
Philadelphia, Pennsylvania

**JON WALKER,** MD
Pasadena, California

**JOHN J. WASENKO,** MD
Department of Radiology
University of Alabama School of Medicine
Birmingham, Alabama

**C.P. WILKINSON,** MD
Clinical Professor
Dean A. McGee Eye Institute
Department of Ophthalmology
University of Oklahoma Health Sciences
 Center
Oklahoma City, Oklahoma

*To our families*

# Preface

This book is intended to bridge the gap between journal manuscripts and the subspecialty texts. Journal articles rarely contain the practical "how to" material—the kind of material highlighted in this book.

Each chapter is written by an expert in the field and is either a review of a disease, treatment, drug, or surgical technique that will be of interest to the practicing ophthalmologist. There are "pro" and "con" contributions, highlighting current areas of controversy, and important contributions from ancillary fields such as anesthesia and pathology. While this book is not intended to be encyclopedic, many important topics in ophthalmology are covered. The editors hope that the readers will find the material accessible, helpful, and interesting.

**Andrew P. Schachat**

# Contents

## PART II
## THE EVOLUTION OF CURRENT PRACTICE—THEN AND NOW

# PART I

# CURRENT PRACTICE

# 1 AIDS and the Eye: New Concepts and Emerging Problems

James P. Dunn, Jr., MD
Gary N. Holland, MD

Ten years ago the acquired immunodeficiency syndrome (AIDS) was unknown and unnamed. Despite intensive research efforts that have identified its cause and epidemiologic features, AIDS has reached epidemic proportions and become a leading cause of morbidity and mortality world wide. Between 1981, when the first case of AIDS was reported, and mid-1990, over 125,000 cases have been reported in the United States alone, and there are an estimated 1 to 1.5 million asymptomatic carriers of the causative agent, human immunodeficiency virus (HIV).

AIDS is the most severe in a spectrum of clinical states caused by HIV infection. Some HIV-infected patients develop a set of debilitating problems such as lymphadenopathy, weight loss, and fevers that do not fulfill criteria for a diagnosis of AIDS; these patients are commonly said to have "AIDS-related complex" (ARC). Recent cohort studies suggest that over half of all infected patients will develop the full AIDS illness within 10 years, and it is believed by many that 99% will eventually do so. Despite fears of extensive spread of AIDS into the general population, AIDS remains primarily associated with the well-known risk factors of male homosexuality or bisexuality, intravenous drug use, transfusion with contaminated blood products, heterosexual intercourse with an infected partner (with greater risk to female partners of HIV-infected males than vice-versa), and congenital infection of children born to HIV-infected mothers. There has been an increase in the number of heterosexuals with AIDS, but they remain for the most part in previously established risk groups, particularly intravenous drug users and their sexual partners.

Most ophthalmologists are now familiar with the more common ocular manifestations of AIDS: cytomegalovirus (CMV) retinitis, cotton-wool spots, and conjunctival Kaposi sarcoma (KS) (see box on p. 2). There are numerous reviews of these manifestations in the ophthalmic literature,[1-4] and it is not the intent of this chapter to review that basic information. Instead this chapter will emphasize recent advances in diagnosis and treatment, discuss atypical manifestations of AIDS-related diseases, and highlight ongoing controversies in the management of ocular disorders among HIV-infected patients.

Although AIDS remains a fatal disease, survival is now longer than in the early years of the epidemic. Advances have been made in treatment of both the HIV infection itself and the secondary infections and malignancies associated with

## Ophthalmic Disorders Associated with the Acquired Immunodeficiency Syndrome

I. Vascular disease
  A. Microvasculopathy
    1. Retina
        a. Cotton-wool spots
        b. Retinal hemorrhages
        c. Microaneurysms
        d. Ischemic maculopathy (rare)
    2. Conjunctiva
        a. Dilated capillaries
        b. Microaneurysms
        c. Vessels of irregular caliber
        d. Isolated vessel segments
        e. Sludging of blood flow
    3. Optic nerve
        a. Ischemic optic neuropathy (rare)
  B. Central retinal vein occlusion
II. Opportunistic ocular infectious diseases
  A. Retinal and choroidal pathogens
    1. Cytomegalovirus
    2. *Cryptococcus neoformans*
    3. *Toxoplasma gondii*
    4. *Mycobacterium avium* complex
    5. Herpes simplex virus
    6. Herpes zoster virus
    7. *Histoplasma capsulatum*
    8. *Candida albicans* (uncommon)
    9. *Pneumocystis carinii*
  B. Ocular surface/external pathogens
    1. Herpes zoster virus
    2. Herpes simplex virus
    3. *Microsporidia species*
    4. Cytomegalovirus
    5. *Candida albicans*
    6. Molluscum contagiosum virus
III. Neoplasms
  A. Kaposi sarcoma
    1. Eyelids
    2. Conjunctiva
    3. Orbit
  B. Burkitt lymphoma
    1. Orbit
IV. Neuroophthalmic signs of intracranial disease
  A. Cranial nerve palsies
  B. Visual field defects
  C. Papilledema
  D. Pupillary abnormalities
  E. Optic atrophy
  F. Abnormal saccades

it. Zidovudine (azidothymidine or AZT) has been shown in controlled trials to prolong survival and decrease the frequency of opportunistic infections in some patients with AIDS or ARC. It appears to delay progression of the disease in HIV-infected patients with early symptoms and in those with no symptoms but with fewer than 500 cells/ml of a specific subset of circulating lymphocytes called CD4 cells. It may have a role in preventing HIV infection following exposure, but failure of zidovudine prophylaxis has been reported. Hematological toxicity, primarily bone marrow suppression, has limited the drug's usefulness. Currently recommended dosages (100 mg PO every 4 hours while awake) appear equally effective, with much less toxicity than the higher doses previously used. Dideoxyinosine (DDI), another drug with activity against HIV, has also been approved by the FDA. DDI is minimally toxic to bone marrow and may emerge as an important treatment for HIV infection.

Increased survival has also resulted from improved therapy for opportunistic infections associated with AIDS. Prophylaxis against *Pneumocystis carinii* pneumonia (PCP) with aerosolized pentamidine or trimethoprim-sulfamethoxazole, both in previously infected patients and in those individuals with fewer than 200 CD4 cells/ml, has reduced mortality from this disease. Fluconazole (Diflucan) appears as effective in the prevention of recurrent cryptococcal meningitis as amphotericin B but has fewer adverse effects. There is even limited evidence that ganciclovir and foscarnet may increase the lifespan of patients infected with CMV.

The longer and more productive lifespan of HIV-infected patients increases the need for prompt recognition and effective treatment of ocular disease. It is anticipated that prolonged survival and use of new drugs will be associated with the emergence of atypical disease patterns and possibly the emergence of entirely new ones. Furthermore, treatments for these diseases will bring about their own problems resulting from side effects of medications. Among the challenges facing ophthalmologists in the 1990s will be the need to keep abreast of developments in AIDS, to recognize its changing manifestations, and to intervene appropriately as new treatments are introduced.

## CMV RETINITIS

CMV retinitis is the only common opportunistic infection of the eye in AIDS patients. It is a necrotizing retinopathy that is seen exclusively in immunosuppressed individuals. For unknown reasons it is more commonly associated with AIDS than with other immunodeficiency states; it is seen in approximately 25% of AIDS patients, and it is the leading cause of blindness in this group. CMV rarely infects ocular tissues other than the retina, and it has not been shown to cause any other diseases of the eye.

The presence of CMV retinitis fulfills CDC criteria for the diagnosis of AIDS, and rarely CMV retinitis will be the presenting manifestation of AIDS. Because of referral bias, however, as many as 10% of patients with CMV retinitis seen in some centers will not yet have a diagnosis of AIDS. Ophthalmologists, therefore, should be alert to other manifestations of AIDS in patients who present with a necrotizing retinopathy.

CMV retinitis is generally both a late manifestation and a poor prognostic sign, reflecting waning immunity in the late stages of the disease. The median time between the diagnosis of AIDS and the onset of CMV retinitis is about 9 to 10 months. The median survival after a diagnosis of CMV retinitis is 7 to 12 months in various series.[5]

Diagnosis of CMV retinitis is based on clinical criteria alone. The high prevalence of past CMV infection, not only in AIDS patients but in the general population as well, means that isolation of CMV from other body sites or the presence of antibodies against CMV does not establish the diagnosis. Conversely, the absence of antibodies does not necessarily rule out CMV because antibody production may wane in later stages of AIDS. Isolation of the virus by endoretinal biopsy is possible in particularly difficult cases, but the risks of the procedure are too great for routine diagnostic use. In certain cases, where the cause of a retinitis in an AIDS patient cannot be ascertained and retinal detachment is present, endoretinal biopsy may be indicated; in situ hybridization has been used to demonstrate infectious organisms in such tissue. In most cases, though, the clinical characteristics of the lesions themselves are sufficient for accurate diagnosis of CMV infection.

## Clinical Features

The classic appearance of CMV retinitis consists of densely opaque retinal lesions with blotchy hemorrhage and vasculitis. In AIDS patients there may be a spectrum to the appearance of lesions. The classic appearance has come to be known as the "fulminant/edematous" type, and is usually found in the posterior pole adjacent to blood vessels (Figure 1-1). The "indolent/granular" type, on the other hand, has less dense opacification, little or no hemorrhage, and no vasculitis. These lesions are more common in the retinal periphery (Figure 1-2).

The common feature of both is a very dry, granular-appearing border. Neither form has much vitreous inflammatory reaction overlying the lesions. Accurate diagnosis of all cases makes it important to recognize that different forms of CMV retinitis lesions may exist, but there does not appear to be any prognostic or other clinical significance to the distinction of different types.

Atypical patterns should suggest other causes of retinitis. Rapidly progressive, deep homogenous retinal opacification without granularity is more likely to be caused by herpes zoster or possibly herpes simplex virus infection (Figure 1-3). A prominent inflammatory reaction should suggest toxoplasmosis (Figure 1-4), fungal infection, or syphilis (Figure 1-5).

A standardized system for the description of CMV retinitis and its response to treatment has been described.[6] It has been useful in studying the efficacy of new treatment regimens and for describing the course of the disease. (Terms used to describe CMV retinitis are listed in the box on p. 8).

## Treatment

Ethical and social considerations have made rigidly controlled, prospective, and randomized trials of different therapies for CMV retinitis very difficult to perform. There has nonetheless developed a consensus that ganciclovir (DHPG), a viral DNA polymerase inhibitor, is effective in controlling CMV retinitis (Figure 1-6).[6,7] On the basis of extensive experience on "compassionate use" protocols, the drug

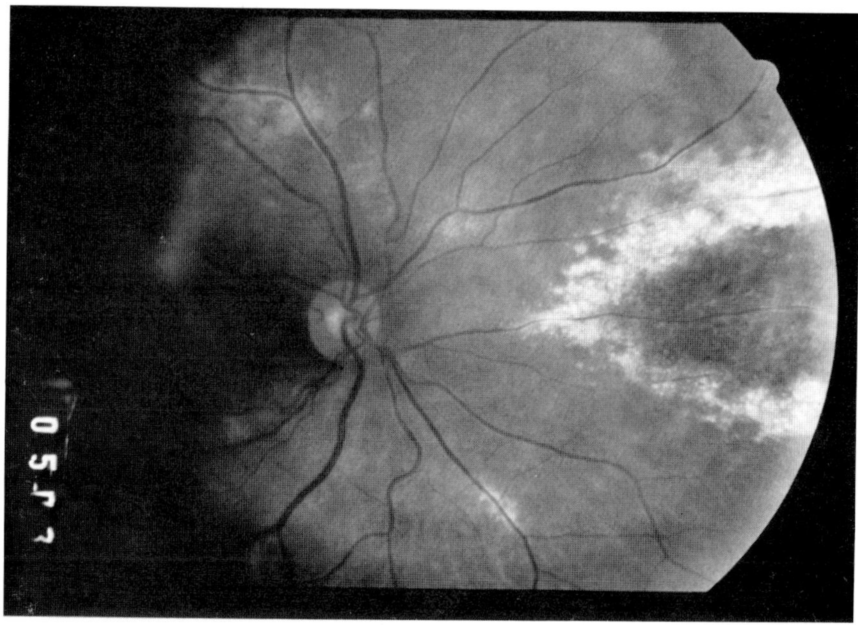

**FIGURE 1-1**    CMV retinitis. The classic appearance of the disease consists of a patch of retinal necrosis and edema with granular-appearing, irregular borders extending along retinal vessels. There may be hemorrhage and vasculitis. The overlying vitreous is clear.

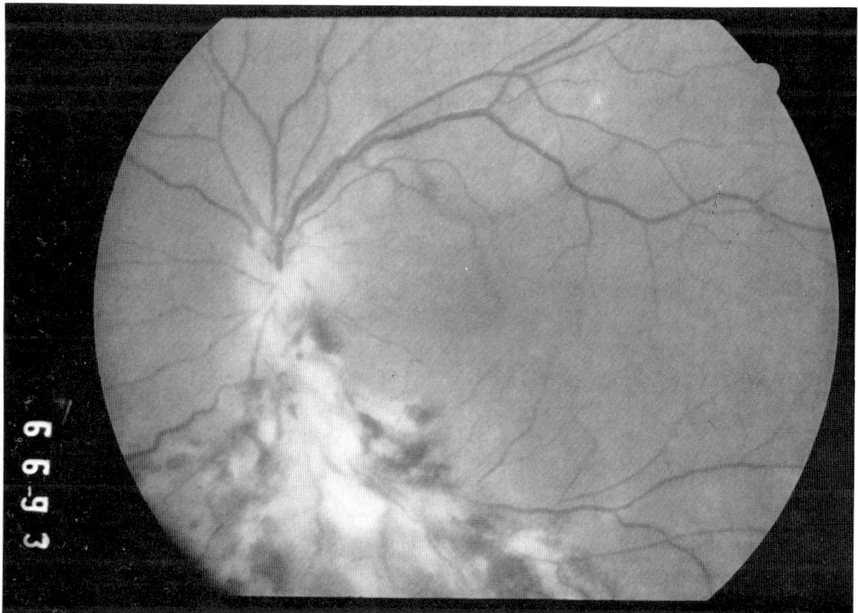

**FIGURE 1-2**    CMV retinitis. Some patients have a more indolent-appearing form of disease, with less retinal whitening and little or no hemorrhage. These lesions have the granular border characteristic of all CMV retinitis lesions. This form of disease is more common in the retinal periphery.

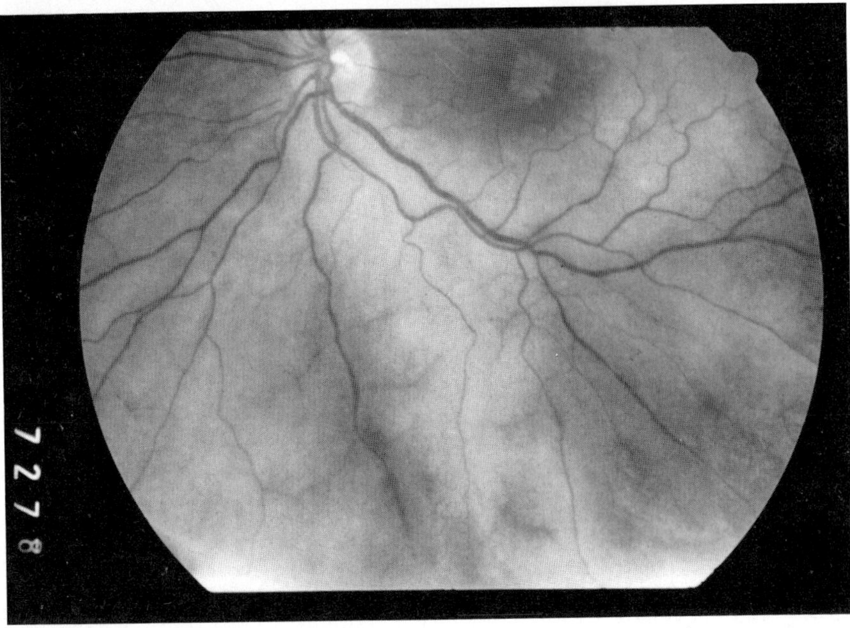

**FIGURE 1-3**     Herpes zoster virus retinitis. This infection progressed to destroy the entire retina over a 2-week period. It was characterized by a deep, homogeneous opacification of the retina.

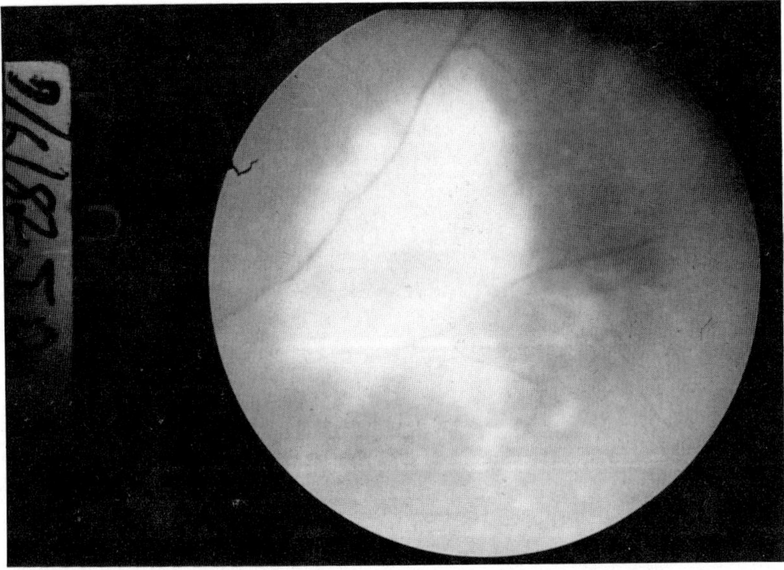

**FIGURE 1-4**     Toxoplasmic retinochoroiditis. This patch of retinal necrosis, caused by *Toxoplasma gondii* infection, is associated with a much greater amount of vitreous inflammation than would be seen with CMV retinitis.

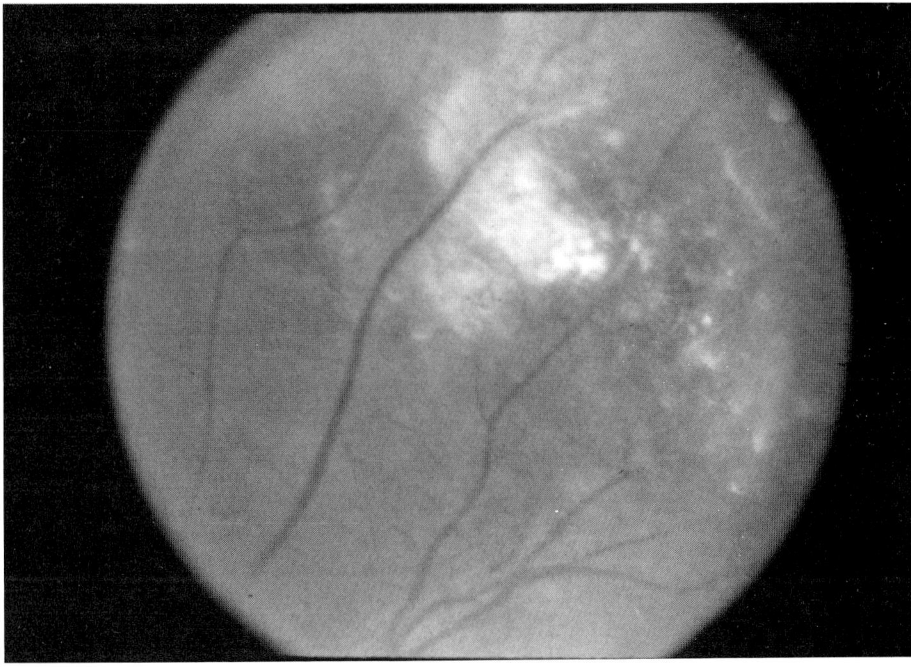

**FIGURE 1-5**    Syphilitic retinitis. This patch of granular retinal infiltration was differentiated from CMV retinitis by the patient's marked vitreous and anterior-chamber inflammatory reaction and positive serological tests for syphilis.

was approved by the Food and Drug Administration for use in the treatment of CMV retinitis in 1989.

Ganciclovir is virostatic only, meaning that recurrence following discontinuation of the treatment will be inevitable. Experience with the drug has led to a standard dosage regimen. An initial course of "induction therapy" (5mg/kg IV twice daily for 2 weeks) is used to bring the retinitis under control, followed by indefinite "maintenance therapy" to prevent reactivation (5 mg/kg IV once daily or, less commonly, 6 mg/kg IV 5 days per week).

Patients are seen regularly to monitor their response to treatment. Patients should be seen before treatment begins, at the end of induction therapy, then periodically during maintenance therapy. Examination 2 weeks after the end of induction and at monthly intervals thereafter is a schedule used by many ophthalmologists who treat large numbers of patients with CMV retinitis. Stabilization of lesions is generally seen by the end of induction, but lesions may not become inactive for 2 to 4 weeks after the start of maintenance therapy. Some lesions never become completely inactive; but a lack of progression, despite some residual whiteness, is still considered successful therapy.

Treatment with intravenous ganciclovir has demonstrated the following:
- Lack of progression by the end of induction therapy in 50% to 80% of patients.[6,7]
- Prevention of or reduced involvement of the second eye in unilateral CMV retinitis.[7]

---

### A Glossary of Terms Used in the Evaluation and Management of CMV Retinitis

| | |
|---|---|
| **Zone 1** | The area 3000 microns from the center of the macula or 1500 microns from the border of the optic nerve head; CMV retinitis in this area is considered to be immediately vision-threatening. |
| **Zone 2** | The area anterior to zone 1 extending to the anterior border of the ampullae of the vortex veins; generally the farthest area anteriorly that can be photographed easily. |
| **Zone 3** | The area anterior to zone 2, extending to the ora serrata. |
| **"Peripheral lesions"** | An inexact term generally used to denote the infection in zones 2 and 3 only. |
| **Active lesions** | Those lesions with opaque or white borders, indicating "active" viral disease. |
| **Inactive lesions** | Those with no opacity of the border. They appear as transparent retina scars with faint pigmentary mottling. |
| **Progression** | Enlargement of prexisting lesions (identified on retinal photographs as advancement of borders into previously uninfected retina) or development of discrete new lesions. |
| **Stabilization** | No progression and no change in border opacification. |
| **Improvement** | Used only for lesions without progression; indicates decreased border opacity and, presumably, decreased viral activity. |
| **Deterioration** | Used only for lesions without progression; indicates increased border opacity and, presumably, increased viral activity. Progression usually follows deterioration after a short period of time. |

Adapted from Holland GN, Buhles WC, Mastre B, Kaplan HJ, the UCLA CMV Retinopathy Study Group. A controlled retrospective study on ganciclovir treatment for cytomegalovirus retinopathy: use of a standardized system for the assessment of disease outcome. Arch Ophthalmol 1989; 107:1759-1766.

---

- Possibly increased survival of patients with CMV retinitis,[5] particularly cases in which lesions became inactive.[7] This effect, if it is in fact real, is probably due to the drug's action against CMV in nonocular sites.

Reactivation and progression of CMV retinitis while patients are on maintenance therapy after initial control (sometimes referred to as "breakthrough") has been reported to occur in 27% to 50% of cases (Figure 1-7). Some investigators believe that all patients will have reactivation of disease if they survive long enough.

The average time between the end of induction therapy and reactivation is significantly longer in patients receiving maintenance therapy than in patients who for some reason do not receive the drug after induction therapy. Reactivation is usually treated with a course of "reinduction" therapy in which the patient is given another 2 week course of twice-daily medication. Many patients can be reinduced multiple times if reactivation occurs repeatedly. Continuous induction levels of medication to prevent any reactivation are believed to be too toxic, however.

Intravenous ganciclovir has a number of side effects, the most serious of which is bone marrow toxicity. Up to 38% of treated patients develop severe

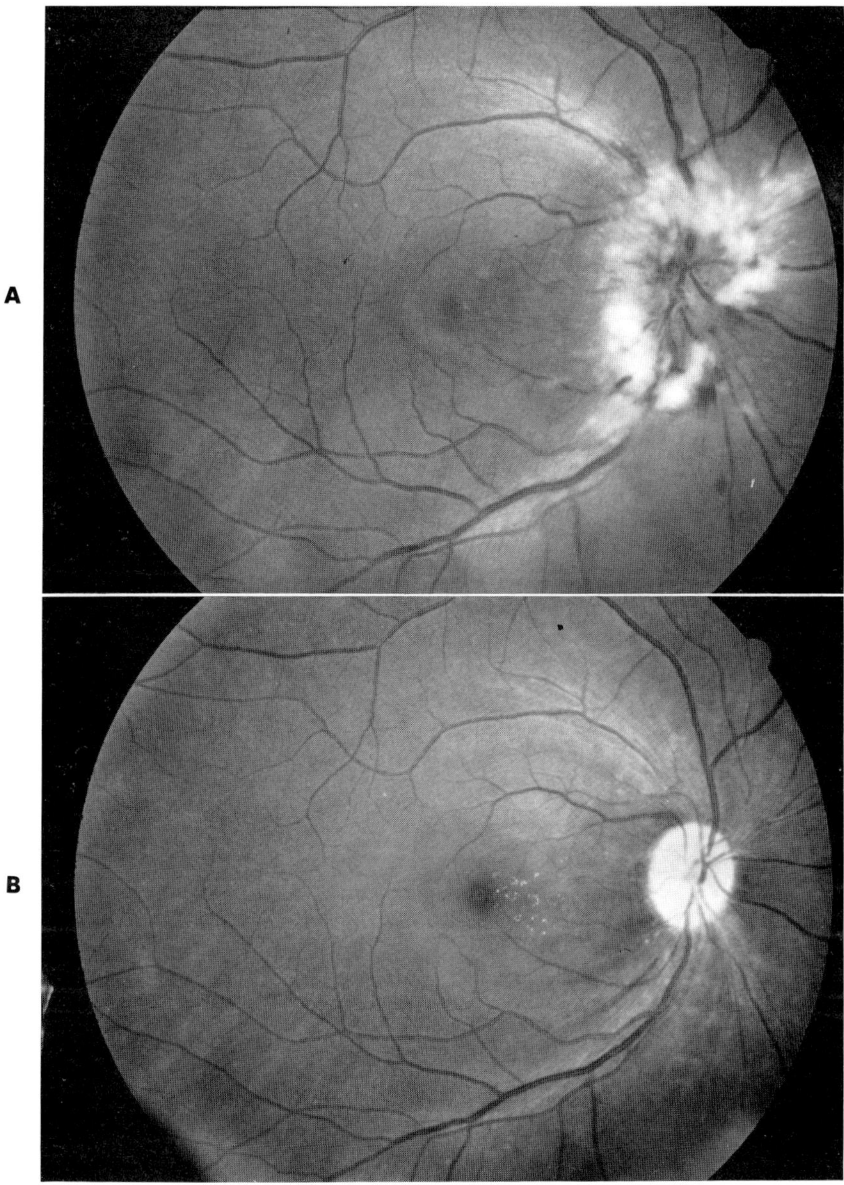

**FIGURE 1-6**     **A,** An untreated focus of CMV retinitis involving the peripapillary retina at the time of diagnosis. **B,** The same eye after one month of ganciclovir therapy. The infection is inactive and the patient retains 20/20 acuity in the eye.

neutropenia, necessitating discontinuation of maintenance therapy. Another disadvantage of its marrow-suppressive effect is that administration of ganciclovir makes it difficult to simultaneously give patients zidovudine, which also causes bone marrow suppression. Thrombocytopenia has also been reported. Granulocyte-monocyte colony stimulating factor (GM-CSF) is an investigational hematologic growth factor that may reduce neutropenia in these cases.

Another problem with ganciclovir therapy is the fact that it can be given only intravenously. Daily therapy for the remainder of a patient's life requires that

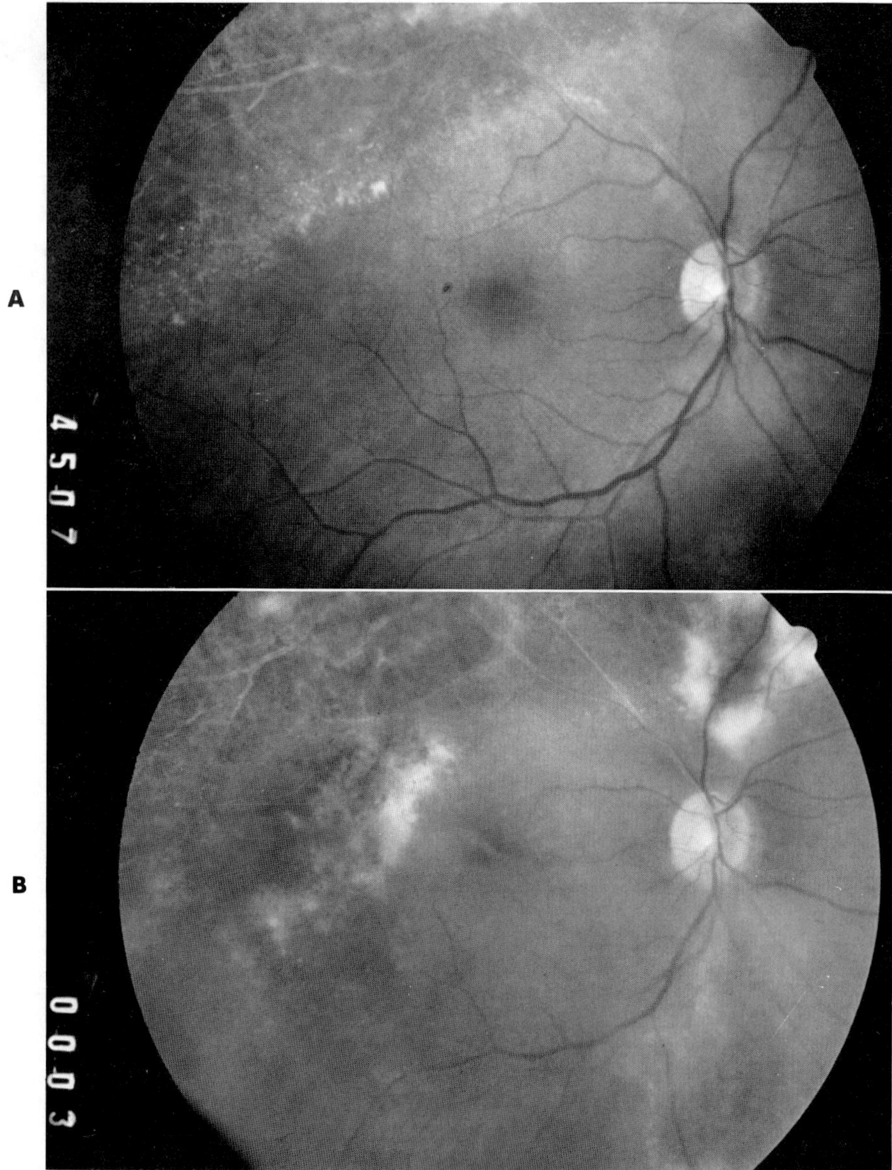

**FIGURE 1-7**    **A,** An eye with a treated focus of CMV retinitis superior and temporal to the fovea. The border of the lesion is seen as a faintly opaque line. **B,** Reactivation of CMV retinitis in the same eye, despite continued ganciclovir maintenance therapy. The border is now more opaque and closer to the optic nerve head and fovea.

an indwelling catheter be placed, and the potential for sepsis from an infected catheter is a constant source of concern. An oral form of ganciclovir, however, is in the early stages of investigation. Currently it is being used only in certain patients who have had successful induction therapy with intravenous ganciclovir.

Concern about the side effects of intravenous ganciclovir has stimulated the search for other approaches to the treatment of CMV retinitis. A regimen of intravitreal ganciclovir (200 micrograms in 0.1 ml injected into the midvitreous twice weekly for induction therapy, followed by once-weekly injections for maintenance therapy) has been successful in some cases.[8] Questions remain about the toxicity of the intravitreal preparation, and the risks of the injection itself include retinal detachment and endophthalmitis. This technique therefore should probably be limited to patients who cannot tolerate intravenous ganciclovir.

Foscarnet (trisodium phosphonoformate) is another viral DNA polymerase inhibitor with in vitro activity against CMV. Like ganciclovir, foscarnet is only virostatic; maintenance therapy is therefore required. Although the optimal dosages remain to be worked out, the drug has shown promise in early trials.[9] Its major advantage is lack of bone marrow suppression, making it compatible with zidovudine. However, it too is a very toxic drug. Its major side effects are renal.

A summary of the various approved and investigational treatment regimens used for CMV retinitis is given in Table 1-1. An important update concerning the results of a multi-center trial comparing foscarnet and ganciclovir appears on p. 31.

There are several reports of CMV retinitis control using zidovudine alone,[10,11] although the effect is observed long after zidovudine therapy is started. This response must be indirect since the drug has no activity against CMV itself. It may reflect the overall improvement in immune status that zidovudine induces, or perhaps it is related to its effect on HIV in the retina, which is believed to facilitate active CMV infection of the retina. Because of the lag in the onset of its effect on CMV retinitis and because it is not particularly effective in most cases, zidovudine should never be considered as a first-line drug for the treatment of CMV retinitis.

Deciding which patients with CMV retinitis should be treated raises several questions. The cost and inconvenience of therapy, the toxicity of the available drugs, and the risk of sepsis from indwelling catheters must be weighed against the need for control of the retinal infection. A few patients choose to leave CMV retinitis untreated if it involves only one eye, particularly if treatment means discontinuation of zidovudine. Untreated patients must be followed closely, however.

Similarly, the progression of peripheral lesions among patients on maintenance therapy does not necessarily mandate reinduction with a higher dose of ganciclovir and its attendant toxicity. A slowing of progression may be sufficient to prevent macular involvement, thereby preserving central vision for the remainder of the patient's life.

When to initiate treatment for peripheral lesions is the most controversial aspect of therapy. Treatment of peripheral lesions minimizes enlargement; since large lesions may be more prone to retinal detachment, early treatment may reduce the incidence of retinal detachment. There is some evidence, however, that the risk of retinal detachment is increased in treated cases of CMV retinitis, possibly because treatment hastens the involutional stage of disease, in which the retina thins and holes form. Treatment reduces the development of new lesions and frequency of bilateral involvement. On the other hand, the fovea is rarely the first site of CMV retinitis and typically the last area involved as the disease spreads. Because peripheral lesions progress slowly, central vision may be maintained in an untreated eye for the duration of a patient's life. Also, treatment may or may not have an effect on certain visual symptoms such as floaters. Finally the effect of treatment for CMV infection on patient survival is undecided. Ultimately, de-

**Table 1-1**   Treatment Options for CMV Retinitis

| Treatment | Status | Indications | Dosage | Management considerations |
|---|---|---|---|---|
| Intravenous ganciclovir (DHPG) | FDA-approved | Immediately vision-threatening lesions in one or both eyes in patients who retain good vision. Possible benefit (efficacy uncertain): 1. Lesions in zones 2,3 ("peripheral disease"); 2. Preservation of remaining vision in patients who already have decreased vision from macular lesions. | Induction therapy: 5.0 mg/kg IV q12h × 14d. Followed by maintenance therapy 5.0 mg/kg IV qd, 7 days/week or 6.0 mg/kg IV qd, 5 days/week. | 1. Appropriate examination schedule: at start of induction, at end of induction, after 2 weeks of maintenance therapy, monthly thereafter if no progression noted. 2. "Reinduction therapy" if new lesions develop or enlargement occurs near zone 1. 3. Major toxicity: bone marrow suppression (neutropenia) |
| Intravitreal ganciclovir | Investigational | Patients with progressive retinitis in one or both eyes who cannot tolerate systematic therapy. | 200 mg in 0.1 cc into midvitreous twice weely until stabilization, then once weekly. | 1. 300 mg injections have been tried in refractory cases. 2. Potential side effects: retinal drug toxicity, retinal detachments, endophthalmitis. |
| Ganciclovir plus granulocyte-monocyte colony stimulating factor (GM-CSF) | Investigational | GM-CSF given to maintain acceptable neutrophil levels despite marrow toxicity of ganciclovir. | Optimal GM-CSF dosage regimen to be determined. | Effect of GM-CSF on CMV retinitis response to ganciclovir therapy not known. |
| Foscarnet | FDA-approved | As for ganciclovir patients with ganciclovir-resistant virus isolates; patients with progression despite maximum tolerated ganciclovir therapy; neutropenia precluding ganciclovir use. | Induction therapy: 60 mg/kg IV q8h × 14d. Followed by maintenance therapy 90 mg/kg IV qd. Dosage must be carefully adjusted for creatinine clearance. | Major side effects: renal toxicity; disruption of calcium, phosphate, magnesium metabolism; anemia; nausea |

cisions concerning therapy require that the ophthalmologist and the primary care provider give the patient a thorough explanation of the risks and benfits of treatment so that he or she can make an informed decision. In our experience, most patients choose to have their CMV retinitis treated regardless of its location.

Retinal detachments occur in 15% to 20% of treated patients.[7,12] Detachments do not seem to occur in patients with lesions confined to the posterior pole. Since the natural course of the untreated disease is one of relentless progression and blindness, the potential for increased risk of retinal detachment with treatment does not necessarily represent a contraindication to therapy. Retinal detachments in treated CMV retinitis, which usually involve multiple breaks, often are best treated with techniques such as vitrectomy and silicone oil.[12]

## ATYPICAL INFECTIONS
### Syphilis

There are many ocular manifestations of acquired syphilis, including iridocyclitis, vitritis, vasculitis, optic neuritis, and chorioretinitis, so that the disease is almost always in the differential diagnosis of ocular inflammation. Several recent reports have noted the coexistence of ocular syphilis and AIDS and have emphasized that concurrent HIV infection alters both the course of disease and response to conventional therapy.[13,14] Because syphilis is a treatable disease, it is essential to make the proper diagnosis. Frequently, however, the possibility of syphilis is overlooked; either syphilis is not even considered or the administration of corticosteroids temporarily reduces the inflammation, suggesting a noninfectious cause.

Syphilis is more aggressive in patients infected with HIV. Vitreal, retinal, and optic nerve involvement appear more commonly than in otherwise healthy patients with syphilis; and bilateral involvement may also be more frequent.[14] Two forms of posterior involvement have been seen in patients with ocular syphilis; some patients have large cream-colored subretinal plaques, while others have areas of grainy-appearing retinal infiltration (see Figure 1-5). The latter form of infection can be confused with CMV retinitis. Ocular syphilis is likely to be associated with a prominent anterior chamber reaction and a red, painful eye, findings that are not present in patients with CMV retinitis, which helps to differentiate these disorders.

Based on spinal fluid findings, there is an increased frequency of neurosyphilis in patients with AIDS; findings include reactive VDRL, lymphocytic pleocytosis, and elevated protein. The natural course of syphilis appears accelerated in HIV-infected individuals; typically late findings such as neurosyphilis may develop only a few months after primary infection occurs.

HIV infection may render the normal serologic pattern of syphilis unpredictable, so that a false negative VDRL may be obtained.[13] Therefore, all patients with syphilis should be tested for HIV antibodies and vice versa. The presence of both mandates examination of the cerebrospinal fluid to rule out neurosyphilis.

Ocular syphilis associated with HIV responds poorly to benzathine penicillin, the standard treatment for secondary syphilis. It is therefore recommended that infected patients be treated as if neurosyphilis is present; intravenous aqueous penicillin 12-24 MU daily for a minimum of ten days is the treatment of choice.

Because of the concern of recurrence, even after this regimen, patients should be examined frequently. Reagin titers should be measured monthly for three months and every six months thereafter.

## Toxoplasmosis

*Toxoplasma gondii* is a common opportunistic pathogen in AIDS patients and a leading cause of AIDS-related mortality. Toxoplasmosis in fact is the most common nonviral intracranial infection associated with AIDS. Ocular involvement in AIDS on the other hand is uncommon. Nevertheless ocular toxoplasmosis is occasionally the first serious disorder to affect an HIV-infected patient, and this may be the first manifestation of life-threatening disseminated *T. gondii* infection.

Ocular toxoplasmosis in AIDS patients differs clinically and histopathologically from that in immunocompetent patients,[15] making the diagnosis difficult in some cases. As with syphilis, a high degree of clinical suspicion is essential. The varied manifestations of AIDS-related toxoplasmic retinochoroiditis include single discrete lesions in one or both eyes, multifocal discrete lesions, and diffuse retinal necrosis (see Figure 1-4). Lesions rarely arise from the borders of preexisting scars, as they do in healthy adults. The retinochoroidal lesions often occur adjacent to retinal blood vessels, suggesting that they result from organisms that reach the eye via hematogenous spread, either in acquired disease or from reactivation in remote sites of the body. Characteristics of HIV-associated ocular toxoplasmosis are compared to those in healthy adults in Table 1-2.

Full-thickness retinal necrosis is usually present, but early lesions may be confined to the inner or outer retinal layers. Hemorrhage is usually minimal, which is one factor that may help to distinguish it from CMV retinitis. Iridocyclitis and vitritis are common and much more severe than in CMV retinitis. A red, painful eye may be the symptom that first brings the patient to the attention of the ophthalmologist.

**Table 1-2**   Characteristics of Ocular Toxoplasmosis in AIDS Patients Compared to Healthy Adults

| Route of infection | Laterality | Lesions | Treatment |
|---|---|---|---|
| **HIV-infected patients** | | | |
| Usually acquired disease or newly disseminated to the eye | May be unilateral or bilateral | May be multifocal May be small, round lesion or diffuse area of retinal necrosis | Antiparasitics No systemic steroids Maintenance therapy required |
| **Healthy adults** | | | |
| Usually recurrent disease | Active disease almost always unilateral (scars may be bilateral) | Almost always single lesion Usually a focus of intense inflammation at border of an atrophic scar | Antiparasitics Systemic steroids Finite course of therapy |

Like CMV retinitis, toxoplasmic retinochoroiditis can be complicated by rhegmatogenous retinal detachments. Lesions tend to enlarge progressively, becoming bigger than those seen in immunocompetent patients.

The differential diagnosis of ocular toxoplasmosis includes CMV retinitis, herpes simplex or herpes zoster virus retinitis, and *Candida* chorioretinitis. CMV retinitis and toxoplasmic retinochoroiditis may coinfect the retina.

Serologic diagnosis may be unreliable in patients with AIDS, since altered antibody responses are common in AIDS, especially late in the disease. IgM titers are usually low or negative; IgG titers are rarely as high as 1:1,024; and convalescent titers may not rise. Biopsy-proven toxoplasmosis with negative serologic tests has been reported.

The best treatment for ocular toxoplasmosis in AIDS is uncertain, but experience suggests that pyrimethamine in combination with at least one other antimicrobial agent such as clindamycin, sufadiazine, or even tetracycline is the treatment of choice. Folinic acid (Leucovorin) must be added to reduce pyrimethamine-induced thrombocytopenia. Corticosteroids, which are often used in immunocompetent individuals in the treatment of ocular toxoplasmosis, are not indicated because of their further immunosuppressive effect and because there is little intraretinal inflammation in areas of necrosis. Recurrence following cessation of therapy is frequent, and patients appear to require maintenance therapy to prevent reactivation. Ideal maintenance regimens have not been determined because of the bone marrow suppression associated with pyrimethamine and the frequent development of allergic reactions to sulfonamides in AIDS patients. In our experience, single-drug maintenance with clindamycin has proved to be one effective and tolerable treatment.

## Herpes Zoster Virus Infections

Herpes zoster ophthalmicus is usually a disease of older individuals. Seeing the disease in younger people should raise the possibility of HIV infection in the mind of the examiner.[16] It can be an early manifestation of HIV infection, before the onset of other disorders. It alone is an insufficient criterion to make a diagnosis of AIDS, but its presence appears to be a likely prognostic sign for development of the full AIDS illness.

When it is associated with HIV infection, zoster ophthalmicus is characterized by severe and prolonged cutaneous lesions, keratitis, and anterior uveitis.[17] Subsequent neurotrophic keratitis and chronic uveitis may be particularly difficult to treat. In otherwise healthy adults with zoster ophthalmicus, the virus can be cultured from the cornea only during the first 48 hours after the onset of acute keratitis. In contrast, a case was reported in an AIDS patient in which the virus was cultured from corneal scrapings 11 weeks after onset, suggesting that immunodeficiency may allow persistence of active viral disease.[18]

Recent reports have confirmed that herpes zoster virus can also infect the retina in patients with AIDS. In many cases it causes the rapidly progressive peripheral retinal destruction seen in the acute retina necrosis syndrome (ARN). An entity clinically distinct from ARN, characterized by patchy choroidal and deep retinal inflammation and edema with little or no vitreal reaction, has been found to be due to herpes zoster virus infection as well. In all cases the lack of dry granular borders and the rapid progression of disease help to distinguish herpes zoster virus infections from CMV retinitis (see Figure 1-3).

Acyclovir is the treatment of choice for herpes zoster virus infections. Oral drug (800 mg five times a day) is used at the onset of skin lesions in the distribution of the first division of the Trigeminal Nerve to reduce the severity and incidence of ocular involvement. Intravenous acyclovir must be used for disseminated infections and retinal infections because of its better bioavailability. Acyclovir ointment, which is not currently available in the United States, may play a role in persistent corneal disease. While topical steroids may be helpful, oral corticosteroids are probably contraindicated. Case reports have cited the usefulness of immune-enhancing agents such as cimetidine, but this observation has not been confirmed in other studies. Finally, antivirals such as trifluridine (Viroptic) and idoxuridine, which are effective against herpes simplex virus, are ineffective against herpes zoster virus.

## Herpes Simplex Virus Keratitis

It is not known whether the incidence of herpes simplex virus keratitis is increased in HIV-infected patients. A limited retrospective study suggested several atypical features of herpetic keratitis in AIDS patients when it does occur.[19] First, there was a predilection for marginal, as opposed to central, epithelial involvement (Figure 1-8). Second, the keratitis appeared to be more resistant to treatment with topical antivirals, with an average healing time of 3 weeks, compared to less than 2 weeks in immunocompetent patients. (This finding may simply reflect the location of the dendrites rather than the immunodeficiency, since peripheral dendrites take longer to heal in immunocompetent patients as well.) Oral acyclovir

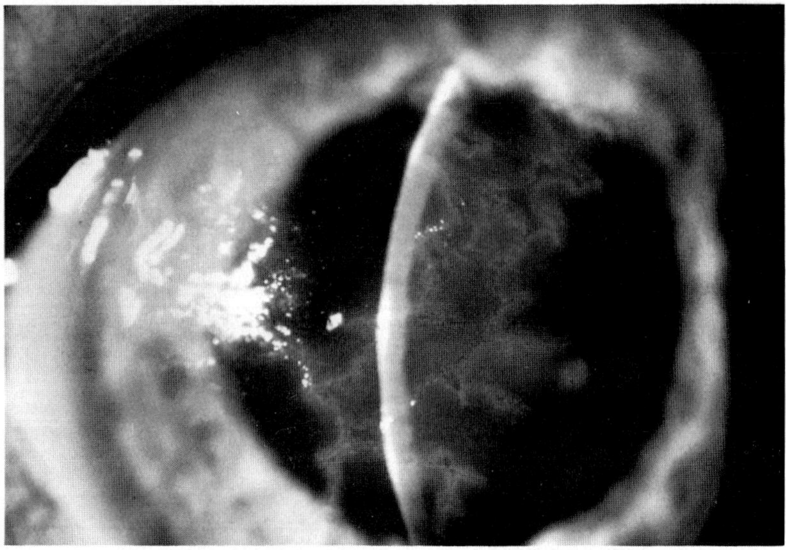

**FIGURE 1-8**     Herpes simplex virus epithelial keratitis. This lesion appeared to arise at the limbus with a large dendrite extending to the central cornea. The location and severity of this lesion are typical of those found in AIDS patients.

may be a useful adjunct to topical antiviral therapy in these patients, although the benefits of such therapy have not been established. Third, recurrences were more frequent in this group of AIDS patients and were lengthier than the original infection.

Severe cutaneous infections in AIDS patients due to HSV-2, which is resistant to conventional therapy are becoming more frequent. Vidarabine and foscarnet therapy may be useful in these cases. Whether ocular involvement with HSV will show the same pattern is unknown.

## Molluscum Contagiosum

In healthy individuals, the virus responsible for molluscum contagiosum causes a self-limited follicular conjunctivitis or keratitis if the lesions involve the eyelid margins. Many therapies, including curettage, can shorten the course of the disease. In the immunosuppressed host, the lesions are of rapid onset, tend to be larger and more numerous, and have a prolonged course (Figure 1-9). In many cases they are resistant to conventional treatments, although anecdotal reports indicate that cryotherapy may be helpful for eyelid margin lesions.

## Other Ocular Infections

Bacterial and fungal infections of the cornea have been reported infrequently in AIDS patients (Figure 1-10). Bacterial corneal ulcers have usually been associated with such predisposing factors as trauma or contact-lens wear. Fungal ulcers, on the other hand, have occurred spontaneously, in contrast to such occurrences in otherwise healthy patients where fungal infection usually follows some form of trauma.

Because of diminished host immune defenses, these infections may be par-

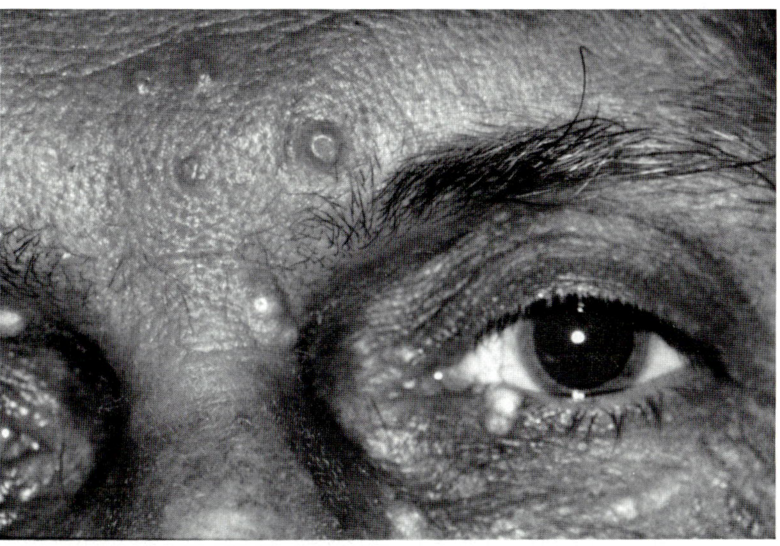

**FIGURE 1-9**  *Molluscum contagiosum.* Numerous nodules are present on the face and eyelids.

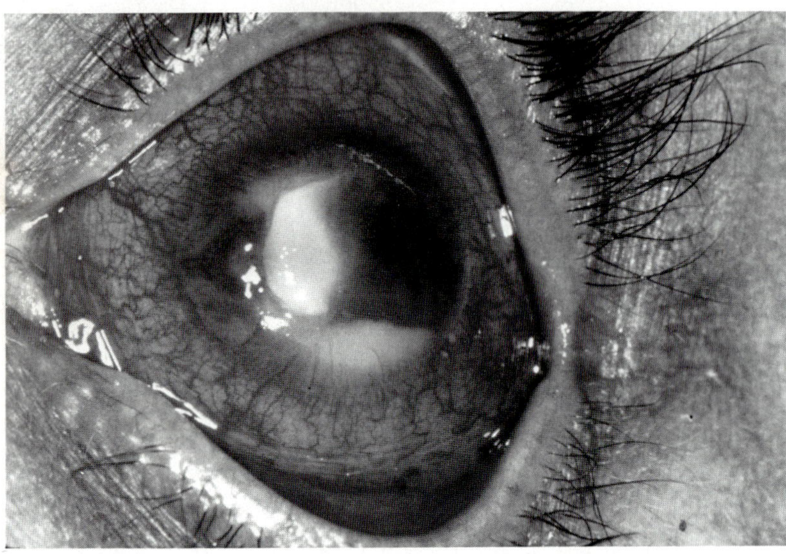

**FIGURE 1-10**    *Candida* corneal ulcer. Fungal and bacterial infections of the cornea are uncommon in patients with AIDS but are difficult to treat when they occur.

ticularly severe. Treatment involves appropriate topical antimicrobials, but the ophthalmologist should be prepared to administer a prolonged course of therapy. Other factors such as dry eyes and keratoconjunctivitis sicca, which appear to be more common in HIV-infected individuals, may contribute to the severity of infections, should they occur.

## Cryptococcosis

As with toxoplasmosis, central nervous system infection by *Cryptococcus neoformans* is quite common in AIDS patients, but direct ocular involvement is rare. When it does occur, intraocular disease usually consists of subclinical infection of the choroid and retina, which is discovered at autopsy. Secondary ocular involvement in the form of papilledema, neuroretinitis, and optic atrophy is more common; in fact cryptococcal meningitis is believed to be the most common cause of papilledema in patients with AIDS. Two cases of rapid, permanent visual loss and bilateral optic atrophy in AIDS patients with cryptococcal meningitis have been reported.[20] There is speculation that this phenomenon is attributable to perineuritic adhesive arachnoiditis, but its mechanism is not fully understood.

## NEWLY REPORTED INFECTIONS
### Pneumocystis Carinii Choroiditis

*Pneumocystis carinii,* an opportunistic organism, is one of the most common infections associated with AIDS, producing life-threatening pneumonia in over 80% of patients. *P. carinii* pneumonia (PCP) is the initial manifestation of AIDS

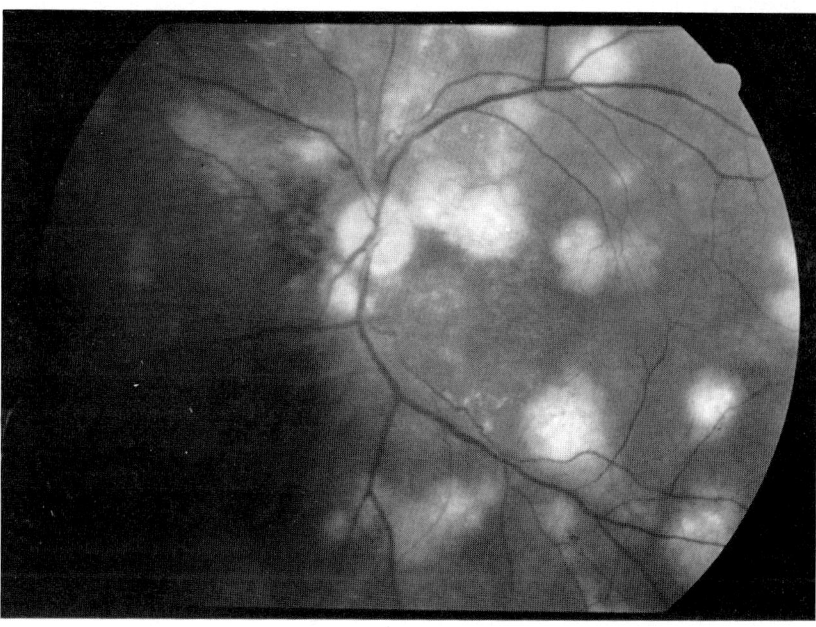

**FIGURE 1-11**  *Pneumocystis carinii* choroiditis. The subretinal patches, which are collections of organisms, enlarge and coalesce slowly without apparent inflammatory reaction.

in over 60% of patients. As noted earlier, aerosolized pentamidine and trimethoprim-sulfamethoxazole have been a major advance in the prophylaxis against recurrent PCP.

Extrapulmonary infections with *P. carinii* have been reported only rarely. One early report noted the presence of *P. carinii* in the ganglion and inner plexiform layers of the retina adjacent to blood vessels, raising the possibility that the organism was associated with cotton-wool spot formation. Subsequent studies cast doubt on these findings, and it was not until recently that *P. carinii* was confirmed to be an ocular pathogen in AIDS patients.

Recent reports have described *P. carinii* choroidopathy.[21,22] Many affected patients have been on prophylaxis with aerosolized pentamidine, which may allow systemic dissemination to occur while suppressing pulmonary infection. It has also been hypothesized that concurrent treatment for other conditions, such as the use of ganciclovir for CMV retinitis, may further depress the patient's immune function, thus allowing dissemination. If true, the increased longevity afforded to AIDS patients by various antibiotics and antineoplastic drugs may be accompanied by an increase in disseminated *P. carinii* infections, including choroiditis. A less likely explanation of extrapulmonary involvement is the development of a more virulent strain of *P. carinii* that can invade pulmonary tissue and spread hematogenously.

The characteristic finding in *P. carinii* choroiditis consists of numerous yellow-white to orange lesions varying in size and shape from round or oval to irregular and confluent groups (Figure 1-11). They may be flat or slightly elevated. An important feature is the absence of vitreal inflammation. Fluorescein angiography shows early hypofluorescence and late staining of the lesions. Involvement under the foveal region causes loss of central vision due to choroidal necrosis. Histopathologic examination reveals densely packed collections of organisms without much inflammation.

The differential diagnosis includes infectious retinitis or choroiditis caused by other uncommon organisms such as atypical mycobacteria, *Candida sp., Aspergillus sp.,* and *Cryptococcus sp.,* and non-AIDS-related conditions such as metastatic carcinoma, sarcoid granulomata, Vogt-Koyanagi-Harada syndrome, sympathetic ophthalmia, and the various multifocal choroidopathy syndromes, such as birdshot choroidopathy. These non-AIDS disorders, however, should be easily ruled out on clinical and historical grounds.

Treatment with intravenous pentamidine has been used with some improvement in lesions, but experience with this disorder is limited. There has been a great deal of interest in this disorder, but disseminated *P. carinii* infections currently remain a very uncommon problem.

## Bacterial Retinitis

Infectious retinitis or choroiditis in patients with AIDS is usually attributed to viruses, protozoa, fungi, or (in the case of syphilis) spirochetes. Although rare cases of bacterial endodphthalmitis due to *Staphylococcus epidermidis* or *Bacillus cereus* have been reported, suppurative bacterial infections of the central nervous system and the eye have not been considered to be prominent features of AIDS.

Davis and associates have reported two patients with similar focal, discrete patches of retinitis that responded to antibiotic treatment.[23] In both cases, the focal lesions progressed slowly, with thickening and exudation; also a moderate vitritis was present. Fluorescein angiography showed dilated retinal vessels over the largest lesions, which leaked profusely. The findings at various times suggested the diagnosis of toxoplasmic retinochoroiditis, viral retinitis, cryptococcal chorioretinitis, and indolent fungal or mycobacterial retinitis. All intraocular cultures were negative. The diagnosis was made in one patient by electron microscopy of a retinal biopsy specimen, which showed unidentified gram-positive bacteria. There was also subsequent response to antibiotics. Diagnosis in the second case was based on clinical features and a good response to empiric antibiotic therapy.

The authors suggest that the causative agent might be *Corynebacterium equi (Rhodococcus equi),* fastidious, gram-positive bacteria known to cause lung abscesses in AIDS patients. Staphylococcal species and *Listeria monocytogenes* were also considered.

The presence of slowly enlarging, multifocal, yellow-white retinal lesions therefore may indicate a metastatic bacterial endophthalmitis in AIDS patients. Cultures of the blood and/or cerebral spinal fluid may assist in diagnosis. Vitreous cultures, on the other hand, are likely to be negative; and empiric antibiotic therapy with doxycycline or vancomycin should be considered before undertaking the risks of a retinal biopsy.

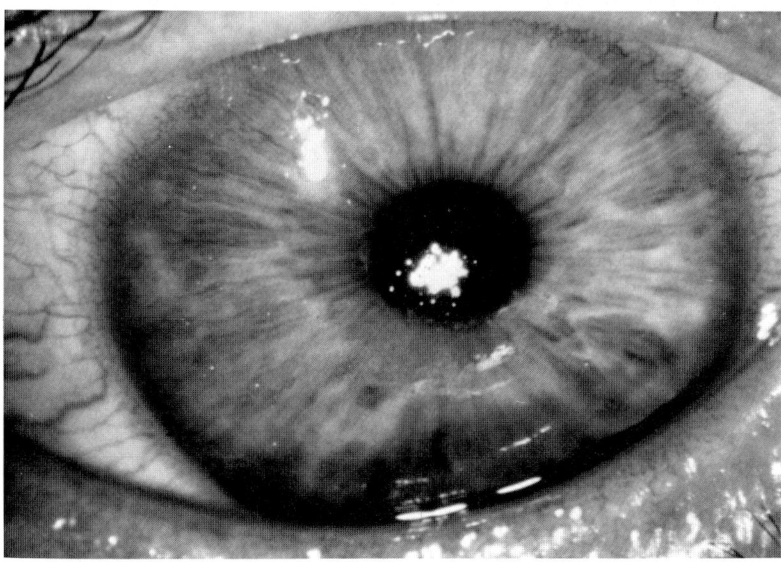

**FIGURE 1-12**    Microsporidial keratopathy. The diffuse infection of the corneal epithelium without much inflammation can be seen to cause distortion of the corneal light reflex. *(Photograph courtesy of Careen Y. Lowder, MD, PhD).*

## MICROSPORIDIAL KERATOPATHY

Microsporidia are ubiquitous intracellular protozoa increasingly recognized as pathogens in immunosuppressed individuals. Enteric involvement is most common, and hepatic and peritoneal infections have also been reported. Several cases involving corneal epithelial infection have also been identified.[24,25]

Cases are characterized by a recalcitrant bilateral epithelial keratitis (Figure 1-12). Routine bacterial and viral cultures are negative. Patients complain of photophobia, dryness, foreign-body sensation, and mild to moderately blurred vision. Typical slit-lamp findings included diffuse punctate epithelial keratopathy and minimal conjunctival inflammation. The absence of destructive stromal disease in these patients, in contrast to corneal microsporidiosis in immunocompetent hosts, represents yet another condition in which the inflammatory responses to infection in AIDS is markedly diminished.

Fecal-oral transmission is probably the route of infection in intestinal microsporidiosis, but the source of ocular infection is unknown. The superficial location of the organisms in the cornea suggests that direct inoculation may occur.

Diagnosis is based on light- and electron-microscopic findings from epithelial scrapings. Gram-positive oval forms are seen within epithelial cells. Ultrastructural features seen with transmission electron microscopy include a cell wall, coiled filaments, a polar vacuole, and single nucleus. Serologic tests are unreliable, and the organism is difficult to recover in culture. There is no known curative therapy, although sulfa drugs may have some effect. Topical lubricants may provide symptomatic relief. The efficacy of lamellar or penetrating kerotoplasty is unclear.

## THE ROLE OF HIV IN OCULAR DISEASE

Although HIV has been recovered from numerous ocular tissues, it apparently does not usually cause clinically apparent ocular disease. Farrell and colleagues reported the case of a 36-year-old male intravenous drug abuser with chronic iridocyclitis who had been found to be HIV-positive 2 months earlier.[26] After 2 weeks of left-eye irritation, examination revealed 20/50 vision, moderate epibulbar injection, anterior-chamber cells and flare, mutton-fat keratic precipitates, and posterior synechiae. Clinical and laboratory evaluation revealed no evidence of mycobacterial infection, syphilis, toxoplasmosis, herpes simplex virus–related uveitis, or CMV infection. After there was no response to topical and oral corticosteroid therapy, the patient underwent anterior chamber parecentesis; HIV was cultured from the aqueous humor. He was started on zidovudine and within two weeks recovered 20/20 vision, with resolution of the keratic precipitates. Other investigators have seen similar cases.

Inflammation in these cases may be the result of unidentified opportunistic pathogens, and the presence of HIV in the aqueous humor may simply be the result of a breakdown in the blood-aqueous barrier. Furthermore, the patient's improvement with zidovudine may have resulted from improved immune function. Nevertheless, the consistent lack of other findings and the rapid response to therapy with zidovudine (which is known to penetrate the blood-brain barrier and is known to have direct benefits in treatment of other HIV-associated diseases such as encephalopathy) support the hypothesis that uveitis in such cases is a direct effect of HIV infection.

There have been other AIDS patients without evidence of secondary intraocular infections who have been found to have decreased vision, vitritis, constricted visual fields, and reduced or extinguished electroretinograms. It is theorized that the findings might represent direct intraocular infection with HIV.

Ophthalmologists should remember that despite these interesting cases, intraocular inflammation in AIDS patients is usually caused by opportunistic infections such as toxoplasmosis, zoster ophthalmicus, syphilis, or fungal endophthalmitis. Only after these disorders are ruled out should HIV-induced uveitis be considered.

## VASCULAR DISEASE

Retinal microvaculopathy in AIDS patients is a very common phenomenon, but its cause remains unknown despite years of study. Its manifestations consist of cotton-wool spots and, less commonly, intraretinal hemorrhages and other associated microvascular changes, such as microaneurysms. These lesions rarely if ever cause visual changes.

Studies have shown that at least 40% to 60% of AIDS patients have cotton-wool spots and hemorrhages, and still higher percentages are noted by fluorescein angiography or at autopsy. It is much more common in patients with AIDS than in those with ARC and uncommon in asymptomatic HIV-infected individuals.[4] Furthermore, the helper-to-suppressor T-lymphocyte ratio is significantly lower in AIDS and ARC patients with signs of microvasculopathy than in those without, suggesting that it is associated with greater degrees of immunosuppression. Thus, the signs of microvasculopathy may have some prognostic significance as originally suspected. However, no association has been identified between the presence of retinal microangiopathy and any specific AIDS-related infection, neoplasm, or the duration of AIDS or ARC.

Trypsin digest preparations of affected retina show loss of pericytes and microaneurysm formation. Histologically, there are thickened vascular walls and lumenal narrowing. Ultrastructural studies show swollen endothelial cells, occluded vascular lumina, and thickened vascular basal lamina. These findings are strikingly similar to vascular changes in diabetic retinopathy.

Conjunctival microvascular changes have also been reported in HIV-infected patients, and they may be present to at least some degree in all AIDS patients.[27] Changes, which are most apparent in the inferior, perilimbal, and bulbar conjunctiva, consist of dilated capillaries, isolated vascular fragments, vessel segments of irregular caliber, and sludging of blood flow. These changes may be due to the same mechanisms that cause the retinal microvasculopathy.

There are several theories regarding the pathogenesis of HIV-associated microvasculopathy. They do not appear to be the result of opportunistic infections of the involved tissues. HIV infection of the endothelial cells with subsequent vascular occlusion has been hypothesized to cause the microvasculopathy, but this does not fully explain all findings of the condition. Two other hypotheses are that deposition of circulating immune complexes injure the vasculature and that rheologic (blood flow) abnormalities contribute to the damage.

Circulating immune complexes are frequently found in patients with AIDS or ARC, and immunoglobulin deposition has been noted in arteriolar walls. The presence of polyclonal B-cell activation, hypergammaglobulinemia, and circulating immune complexes characterizes not only AIDS but also collagen vascular diseases that have similar microvasculopathies.

Engstrom and associates found an association between fibrinogen levels and both conjunctival microvasculopathy and cotton-wool spots in HIV-infected patients.[27] The cause of the increased fibrinogen is unknown. The authors theorized that increased fibrinogen causes increased red cell aggregation and blood flow sludging; this abnormality in turn causes vascular hypoxia that contributes to the development of the microvasculopathy. Anemia and other factors may contribute to the hypoxia and vessel damage as well. In these studies, circulating immune complex levels did not correlate strongly with microvasculopathy.

Central retinal vein occlusion has been recognized by several investigators to be more frequent in HIV-infected patients. It generally is not associated with evidence of other retinal or optic nerve disease. These cases indicate large-vessel disease can occur as well as microvasculopathies. Abnormal blood flow may be a common factor in these various disorders.

Perivascular sheathing not associated with infectious retinitis is another vascular abnormality that has been associated with AIDS. In fact, it was found in one patient described in the first report of the ocular manifestations of AIDS. It has not turned out to be a common manifestation of the syndrome in the United States, but interestingly, it is a common finding in African patients with AIDS, particularly in African children with AIDS. The cause of this disorder and the reason for its geographic distribution is not known.

## KAPOSI SARCOMA

Kaposi sarcoma (KS) is a highly vascularized, malignant tumor of mesenchymal origin that can occur on skin, mucous membranes, and visceral organs. It is seen in about one-fourth of AIDS patients, and it may be the first clinical sign of the disease. Studies indicate that 20% of patients with AIDS-related KS have ocular involvement, and in fact KS may make its first appearance on or around the eye.[28]

The most commonly involved ophthalmic tissues are, in decreasing order, eyelids, conjunctiva, and orbit. Orbital involvement has been reported rarely. Conjunctival tumors are most common in the inferior fornix, where they can be missed if the lower eyelids are not pulled down. Bilateral disease is frequent. Conjunctival lesions, which are deep red or violaceous, may initially be mistaken for chronic subconjunctival hemorrhages (Figure 1-13). Eyelid lesions may be misdiagnosed as persistent hordeola, foreign body granulomata, or cavernous hemangiomas (Figure 1-14). If the diagnosis is in doubt, biopsy is appropriate.

Eyelid and conjunctival tumors may be asymptomatic, or they may cause irritation, recurrent hemorrhage, or cosmetic disfigurement. Eyelid lesions may result in entropion formation or trichiasis and may become secondarily infected.

KS lesions typically progress slowly; only occasionally will rapid enlargement be seen, and conjunctival lesions are noninvasive. Because AIDS-related KS is a multifocal neoplasm, therapy is usually directed at palliation of focal lesions. In contrast to KS in the pre-AIDS era, excision will not be curative; there is a high recurrence rate following excision of eyelid or conjunctival lesions.

Therapy of conjunctival lesions is rarely necessary because of the tumor's slow growth and lack of invasiveness. Eyelid margin lesions, on the other hand, are more commonly treated to prevent development of complications such as entropion formation with trichiasis or ulceration of the eyelid margin with secondary infection. Systemic chemotherapy, with single-agent or combination therapy using drugs such as bleomycin sulfate, vinblastine sulfate, and doxorubicin hydrochloride (Adriamycin), has had good results in small series of patients, but recurrence following discontinuation of chemotherapy is common. For local ocular therapy when systemic treatment is not planned, the most common treatments include radiation therapy and cryotherapy. The indications for therapy and suggested treatment strategies suggested by Shuler and associates are summarized in the box (top of p. 26).

## REPORTED DISEASE ASSOCIATIONS OF UNCERTAIN SIGNIFICANCE

There is little doubt about the association between HIV infection and the disorders discussed above, because of the large number of reported cases and the fact that they are seen by many different investigators in different geographic areas over time. The significance of isolated case reports or single reports of very small patient series, on the other hand, is less certain. Isolated case reports of HIV-related ocular diseases do provide a framework on which other investigators can elaborate, but obviously, not all case reports will stand the test of time. Some may simply be fortuitous associations and not the sequelae of the immunodeficient state, while others may be so rare that cause-and-effect relationships are hard to establish. Others, however, may be the first indication of an emerging problem.

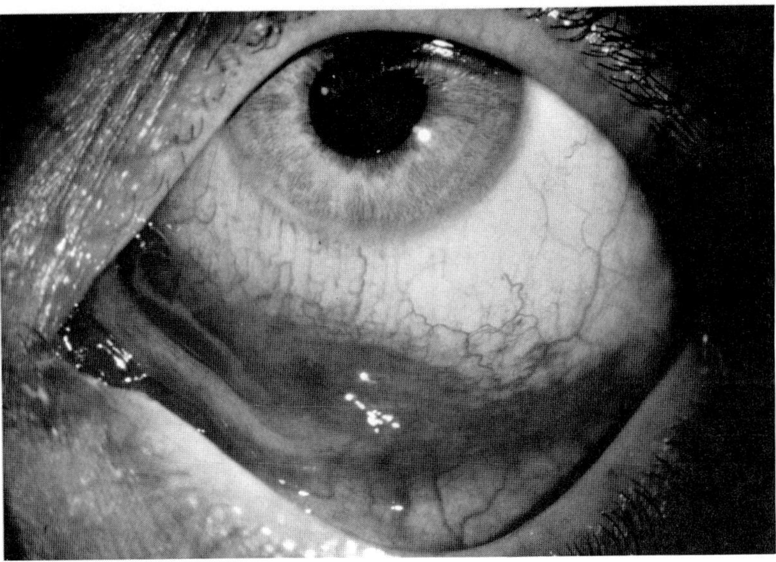

**FIGURE 1-13**    Kaposi sarcoma of the conjunctiva. The diffuse, red lesion is located in the inferior fornix, the most common site for this AIDS-related tumor.

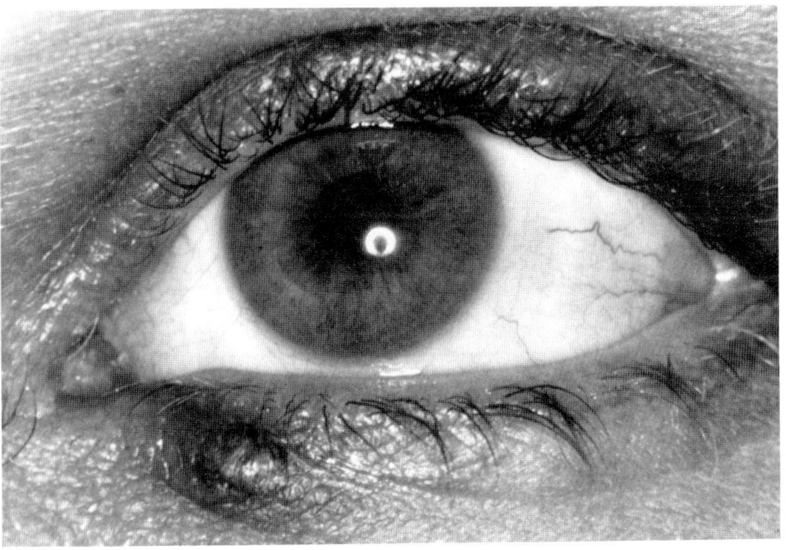

**FIGURE 1-14**    Kaposi sarcoma of the eyelids. The patient has a nodular tumor on the medial aspect of the lower eyelid and diffuse involvement of the upper eyelid.

Thus all such cases are viewed with interest. In this section a number of such disorders are described. All have been reported in HIV-infected patients; with time they may be found to be important AIDS-related problems — or they may eventually be disregarded as being of little or no significance (see box, bottom of p. 26).

Bilateral angle-closure glaucoma due to ciliochoroidal effusions of unknown cause has been reported in patients with AIDS.[29,30] They present with corneal

### Management of Ophthalmic Kaposi Sarcoma

I. Indications for treatment
  A. Cosmesis
  B. Bulky conjunctival lesions
  C. Entropion formation, trichiasis from large eyelid margin lesions
  D. Ulceration of eyelid margin lesions
  E. Prophylactic treatment of eyelid margin lesions to prevent complications from enlargement
II. Treatment
  A. Systemic treatment alone
    1. Indications
      a. Multifocal disease with nonphthalmic lesions
      b. If immediate response *not* required
  B. Local therapy
    1. Indications
      a. If systemic therapy not planned
        (1) Eyelids or conjunctiva only site of disease
        (2) Intolerance to systemic therapy
      b. Failure of systemic therapy
      c. If immediate response required (with or without systemic treatment)
    2. Treatment regimens
      a. Radiation therapy: 2000-3000 centiGrays (cGy) in 200-300 cGy fractions over 2-3 weeks
      b. Cryotherapy (little reported experience)

Adapted from Shuler JD, Holland GN, Miles SA, Miller BJ, Grossman I: Kaposi sarcoma of the conjunctiva and eyelids associated with the acquired immunodeficiency syndrome. Arch Ophthalmol 1989; 107:858-862.

### Ocular Disorders in HIV-Infected Patients
### Associations of Uncertain Significance

I. Ocular surface
  A. Culture-negative keratoconjunctivitis
  B. Peripheral corneal melting
  C. Lymphogranuloma venereum
  D. Reiter syndrome
  E. Atypical conjunctival squamous cell carcinoma
II. Intraocular
  A. Retinal vasculitis
  B. Vitritis
  C. Choriodal effusion, anterior rotation of ciliary body, and angle closure glaucoma
  D. Reduced or extinguished electroretinogram
III. Orbit
  A. Orbital pseudotumor
  B. Eosinophilic granuloma

bedewing, markedly elevated intraocular pressure, deep central chambers, and occluded peripheral angles without iris bombe. Ultrasonography demonstrates bilateral thickening of the choroid and sclera and ciliochoroidal effusions consistent with posterior scleritis. Reported cases have not responded to medical management with pilocarpine and iridotomies, although improvement with cycloplegic therapy has been observed. Drainage of the suprachoroidal effusions may be necessary. Although reported by more than one group of investigators, this disorder has not turned out to be a common problem, and its cause and association to HIV infection remain unclear.

Lymphogranuloma venereum (LGV) is a sexually transmitted disease caused by serotypes L1-3 of *Chlamydia trachomatis*. Ocular involvement in this rare infection can cause Parinaud oculoglandular syndrome, keratoconjunctivitis, episcleritis, uveitis, papilledema, and retinal hemorrhages. Fleshy vascularized superior limbal conjunctival lesions, marginal corneal infiltrates, and full-thickness crescentic corneal infiltrates have also been reported. Corneal perforation, however, was not described as a sequelae of LGV until a recent case reort of the disease in an HIV-infected patient. This situation appears to be another where HIV-infection does not necessarily increase the risk of developing a disorder, as it does with opportunistic organisms, but can make the disorder much more severe when it does occur as a coincident infection.

Eosinophilic granuloma involving the cavernous sinus and orbital apex has recently been described in a patient with AIDS. Eosinophilic glanuloma is one of the diseases collectively known as histiocytosis-X. The abnormal histiocytes that proliferate in the tumor are derived from Langerhans cells. Both histiocytes and Langerhans cells express a receptor for HIV and are, therefore, susceptible to infection. Since other tumors, such as lymphomas, in AIDS patients are believed to be caused by malignant transformation of HIV-infected lymphoid cells, it is theorized that a similar maligant transformation and proliferation of histiocytic cells could explain this rare tumor.

Squamous cell carcinoma has been associated with HIV infection, usually in the oral cavity or anorectum, but also in the lungs and skin. Conjunctival squamous cell carcinoma has also been reported in an HIV-infected individual. It was an atypical tumor, occurring in a relatively young individual, characterized by rapid growth and a high degree of mitotic activity. It is possible that HIV infection increases the risk of this tumor and results in a more aggressive course.

Corneal diseases of uncertain cause have been reported in several cases. Peripheral corneal ulceration in a patient with ARC has been seen. The ulcer extended almost 360 degrees with absent epithelium and clear stroma. A 10% hypopyon was present. Evaluation revealed no evidence of infection. Successful resolution was obtained following a 360-degree conjunctival resection, application of cyanoacrylate glue, and placement of a bandage soft contact lens. Peripheral corneal ulceration resulting from limbal immune complex deposition, complement activation, and neutrophil invasion has been noted in a variety of immunologic disorders, including rheumatoid arthritis and Mooren ulcer. The success of conjunctival resection in some of these cases has been attributed to debulking of the immune complex load. The high levels of circulating immune complexes frequently found in patients with AIDS may therefore predispose them to peripheral corneal problems. Nevertheless, peripheral corneal ulcerations in AIDS patients are not frequently seen; perhaps the diminished inflammatory response in AIDS patients is protective.

Reiter syndrome, which consists of seronegative asymmetric arthropathy, nongonococcal urethritis, conjunctivitis and/or iritis, and skin disease (keratoderma blennorrhagicum) that is indistinguishable from psoriasis, has been reported in association with AIDS. Whether this syndrome can be induced by HIV infection or its course altered by the associated immunodeficiency is not known.

There is little doubt that some isolated case reports describe definite HIV-associated problems; orbital Burkitt lymphoma and retinal infection with disseminated *Histoplasma capsulatum* are 2 examples. Neither of these disorders, described several years ago, has turned out to be a major problem in American patients with AIDS.

## PRECAUTIONS IN CARING FOR AIDS PATIENTS WITH EYE DISEASE

There is no evidence that HIV can be transmitted by casual contact, but there has been much concern and much has been written about the potential for HIV transmission in the workplace. The presence of virus in corneal tissue, tears, and even contact lenses worn by patients with HIV infection raises special concerns for ophthalmologists and allied health care professionals. Special emphasis has been placed on the potential for disease transmission via contaminated tonometer tips. To date, there are no reports of HIV transmission related to the practice of ophthalmology. Because the actual risk is not fully known, however, it is prudent to take precautions to minimize any potential risk. Infectious disease guidelines will also reduce the spread of secondary pathogens, such as herpes simplex virus, that may be present in AIDS patients. A summary of guidelines for ophthalmologists is presented in the box on p. 29.

Because HIV infection is often asymptomatic and because patients may be unaware of their serologic status or deny their HIV infection and risk factors, precautions should be used for all patients. The assumption that any patient may be infected gives rise to the approach termed "universal precautions." Gowns and masks are rarely required, unless there is potential for contamination with blood or other body fluids. Masks are required only in those situations where the patient has a secondary respiratory infection, such as tuberculosis.

Gloves are unnecessary for the usual ophthalmic examination. Some ophthalmologists prefer to wear disposable gloves during indirect ophthalmoscopy or in other situations where the lids are manipulated and tearing can be expected. Gloves are specifically recommended in such situations if the examiner has open or weeping lesions on the hands. Some ophthalmologists wear gloves while administering retrobulbar anesthesia; although the gloves will not prevent needlestick injuries, they will prevent direct contact with blood that may leak from the needle tip. If gloves are worn, they should be changed after each patient has been treated. There is some evidence that latex gloves offer more protection than vinyl gloves. For most situations, thorough handwashing before and after every examination is probably sufficient.

Any contaminated device can be disinfected against HIV by a 10-minute soak in one of the following solutions: fresh 3% hydrogen peroxide, 70% isopropyl alcohol, 70% ethanol, or a 0.525% sodium hypochlorite solution (a 1:10 dilution

---

### Guidelines for Prevention of Disease Transmission

---

Guidelines should be used for all patients, whether or not HIV infection is known ("universal precautions").

Caution with needles and other sharp objects with *all* patients.

Gloves: optional for most examination procedures. Should be worn if there are open sores on the examiner's hands.

Gowns: not necessary unless contamination with body fluids expected.

Masks: not necessary unless secondary respiratory infection (e.g., tuberculosis) is present in a coughing patient.

Goldmann tonometer tips: wipe tips with 70% isopropyl alcohol swabs and air dry.

Other contaminated devices: physically remove any particulate matter, then soak for 10 minutes in one of the following solutions:

a. Fresh 3% hydrogen peroxide.
b. 70% isopropyl alcohol.
c. 70% ethanol.
d. 0.525% sodium hypochlorite (1:10 dilution of household bleach).

Surgical instruments: sterilize by routine methods.

Surfaces contaminated with body fluids: wipe immediately with disinfectant such as Amphyl.

Contact lenses: all lenses from fitting sets should be sterilized by hydrogen peroxide or heating techniques.

---

of household bleach). Recent studies by Pepose and associates have also shown that Goldmann tonometer tips can be disinfected against HIV and HSV simply by wiping with a 70% isopropyl alcohol swab followed by air drying.[31] Only the tip need be treated, thus avoiding dissolution of the side markings. It is important in such disinfection procedures to physically wipe any debris from the contaminated device.

Contact lenses are effectively disinfected against HIV with either hydrogen peroxide or thermal disinfection. One or the other of these techniques can be used on any available rigid or soft contact lens; recommendations can be obtained from the manufacturer. The efficacy of various commercially available chemical disinfection systems against HIV in the clinical setting has not been established.

Although routine patient contact poses little or no risk of HIV transmission, it has been well established that transmission can occur by needlestick injuries. Seroconversion occurs in less than 1% of needlestick injuries. Nevertheless, extreme caution is warranted when handling any sharp object that has been contaminated with blood. Most needlestick injuries occur when used needles are resheathed before disposal. It is therefore recommended that a puncture-resistant disposable container be available for placement of unsheathed needles immediately after use.

Concern has been raised about transmission of HIV via penetrating keratoplasty, since transmission has occurred with other procedures such as kidney transplantion. CMV has never been isolated from the cornea, so the risk of transmitting that virus appears minimal. The transmission of other viruses, such as the agents responsible for rabies and hepatitis B, with corneal transplantation is well documented; but despite intensive study, there is no evidence that HIV transmission occurs by this route. In 1987, Pepose reported several cases in which corneal donors were found in retrospect to be HIV infected.[32] None of the recipients had developed antibodies to HIV at the time of the report. Many of them are still being followed, and none have seroconverted, with followup periods as long as 3 years (J.S. Pepose, MD, PhD, personal communication). Failure to become infected with HIV may reflect the low viral load that corneal transplantion presents, compared to that of a blood transfusion or sexual intercourse.

Although there appears to be little or no risk of HIV transmission by corneal transplantation, many potential donors, such as coroners' cases, will be from groups at high risk for HIV infection. Therefore, the Eye Bank Association of America now routinely screens all potential donors for HIV antibodies. Because seroconversion may not occur immediately after HIV infection, individuals are not accepted as donors if they are definitely known to have specific risk factors.

## CONCLUSIONS

The increasing numbers and survival of AIDS patients mean that the ocular disorders associated with this syndrome will become more frequent problems for the ophthalmic community. For several reasons, general ophthalmologists should become familiar with the syndrome and its various manifestations. The first clinical appearance of an opportunistic infection or of KS may be in or on the eye, and occasionally ocular disease is the first manifestation of AIDS. Given the success of some prophylactic treatments and evidence that zidovudine prolongs life in the early stages of HIV infection, ophthalmologists can provide a valuable service to patients by prompt and appropriate referral to other specialists for evaluation and management of nonocular disease.

Some HIV-infected patients decline either to enter double-blind, randomized clinical drug trials or to be followed in the university setting. Out of desperation, many of these patients also seek alternative therapies, the efficacies and side effects of which are not known. The accumulated experience of community-based ophthalmologists in these situations can provide valuable information in the absence of controlled trials.

Although screening of HIV-infected patients may allow earlier recognition of ocular disease, it is not known whether such screening will ultimately reduce visual loss. Vision-threatening disorders usually occur late in the course of AIDS; it is therefore more appropriate to follow patients with advanced systemic disease or low CD4 counts more closely than asymptomatic HIV-infected patients or patients with ARC. In all cases where a patient experiences visual loss, a sudden increase in floaters, blind spots, redness, or ocular pain, prompt evaluation is necessary.

The ocular manifestations of AIDS and HIV infection are often difficult to diagnose accurately and manage effectively. Nevertheless, all ophthalmologists should at least be aware of the differential diagnosis of intraocular disease in patients with HIV infection to facilitate appropriate laboratory evaluations or referrals to subspecialists and to avoid the institution of improper or even dangerous therapies. Recognition of treatable diseases, such as syphilis, fungal infections, and toxoplasmosis should be foremost in the ophthalmologist's mind. As management for the ophthalmic disorders associated with HIV infection improves, ophthalmologists can add significantly to the quality of life for patients with AIDS.

Since the preparation of this manuscript, the results of a multi-center, NIH-sponsored trial comparing foscarnet and ganciclovir in the treatment of CMV retinitis have been announced.[33] No difference was found between the two drugs for major ophthalmic outcomes, including time to reactivation of disease and final central visual acuity. There was a statistically significant difference in mortality; median survival in the foscarnet-treated group was 12.6 months compared to 8.5 months in the ganciclovir-treated group. Use of anti-retroviral therapy was not controlled in the study.

The cause of the difference in mortality is not known. Until this issue is resolved, the choice of treatment for CMV retinitis should remain up to the patient and the physician. The decision should be based on the patient's overall health, tolerance of side effects, and possible increased life span associated with foscarnet.

---

## References


1. Holland GN, Pepose JS, Pettit TH, Gottlieb MS, Yee RD, Foos RY. Acquired immune deficiency syndrome: ocular manifestations. Ophthalmol 1983; 90:859-872.
2. Palestine AG, Rodriquez MM, Macher AM, et al. Ophthalmic involvement in acquired immune deficiency syndrome. Ophthalmol 1984; 91:1092-1099.
3. Schuman JS, Orellana J, Friedman AH, Teich SA. Acquired immunodeficiency syndrome (AIDS). Surv Ophthalmol 1987; 31:384-410.
4. Jabs DA, Green WR, Fox R, Polk BF, Bartlett JG. Ocular manifestations of acquired immune deficiency syndrome. Ophthalmol 1989; 96:1092-1099.
5. Holland GN, Sison RF, Jatulis DE, et al. Survival of patients with the acquired immune deficiency syndrome after development of cytomegalovirus retinopathy. Ophthalmol 1990; 97:204-211.
6. Holland GN, Buhles WC, Mastre B, Kaplan HJ, the CMV Retinopathy Study Group. A controlled retrospective study on ganciclovir treatment for cytomegalovirus retinopathy: use of a standardized system for the assessment of disease outcome. Arch Ophthalmol 1989; 107:1759-1766.
7. Jabs DA, Enger C, Bartlett JG. Cytomegalovirus retinitis and acquired immunodeficiency syndrome. Arch Ophthalmol 1989; 107:75-80.
8. Heinemann M-H. Long-term intravitreal ganciclovir therapy for cytomegalovirus retinopathy. Arch Ophthalmol 1989: 107:1767-1772.
9. LeHoang P, Girard B, Robinet M, et al. Foscarnet in the treatment of cytomegalovirus retinitis in acquired immune deficiency syndrome. Ophthalmol 1989; 96:865-874.
10. Guyer DR, Jabs DA, Brant AM, Beschnorner WE, and Green WR. Regression of Cytomegalovirus retinitis with zidovudine. A clinicopathologic correlation. Arch Ophthalmol 1989; 107:868-874.
11. Fay MT, Freeman WR, Wiley CA, Hardy D, Bozzette S. Atypical retinitis in patients with the acquired immunodeficiency syndrome. Am J Ophthalmol 1988; 105:483-490.
12. Freeman WR, Henderly DE, Wan WL, et al. Prevalence, pathophysiology, and treatment of rhegmatogenous retinal detachment in treated cytomegalovirus retinitis. Am J Ophthalmol 1987; 103:527-536.
13. Passo MS, Rosenbaum JT. Ocular syphilis in patients with human immunodeficiency virus infection. Am J Ophthalmol 1988; 106:1-6.
14. Becerra LI, Ksiazek SM, Savino PJ, et al. Syphilitic uveitis in human immunodeficiency virus-infected and noninfected patients. Ophthalmol 1989, 96:1727-1730.
15. Holland GN, Engstrom RE, Glasgow BJ, et al. Ocular taxoplasmosis in patients with the acquired immunodeficiency syndrome. Am J Ophthalmol 1988; 106:653-667.
16. Sandor EV, Millman A, Croxson TS, Mildvan D. Herpes zoster ophthalmicus in patients at risk for the acquired immune deficiency syndrome (AIDS). Am J Ophthalmol 1986; 101:153-155.
17. Cole EL, Meisler DM, Calbrese LH, Holland GN, Mondino BJ, Conant MA. Herpes zoster ophthal-

micus and acquired immune deficiency syndrome. Arch Ophthalmol 1984; 102:1027-1029.

18. Engstrom RE, Holland GN. Chronic herpes zoster virus keratitis associated with the acquired immunodeficiency syndrome. Am J Ophthalmol 1988; 105:556.

19. Young TL, Robin JB, Hendricks RL, Engstrom RE, Holland GN, Sugar J. Herpes simplex keratitis in AIDS patients. Ophthalmol 1989; 96:1476.

20. Lipson BK, Freeman WR, Beniz J, et al. Optic neuropathy associated with cryptococcal arachnoiditis in AIDS patients. Am J Ophthalmol 1989; 107:523-527.

21. Rao NA, Zimmerman PL, Boyer D, et al. A clinical, histopathologic, and electron microscopic study of *Pneumocystis carinii* choroiditis. Am J Ophthalmol 1989; 107:218-228.

22. Freeman WR, Gross JG, Labelle J, Oteken K, Katz B, Wiley CA. *Pneumocystis carinii* choroidopathy. Arch Ophthalmol 1989; 107:863-867.

23. Davis JL, Nussenblatt RB, Bachman DM, Chan CC, Palestine AG. Endogenous bacterial retinitis in AIDS. Am J Ophthalmol 1989; 107:613-623.

24. Friedberg DN, Stenson SM, Orenstein JM, Tierno PM, Charles NC. Microsporidial keratoconjunctivitis in acquired immunodeficiency syndrome. Arch Ophthalmol 1990; 108:504-508.

25. Lowder CY, Meisler DM, McMahon JT, Longworth DL, Rutherford I. Microsporidia infection of the cornea seropositive for human immunodeficiency virus. Am J Ophthalmol 1990; 109:242-244.

26. Farrell PL, Heinemann MH, Roberts CW, Polsky B, Gold JWM, Mamelok A. Response of human im-

munodeficiency virus–associated uveitis to zidovudine. Am J Ophthalmol 1988; 106:7-10.

27. Engstrom RE, Holland GN, Hardy WD, Meiselman JH. Hemorheologic abnormalities in patients with human immunodeficiency virus infection and ophthalmic microvasculopathy. Am J Ophthalmol 1990; 109:153-161.

28. Shuler JD, Holland GN, Miles SA, Miller BJ, Grossman I. Kaposi sarcoma of the conjunctiva and eyelids associated with the acquired immunodeficiency syndrome. Arch Ophthalmol 1989; 107:858-862.

29. Ullman S, Wilson RD, and Schwartz LS. Bilateral angle-closure glaucoma in association with the acquired immune deficiency syndrome. Am J Ophthalmol 1986; 101:419-424.

30. Williams AS, Williams FC, O'Donnell JJ. AIDS presenting as acute glaucoma. Arch Ophthalmol 1988; 106:311-312.

31. Pepose JS, Linette G, Lee SF, MacRae S. Disinfection of Goldmann tonometers against human immunodeficiency virus type 1. Arch Ophthalmol 1989; 107:983-985.

32. Pepose JS, MacRae S, Quinn TC, Ward JW: Serologic markers after the transplantation of corneas from donors infected with human immunodeficiency virus. Am J Ophthalmol 1987; 103:798-801.

33. The Studies of Ocular Complications of AIDS (SOCA) Research Group collaboration with the AIDS Clinical Trial Group (ACTG): Mortality in patients with AIDS treated with either foscarnet or ganciclovir for CMV retinitis. N Engl J Med 1992; 326:213-220.

# 2 Corneal Alkali Burns

Mark A. Pavilack, MD
Patricia C. Chang, MD
H. Kaz Soong, MD

Exposure to alkali can produce severe destruction of the eye and result in permanent blindness. Most alkali injuries occur in industrial, agricultural, and home accidents or as the result of assault.[1] Patients with ocular alkali burns typically have a protracted clinical course which can be associated with many secondary complications, including delayed epithelial healing, ulceration, and scarring. Unfortunately, numerous clinical and experimental investigations have made only limited progress in improving visual recovery following severe alkali burns.

## TYPES OF ALKALI

Alkalies, including ammonia ($NH_3$), lye (NaOH), lime [$Ca(OH)_2$] and other hydroxides [KOH, $Mg(OH)_2$], are commonly used in fertilizer, plaster, cement, and various household agents, (e.g., cleaning solutions and drain openers [Figure 2-1]).[2] Within minutes to hours after contact with alkali, corneal tissue undergoes varying degrees of destruction in proportion to the biological activity of the chemical. The severity of alkali burns is determined by the volume and concentration (pH) of the alkali solution and duration of exposure to the alkali.[3] In addition, the speed and degree of tissue penetration is a function of the associated cation.[3] Ammonia, which combines with water to form ammonium hydroxide, is capable of causing severe corneal damage often associated with iris, trabecular meshwork, and lens injury. Therapeutic irrigation after ammonia exposure is often only of limited success, due to ammonia's high lipid solubility and rapid penetration into the eye. Lye and potassium hydroxide can similarly penetrate rapidly into the eye, causing severe burns.[4] In contrast, lime reacts with epithelial membranes to form calcium soaps that precipitate and thus limit further penetration and injury.[5] Ocular burns from magnesium hydroxide, found in sparklers and flares, are often additionally complicated by thermal injury.[4]

## ALKALI VERSUS ACID

Alkalies and acids differ most in their reactivity with tissues. Alkalies generate hydroxyl ions which denature collagen, hydrolyze intracellular glycosaminoglycans, and saponify fatty acids in cell membranes, ultimately leading to cell disruption.[4] Deep intraocular penetration of alkali can cause damage of the trabecular meshwork, iris, lens, ciliary body, and retina (Figure 2-2).[3] Injury is further enhanced by the binding of basic cations to mucoproteins and collagen in the corneal stroma. Stromal retention of chemicals allows even low concentrations of alkali to cause slow and continuous breakdown of collagen, prolonged inflammatory mediator release, and increased leukocyte infiltration.[6,7] The production of proteolytic enzymes, including collagenase, by leukocytes may result in the enzymatic degradation of stromal collagen and can promote corneal perforation.[8] Stromal keratocytes and corneal epithelial cells have also been implicated as possible additional sources of collagenase.[9,10] In contrast, acid coagulates proteins, creating a superficial barrier in the tissues which prevents further chemical penetration.

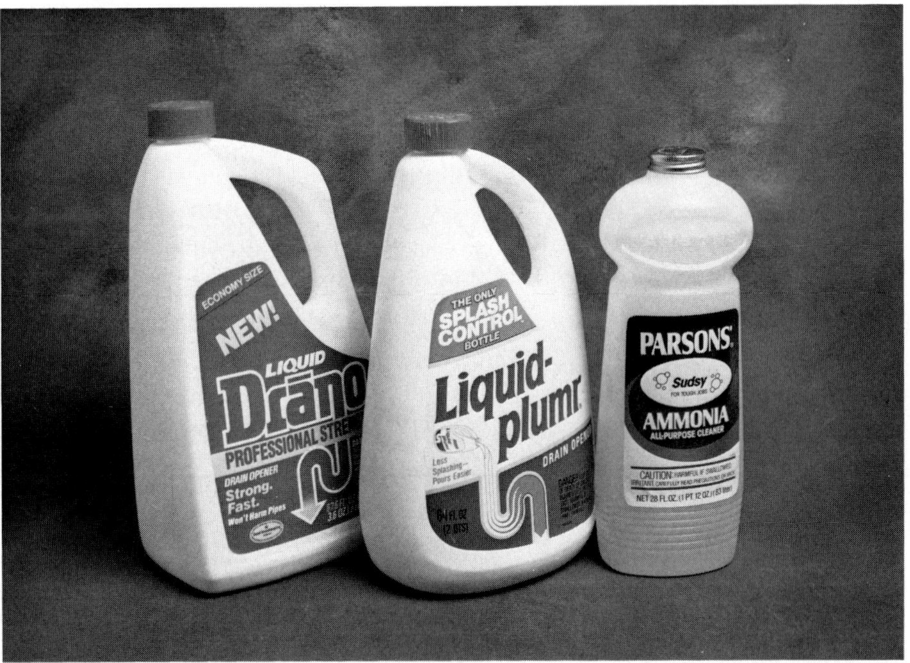

**FIGURE 2-1**     Common alkali-containing household cleaning solutions.

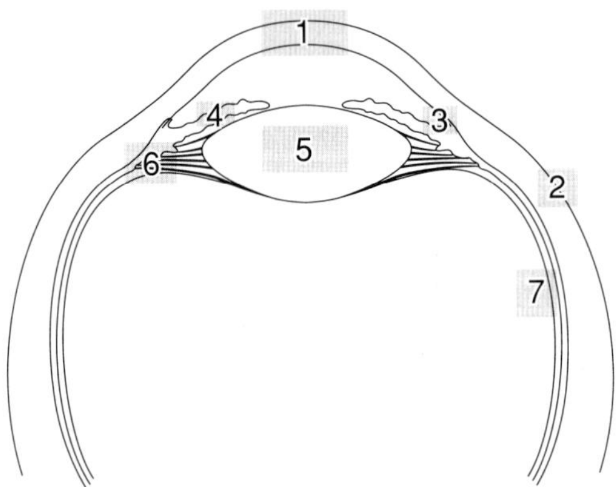


**FIGURE 2-2**     Potential sites of ocular damage following alkali burn: (1) cornea; (2) conjunctiva/sclera; (3) trabecular meshwork; (4) iris; (5) lens; (6) ciliary body; and (7) retina.

The higher resistance of mucopolysaccharides and collagen to acid,[11] the limiting tissue barrier, and the better buffering capacity of tissues and aqueous humor against acid are mutually synergistic in reducing tissue damage from acid.[12]

## CLASSIFICATION OF ALKALI BURNS

A classification scheme for the severity of ocular damage from alkali exposure was originally proposed by Hughes[13] and later modified by others. Hughes's initial classification divided patients into 3 groups, using the degree of corneal clouding and limbal conjunctival blanching as indicators both of the extent of chemical penetration and for the prognostication of the final visual acuity after treatment.[13] Previous classification systems for alkali burns were expanded by Pfister to include several more variables, which together better correlate with final prognosis.[14] This new classification divides patients into five groups:

1. Mild burn (Figure 2-3)
   Corneal epithelial erosion
   Faint anterior stromal haziness
   No coagulation necrosis of perilimbal conjunctiva and sclera
   *Prognosis: healing with little or no corneal scarring*

2. Moderate burn (Figure 2-4)
   Moderate corneal opacity
   Little or no significant coagulation necrosis of perilimbal conjunctiva
   *Prognosis: slow healing of epithelium with moderate scarring and peripheral corneal vascularization*

3. Moderate to severe burn (Figure 2-5)
   Corneal opacity blurring iris details

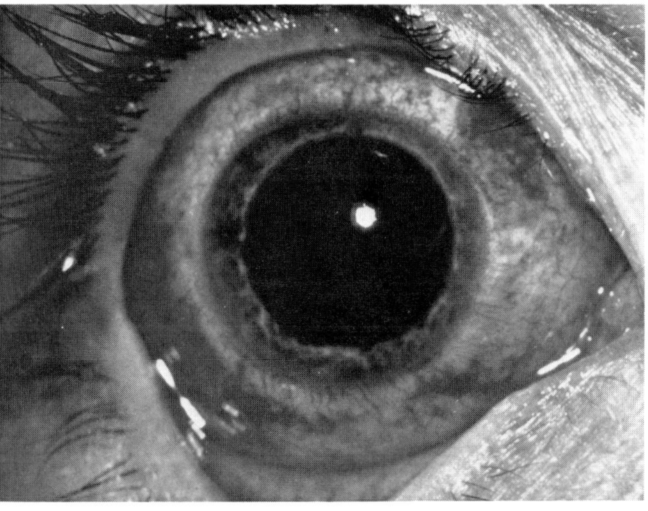

**FIGURE 2-3**    Mild ocular alkali burn.

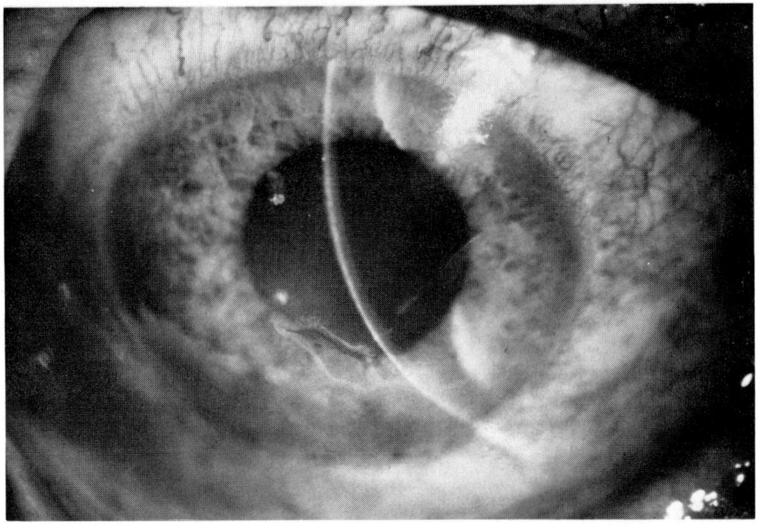

**FIGURE 2-4**     Moderate ocular alkali burn.

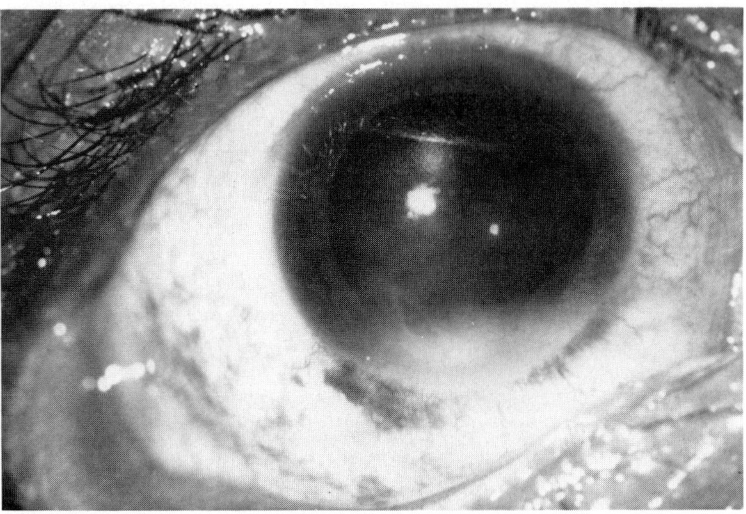

**FIGURE 2-5**     Moderate to severe ocular alkali burn.

Coagulation necrosis of conjunctiva limited to less than one-third of perilimbal conjunctiva

*Prognosis: prolonged corneal healing with significant corneal neovascularization and scarring*

4. Severe burn (Figure 2-6)
Blurring of pupillary outline
Ischemia of approximately one-third to two-thirds of perilimbal conjunctiva
Cornea often marbleized

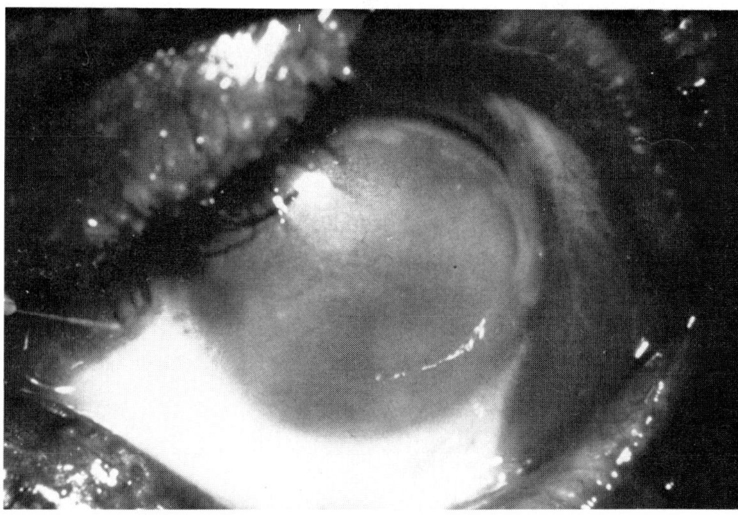

**FIGURE 2-6**  Severe ocular alkali burn.

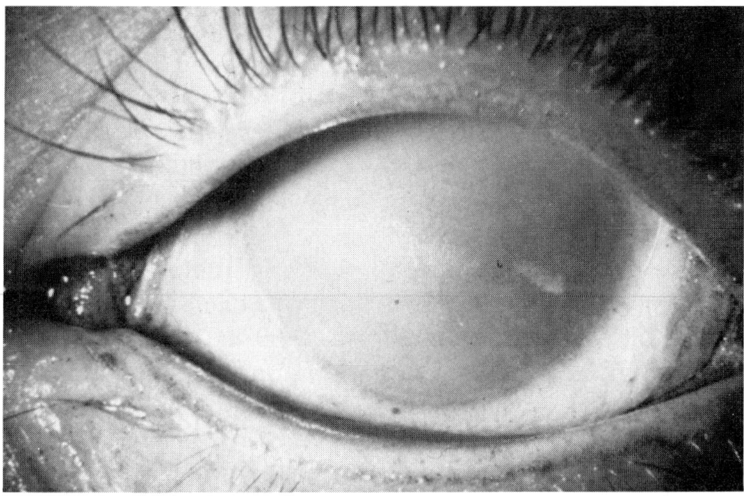

**FIGURE 2-7**  Very severe ocular alkali burn.

*Prognosis: very prolonged corneal healing with inflammation and high inci-dence of corneal ulceration and perforation*

5. Very severe burn (Figure 2-7)
   Pupil not visible
   Greater than two-thirds ischemia of perilimbal conjunctiva
   Completely marbleized cornea

   *Prognosis: healing very prolonged, with frequent conversion of corneal stroma into necrotic sequestra; ulceration and perforation frequent; very severe cor-neal vascularization and scarring; phthisis bulbi may occur with or without ulceration or perforation.*

The amount of corneal epithelial loss and degree of limbal injury influence the prognosis for subsequent epithelial healing and could be used to predict the success of both medical and surgical treatment.[14] To improve the accuracy of the early clinical assessment and the projected prognosis, grading of some alkali burns should be delayed for 48 to 72 hours.

Kinoshita divided late corneal scarring into two types, which differ in prognosis following keratoplasty.[15] Type A scarring, characterized by scarring with the retention of most of the corneal epithelium, is associated with reasonable success after penetrating keratoplasty. Type B scarring, on the other hand, is more frequently associated with epithelial healing difficulties and graft failure; it is characterized by superficial vascularization and coverage of the cornea by conjunctival epithelium.

## ALKALI BURN WOUND HEALING

Healing of the alkali-burned cornea depends on epithelial, stromal, and endothelial wound healing. Alkali burns cause the epithelium to undergo prolonged enzymatic debridement. Basal epithelial cells release plasminogen activator in response to fibrin and fibronectin, both of which are deposited in tissues after alkali injuries.[16] Active plasmin promotes corneal stromal melting by degrading fibronectin, by increasing the production and activity of collagenase, and by attracting polymorphonuclear leukocytes which, in turn, may release other collagenolytic enzymes. The resultant breakdown of fibronectin from underneath the healing epithelium may promote the formation of epithelial defects by preventing epithelial adhesion before hemidesmosomes are reformed.[16]

Rapid corneal reepithelialization is essential to preserving the underlying stroma and maintaining an effective barrier against infection. Corneal epithelial healing begins with early cellular spreading and migration and is followed by late cellular proliferation and substrate adhesion.[17] After cellular regeneration, the substrate adhesion of the epithelium depends on basal hemidesmosomes and anchoring fibrils. Alkali-induced damage retards epithelial healing by interfering with the cellular adherence required for maintenance of epithelial polarity. Severe damage to the basement membrane may be detected as early as one day after alkali burns and may progress to complete disappearance of the basement membrane over the ensuing 72 hours. Once destroyed, the corneal epithelial basement membrane requires about 6 weeks to reform. Formation of subepithelial bullae may lead to further epithelial breakdown.

When the corneal epithelium is injured, limbal corneal epithelial cells migrate centripetally and then proliferate to restore an intact corneal surface. With large corneal epithelial defects, conjunctival epithelium migrates onto the cornea; in such cases, healing tends to be slower and often incomplete.[19] Extensive corneal surface vascularization appears to inhibit the orderly transdifferentiation of conjunctival epithelium into functional corneal epithelium. Furthermore, transdifferentiation itself may take 3 months to complete. Abnormalities in this process may lead to recurrent epithelial erosions, defects, and neovascularization before corneal epithelial healing is complete.[20]

The stroma consists primarily of water, collagen fibrils, keratocytes, and ground substance. The collagen fibrils, embedded in glycosaminoglycans, are uniform and arranged in regular arrays to maintain corneal transparency. Alteration of the glycosaminoglycan "sheath" surrounding the collagen fibrils by alkali injury increases collagen breakdown by collagenases.[18,21] If the collagen destruction is greater than its regeneration, corneal ulceration results.

Stromal ulceration does not appear to result from the direct action of alkali; it is usually not seen before 7 days after injury.[22] Many enzymes, including nonspecific proteases and hydrolases, have been suggested as contributing to stromal ulceration in the alkali-burned cornea.[23] Stromal breakdown and perforation correlate with the increased collagenase activity; the period of highest enzymatic activity occurs 3 to 4 weeks after injury.[24] Regenerating epithelium, infiltrating neutrophils, and damaged stromal keratocytes have been proposed as sources of collagenase release.[9] If untreated, stromal ulceration may progress to descemetocele formation or perforation. With sensitive biochemical assays, collagenase activity has been detected in alkali-burned corneas as early as 9 hours after injury[10] and in nonulcerated, vascularized corneas as long as 2 years after injury.[25]

By the second week after alkali injury, corneal neovascularization begins from the periphery. In severe burns, extensive neovascularization may occur over a period of weeks. Corneal scarring and neovascularization may stabilize the cornea if perforation has not occured by 3 weeks after injury. Corneal perforations tend to occur most often in avascular, acellular regions devoid of infiltrating fibroblasts and in regions where protective epithelium is absent.[26] Neovascularization may enhance the infiltration of inflammatory cells into the alkali-burned cornea. Topical corticosteroids applied within 6 weeks after alkali burn have the potential to inhibit corneal neovascularization.[26] On the one hand, neovascularization (Figure 2-8) reduces the risk of acute perforation; on the other hand, it may unfavorably affect the prognosis of future penetrating keratoplasty.

After severe alkali burns, corneal endothelial cells are often lost. Human corneal endothelium has limited mitotic capacity and heals primarily by migration and enlargement of the remaining endothelial cells. Therefore, when all the

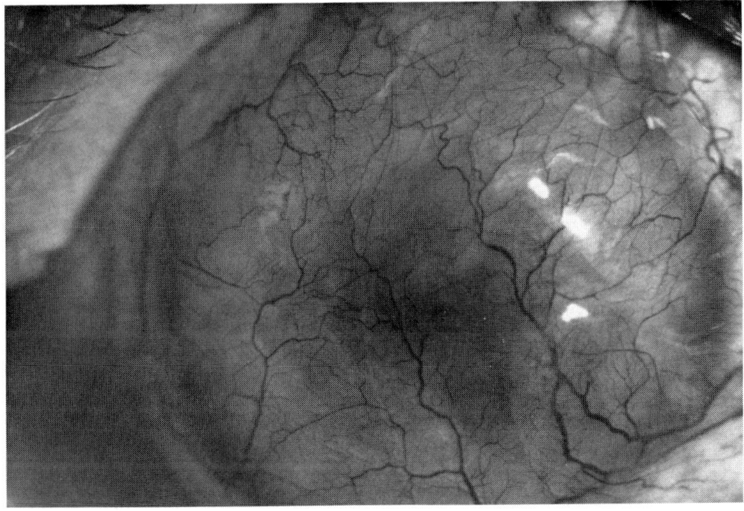

**FIGURE 2-8**     Corneal surface neovascularization after alkali burn.

endothelial cells are destroyed, a retrocorneal membrane may replace the endothelium. Even in corneas with subtotal endothelial destruction, delayed endothelial healing from alkaline pH changes, depressed aqueous glucose levels, and persistent anterior segment inflammation may promote retrocorneal membrane formation in the late healing phases.[27]

## TREATMENT

Clinical approaches to the treatment of alkali burns have been directed primarily towards improving corneal epithelial healing, inhibiting collagenase, enhancing collagen biosynthesis, and reducing leukocyte infiltration. Approaches to therapy may be divided into first acute and intermediate management, then chronic ocular rehabilitation.

## ACUTE AND INTERMEDIATE MANAGEMENT

After acute alkali exposure, immediate irrigation of the eye with water or saline should be started at the accident scene (Figure 2-9) if possible. Upon the patient's arrival at a medical facility, copious irrigation should be continued in order to

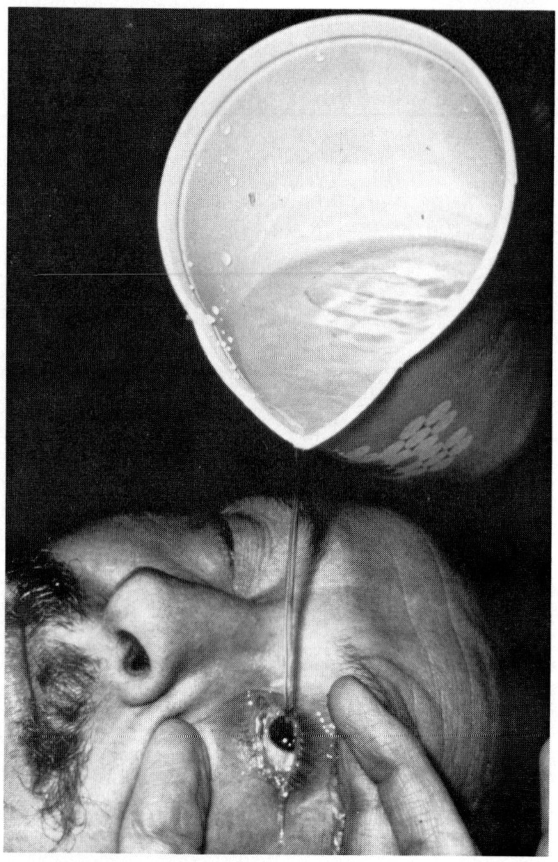

**FIGURE 2-9**    Immediate ocular irrigation at accident scene.

dilute and wash away any remaining alkali.[4] Typically, irrigation consists of at least 2 liters of solution given over a minimum of 30 minutes, but longer treatment may be required in severe cases. While irrigating scleral lenses and other delivery devices are available, effective irrigation can be achieved by applying a steady stream of irrigant via intravenous tubing. Only after copious irrigation has been given, litmus paper may be touched to the inferior palpebral conjunctiva to determine the baseline pH. In general, however, early baseline pH measurements should be eschewed if such measurements may cause any undue delay or interruption of irrigation. Irrigation should continue until the ocular surface has been neutralized as confirmed by repeated pH measurements. Residual chemical material embedded under the eyelids (Figure 2-10) should be removed mechanically and/or by chelation with 0.01-0.05 M sodium ethylenediamine tetraacetic acid (EDTA) to eliminate sources of continued alkali release.[5] Attempts at lowering the intraocular pH by paracentesis and irrigation of the anterior chamber with buffers have shown only marginal success (despite the risks) in reducing injury following alkali burns.[28] In severe burns, however, removal of the alkaline aqueous humor may eliminate a source of continuing intraocular cauterization. Immediate surgical intervention is advocated by a few clinicians; such intervention is limited to simple debridement of necrotic conjunctiva and corneal epithelium, both being potential sources of collagenase production.[21] Symblepharon formation may be reduced by removing or lysing fibrinous bulbar-palpebral adhesions. Special plastic symblepharon rings may also be used to reduce formation of synechiae.

Following the initial injury, treatment should also be directed towards managing any resulting tear insufficiencies and preventing secondary infection and toward controlling inflammation and detrimental tissue responses. Topical antibiotic drops or ointments may be used prophylactically. Cycloplegia with atropine 1% twice daily or 1% cyclopentolate three or four times daily may lessen posterior synechiae formation and reduce discomfort from ciliary spasm. In the late phases following alkali burns, the intraocular pressure may be decreased, normal, or

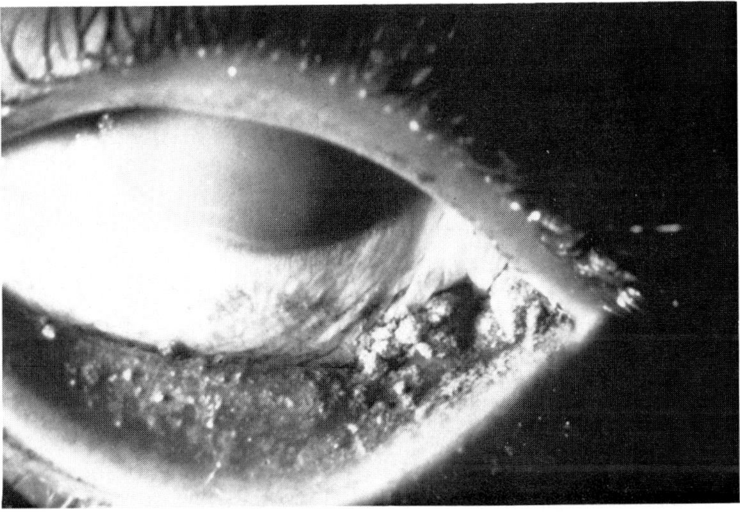

**FIGURE 2-10**     Retained chemical particulate material under eyelid.

increased, depending on the relative predominance of aqueous humor production versus trabecular meshwork outflow. Acutely with severe burns, there is a spiking rise in the intraocular pressure putatively caused primarily by collagen shrinkage; this is followed by a more gradual, prolonged elevation in pressure that is possibly due to prostaglandin release.[29] Elevated intraocular pressure should be treated aggressively with systemic carbonic anhydrase inhibitors and/or topical antiglaucoma medications.

The indications for corticosteroid use in the management of corneal alkali burns remain controversial. Topical corticosteroids are frequently used to reduce posttraumatic inflammation. However, they also have the potential to increase collagenase activity[30] and to retard epithelial regeneration and stromal wound healing.[31] Corneal stromal ulceration may be accelerated if corticosteroids are continued longer than 10 days after injury, especially in the setting of a persistent epithelial defect.[32] If corneal reepithelialization does not occur by 10 to 14 days following the alkali burn, it may be safer to taper the steroids in order to reduce the risk of potentiating collagen breakdown and ulceration. Steroids may be continued as needed if the epithelium remains intact. Other previously reported therapies include subconjunctival injections of heparin and serum, topical vasodilators, and glued-on contact lenses.[4] While systemic immunosuppressives may be useful in several chronic ocular inflammatory disorders, their use in the treatment of alkali burns remains experimental and controversial.[33]

Topical sodium citrate has been demonstrated to inhibit corneal neutrophil infiltration and to reduce the incidence of corneal ulceration and perforation following alkali burns in animal models.[34] Citrate blocks several neutrophil functions, including migration, phagocytosis, and enzyme release, by chelating the necessary calcium ions.[34] Penicillamine, EDTA, and 10% to 20% acetylcysteine (Mucomyst) nonspecifically inhibit collagenase following alkali burns by chelating essential ions, as well as by reducing leukocytic infiltration.[35,36] Due to its wider availability and lower toxicity, 10% to 20% acetylcysteine is frequently used clinically and may be applied every 2 hours while the patient is awake. It has been shown to decrease the incidence of perforation of alkali-burned corneas in animal studies,[36] but its use is partially limited because of its unpleasant odor and its need for refrigeration. L-cysteine (0.2 M) has also been shown to reduce the incidence of corneal perforation.[36] Since it has been observed that the corneal epithelial basement membrane generally remains intact in mild to moderate alkali burns for the first week after injury, collagenase inhibitors are often withheld unless there is evidence of significant collagen breakdown.[4] However, as delayed stromal ulceration may sometimes occur after the second and third week in severe injuries, it may be advisable to begin collagenase inhibitor treatment immediately after the acute injury phase.[4]

Other inhibitors of collagenase include medroxyprogesterone (Provera) and tetracycline. Topical or parenteral administration of medroxyprogesterone may reduce the incidence of deep ulceration and perforation in alkali-burned corneas by suppressing inflammation and tissue collagenase activity.[37] Similarly, systemic tetracycline may improve corneal wound healing by inhibiting collagenase. Tetracycline also blocks neutrophil phagocytosis and chemotaxis, thus lessening corneal destruction from the inflammatory and reparative responses.[38]

Ascorbic acid (vitamin C) is essential to the biosynthesis of collagen and proteoglycans and functions as a scavenger of harmful superoxide radicals.[39] It is a cofactor in the hydroxylation of proline and facilitates the maturation of fibroblasts in wound healing. While the replacement of ascorbic acid after alkali injury may be important if aqueous levels are decreased, ascorbic acid supplementation may actually promote stromal ulceration under conditions in which aqueous levels are normal.[40] In rabbits with severe alkali burns, supplemental ascorbate is associated with a reduced incidence of corneal ulceration.[41] Clinical trials of oral and topical ascorbate in the treatment of human alkali burns are still being conducted.[42]

Epidermal growth factor (EGF) and attachment glycoproteins, such as fibronectin, have been used topically to promote epithelial healing. EGF is a naturally occurring, mitogenic polypeptide which increases epithelial proliferation and stimulates repair of corneal epithelial defects.[43] It also increases synthesis of fibronectin, further enhancing corneal epithelial spreading and healing.[44] Topical application of exogenous fibronectin may help maintain epithelial adherence and assist in hemidesmosome formation.[45] Neither EGF nor fibronectin is apparently effective in preventing recurrent corneal epithelial erosions and breakdown following corneal alkali burns.[46]

Therapeutic soft contact lenses may be applied after alkali burns in order to facilitate epithelialization in recalcitrant cases. Although therapeutic contact lenses can be applied acutely, their use may be deferred until there is clinical evidence that epithelialization is not progressing. Topical medications can often be instilled directly over the lens. Whenever necessary, the contact lens should be moved aside or be removed for the evaluation of the underlying epithelial defect with fluorescein. The lens may be left in place for 6 to 8 weeks after the epithelium has healed, thus allowing the reestablishment of hemidesmosomes and strong epithelial adhesion. Collagen shields and collagen bandage lenses also appear to have promise in the treatment of alkali burns by aiding epithelialization and serving as a drug delivery system.[47,48]

## CHRONIC, LONG-TERM CARE AND REHABILITATION

The ocular surface usually begins to stabilize by 3 to 4 weeks after the initial injury. Topical antibiotics, cycloplegics, and glaucoma medications may often be discontinued. Unfortunately, even at this late stage, epithelial defects may persist and contribute to the development of recalcitrant stromal ulceration. Artificial tears and ointments may be of limited benefit in preventing epithelial breakdown. Recurrent epithelial erosions threaten visual recovery by predisposing the cornea to infection or ulceration. Topical echothiophate iodide (phospholine iodide) may stimulate epithelial proliferation and can be considered if treatment with contact lenses and/or collagen shields fails.[4] Eyelid problems, such as lagophthalmos and trichiasis, may also retard epithelial healing. Symblepharon formation is common after alkali burns and typically recurs following manual synechiolysis. Formation of symblepharon can sometimes be inhibited by the use of scleral lenses or conformer rings. Reconstruction of shortened conjunctival fornices may require transplantation of oral mucous membrane grafts; however, oral mucosa do not function as normal conjunctival epithelium.[49] Topical vitamin A derivatives may also improve the ocular surface condition and reduce keratinization.[50]

Conjunctival flaps are effective in protecting the integrity of the eye if stromal ulceration continues in spite of aggressive medical approaches. However, if severe conjunctival scarring is present, adequate mobilization of a conjunctival flap for corneal coverage may not be possible. An experimental technique of photo-thrombosis has been recently described using intravenous rose bengal and argon laser irradiation for selective occlusion of blood vessels which might promote the induction of conjunctival transdifferentiation.[51] When applied to conjunctival flaps, this technique shows potential for improvement of the new ocular surface.[52]

Following unilateral injuries, autologous conjunctival or limbal transplantation from the uninvolved eye may be combined with superficial keratectomy in order to improve the resurfacing and clarity of the burned cornea.[53,54] Limbal transplantation, a modified method of conjunctival transplantation, includes limbal epithelium containing corneal epithelial stem cells. Both types of conjunctival transplantation can lead to prompt healing of the corneal epithelial defects, long-term stabilization of the new epithelial surface, regression of corneal vascular-ization, and improvement of visual acuity.[54,55] When performed prior to penetrating keratoplasty, conjunctival transplantation may improve the prognosis of graft survival.[53] In cases in which inadequate conjunctival tissue remains, a thick conjunc-tiva-Tenon advancement flap or Tenon-plasty may be performed, although the results may not be as satisfactory as in conjunctival transplantation.[53] Keratoepi-thelioplasty, as originally developed by Thoft,[56] has also been modified to encom-pass limbal epithelium from an allograft source for treatment of chronic ocular surface disorders.[57] Keratoepithelioplasty may prove to be useful in resolving persistent epithelial defects after chemical injuries.[57]

Although prevention is the best treatment for corneal ulceration and per-foration (Figure 2-11), quite often these complications occur despite the best efforts. For small corneal perforations, cyanoacrylate tissue adhesives[58] may be

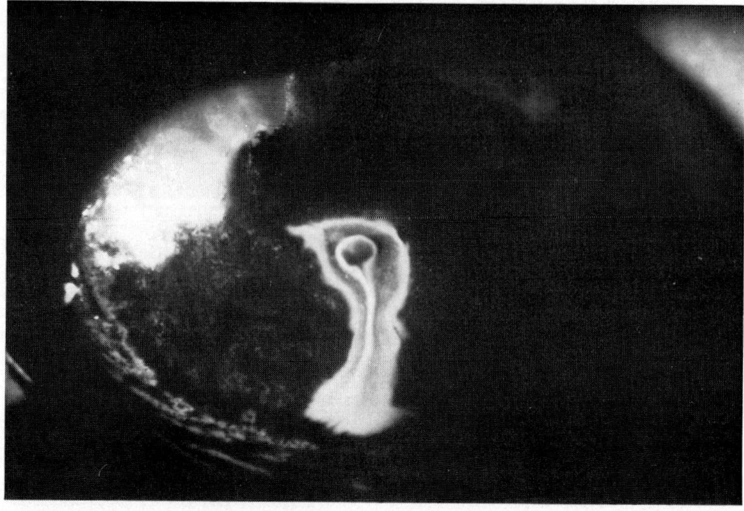

**FIGURE 2-11**     Corneal perforation showing spontaneous Seidel test with fluorescein.

used to seal the perforation. The cyanoacrylates may also retard corneal melting by excluding infiltrating leukocytes and protecting against Gram positive bacterial infections.[8,59] A lamellar keratoplasty using either a surgeon-prepared donor patch graft or Keratopatch lenticle (American Medical Optics) is often necessary for large descemetoceles or perforations. Penetrating keratoplasty is sometimes necessary to preserve or improve vision following moderate to severe alkali burns, but it should be delayed 1 to 2 years to allow the eye to heal fully and for inflammation to subside.[60] Alkali-burn-related complications, such as eyelid problems, symblepharon formation, glaucoma, and retinal damage, contribute to an unfavorable keratoplasty result.[61] If the integrity of the posterior segment of the eye could not be assessed ophthalmoscopically prior to keratoplasty, B-scan echography should be performed.

Frequent followup examinations and good patient compliance have been shown to be essential to achieving a successful keratoplasty following alkali burns.[1] Aggressive postoperative topical steroids should be used to suppress inflammation. Intraocular pressure should be closely monitored following keratoplasty. Scarring of the conjunctiva often precludes successful trabeculoplasty; therefore, cyclo-destructive procedures may be necessary for intraocular pressure control in cases of intractable glaucoma. HLA-matching and topical cyclosporine A may possibly reduce the chances of immune graft rejection in highly vascularized recipient corneas.

In some patients in whom repeated keratoplasty has failed, a keratoprosthesis may be considered. Most keratoprotheses are composed of a methymethacrylate stem attached to a supporting anchoring plate placed in the corneal stroma and are of nut-and-bolt, collar-button, or through-and-through design (Figure 2-12).[62,63] The major complication associated with all types of keratoprotheses is ulceration around the stem leading to extrusion, infection, and retinal detachment.[63] Therefore, these devices should not be considered in unilateral alkali burns or in eyes with relatively good vision.

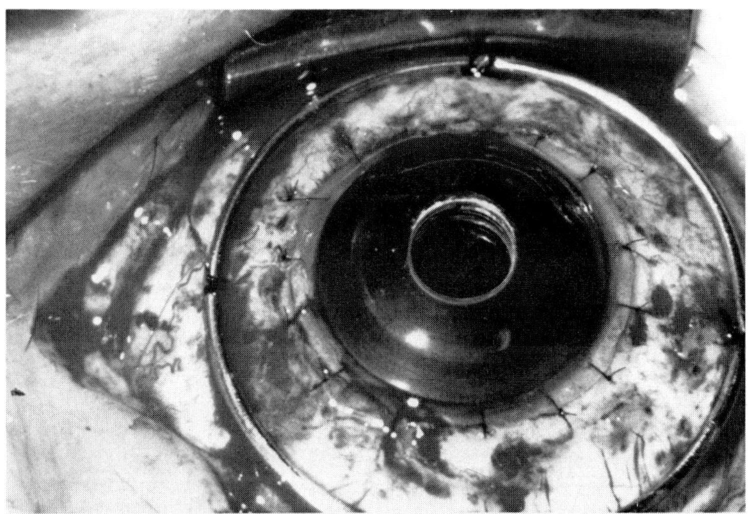

**FIGURE 2-12**   Keratoprosthesis.

## SUMMARY

The recovery of visual function following corneal alkali burns is dependent on the degree of epithelial loss and resultant scarring as graded by previously described classifications. The amount of corneal tissue destruction will affect the epithelial, stromal, and endothelial healing responses. Several therapeutic approaches, both medical and surgical, have been developed to improve corneal healing and retard unfavorable reparative responses. Treatments have been directed toward: (a) reducing acute tissue damage, (b) inhibiting leukocyte infiltration, (c) reducing collagenolytic enzyme production and activity, (d) increasing corneal collagen production, (e) promoting adhesion between the epithelium and the underlying stroma, (f) replacing healthy epithelial cells and enhancing the regeneration of epithelial cells, and (g) reducing secondary complications (Figure 2-13). Penetrating keratoplasty can occasionally be successful following alkali burns, but it should be delayed when possible to allow surface epithelium

Irrigate

Remove embedded chemical material

Check pH; if still elevated then check for retained particulate material

Consider: EDTA application
Simple debridement
Paracentesis/anterior chamber washout

Topical medical treatment:
Aggressive lubricants
Antibiotic prophylaxis
Antiglaucoma medications (if needed)
Cycloplegics
Corticosteroids

Consider: Stop or taper corticosteroids after 10-14 days if persistent epithelial defects

Collagenase inhibitors if severe injury or if significant collagen breakdown

Therapeutic soft contact lens if epithelialization is not progressing

Consider: Collagen shields/collagen bandage lens
Epidermal growth factor (ECG)
Fibronectin
Vitamin A ointment if marked keratinization

Surgical treatment:
Cyanoacrylate glue
Lamellar keratoplasty/keratopatch
Conjunctival/limbal transplantation
Keratoepithelioplasty
Penetrating keratoplasty
Keratoprosthesis

Consider: HLA matching and/or cyclosporine for high risk keratoplasty

**FIGURE 2-13**     Alkali burn treatment algorithm.

to heal and inflammation to subside. In spite of all the recent advancements in the management of corneal alkali burns, prevention through public education is still the best treatment.



## References

1. Klein R, Lobes LA, Jr. Ocular alkali burns in a large urban area. Ann Ophthalmol 1976; 8:1185-1188.
2. Morgan SJ. Chemical burns of the eye: causes and management. Br J Ophthalmol 1987; 71:854-857.
3. Hughes WF, Jr. Alkali burns of the eye: I. Review of the literature and summary of present knowledge, Arch Ophthalmol 1946; 35:423-449.
4. McCulley JP. Chemical injuries. In Smolin G, Thoft RA, eds. The cornea: scientific foundations and clinical practice, ed 2, Boston: Little, Brown & Co, 1987:527-542.
5. Grant WM, Kern HL. Action of alkalies on the corneal stroma. Arch Ophthalmol 1955; 54:931-939.
6. Pfister RR, Haddox JL, Dodson RW, Harkins LE. Alkali-burned collagen produces a locomotory and metabolic stimulus to neutrophils. Invest Ophthalmol Vis Sci 1987; 28:295-304.
7. Berry SM, Hong BS, Lam KW. Degeneration of bovine corneal collagen by alkali. Cornea 1989; 8:150-154.
8. Kenyon KR, Berman M, Rose J, Gage J. Prevention of stromal ulceration in the alkali-burned rabbit cornea by glued-on contact lens. Evidence for the role of polymorphonuclear leukocytes in collagen degradation. Invest Ophthalmol Vis Sci 1979; 18:570-587.
9. Friend J. Physiology of the cornea; metabolism and biochemistry. In Smolin G, Thoft RA, eds. The cornea: scientific foundations and clinical practice, ed 2. Boston: Little Brown & Co, 1987:16-38.
10. Pfister RR, McCulley JP, Friend J, Dohlman CH. Collagenase activity of intact corneal epithelium in peripheral alkali burn. Arch Ophthalmol 1971; 86:308-313.
11. Flynn WJ, Mauger TF, Hill RM. Corneal burns: a quantitative comparison of acid and base. Acta Ophthalmol (Copenhagen) 1984; 62:542-548.
12. Obenberger J, Babicky A. Distribution of $^{24}NaCl$ in tissues of alkali-and acid-burned rabbit eyes. Exp Eye Res 1975; 20:195-206.
13. Hughes WF, Jr. Alkali burns of the eye II. clinical and pathologic course. Arch Ophthalmol 1946; 36:189-214.
14. Pfister RR. Chemical corneal burns. Int Ophthalmol Clin 1984; 24:157-168.
15. Kinoshita S, Manabe R. Chemical burns. In Brightbill FS, ed. Corneal surgery: theory, technique, and tissue. St. Louis: C.V. Mosby Co, 1986:370-379.
16. Berman MB, Kenyon KR, Hayashi K, L'Hernault N. The pathogenesis of epithelial defects and stromal ulceration. In Cavanagh HD, ed. The cornea: transactions of the World Congress on the Cornea III, New York: Raven, 1988:35-43.
17. Khodadoust AA, Silverstein AM, Kenyon KR, Dowling JE. Adhesion of regenerating corneal epithelium: the role of basement membrane. Am J Ophthalmol 1968; 65:339-348.
18. Francois J, Feher J. Collagenolysis and regeneration in corneal burnings. Ophthalmologica 1972; 165:137-152.
19. Friend J, Thoft RA. Functional competence of regenerating ocular surface epithelium. Invest Ophthalmol Vis Sci 1978; 17:134-39.
20. Kinoshita S, Friend J, Thoft RA. Ocular surface epithelial regeneration and disease. Int Ophthalmol Clin 1984; 24:169-177.
21. Gnadinger MC, Itoi M, Slansky HH, Dohlman CH. The role of collagenase in the alkali-burned cornea. Am J Ophthalmol 1969; 68:478-483.
22. Brown SI, Weller CA, Wassermann HE. Collagenolytic activity of alkali-burned corneas. Arch Ophthalmol 1969; 81:370-373.
23. Berman M, Leary R, Gage J. Collagenase from corneal cell cultures and its modulation by phagocytosis. Invest Ophthalmol Vis Sci 1979; 18:588-601.
24. Anderson RE, Kuns MD, Dresden MH. Collagenase activity in the alkali-burned cornea. Ann Ophthalmol 1971; 3:619-621.
25. Brown SI, Weller CA, Akiya S. Pathogenesis of ulcers of alkali-burned cornea. Arch Ophthalmol 1970; 83:205-208.
26. Brown SI, Wassermann HE, Dunn MW. Alkali burns of the cornea. Arch Ophthalmol 1969; 82:91-94.
27. Renard G, Hirsch M, Pouliquen Y. Corneal changes due to alkali burns. Trans Ophthalmol Soc UK 1978; 98:379-382.
28. Burns RP, Hikes CE. Irrigation of the anterior chamber for the treatment of alkali burns. Am J Ophthalmol 1979; 88:119-120.
29. Paterson CA, Pfister RR. Intraocular pressure changes after alkali burns. Arch Ophthalmol 1974; 91:211-218.
30. Brown SI, Weller CA, Vidrich AM. Effect of corticosteroids on corneal collagenase of rabbits. Am J Ophthalmol 1970; 70:744-747.
31. Sugar J, Chandler JW. Experimental corneal wound strength: effect of topically applied corticosteroids. Arch Ophthalmol 1974; 92:248-249.

32. Donshik PC, Berman MB, Dohlman CH, Gage J, Rose J. The effect of topical corticosteroids on ulceration in alkali-burned corneas. Arch Ophthalmol 1978; 96:2117-2120.

33. Foster CS, Zelt RP, Mai-Phan T, Kenyon KR. Immunosuppression and selective inflammatory cell depletion: studies in a guinea pig model of corneal ulceration after ocular alkali burning. Arch Ophthalmol 1982; 100:1820-1824.

34. Pfister RR. The effects of chemical injury on the ocular surface. Ophthalmol 1983; 90:601-609.

35. Francois J, Cambie E, Feher J, Van Den Eeckhout E. Collagenase inhibitors (penicillamine). Ann Ophthalmol 1973; 5:391-408.

36. Slansky HH, Berman MB, Dohlman CH, Rose J. Cysteine and acetylcysteine in the prevention of corneal ulcerations. Ann Ophthalmol 1970; 2:488-491.

37. Newsome DA, Gross J. Prevention by medroxyprogesterone of perforation in the alkali-burned rabbit cornea: inhibition of collagenolytic activity. Invest Ophthalmol Vis Sci 1977; 16:21-31.

38. Seedor JA, Perry HD, McNamara TF, Golub LM, Buxton DF, Guthrie DS. Systemic tetracycline treatment of alkali-induced corneal ulceration in rabbits. Arch Ophthalmol 1987; 105:268-271.

39. Nirankari VS, Varma SD, Lakhanpal V, Richard RD. Superoxide radical scavenging agents in treatment of alkali burns: an experimental study. Arch Ophthalmol 1981; 99:886-887.

40. Foster CS, Zelt R, Kenyon KR, Chakrabarti B. Ascorbate therapy for experimental thermal corneal burns. Invest Ophthalmol Vis Sci 1980; 19:227.

41. Pfister RR, Paterson CA, Hayes SA. Effect of topical 10% ascorbic solution on established corneal ulcers after severe alkali burns. Invest Ophthal Vis Sci 1982; 22:382-385.

42. Pfister RR. Diseases of the external eye: Alkali burns. In Clinical signs in ophthalmology. St. Louis: C.V. Mosby Co, 1986; 8(2):2-11.

43. Frati L, Daniele S, Delogu A, Covelli I. Selective binding of the epidermal growth factor and its specific effects on the epithelial cells of the cornea. Exp Eye Res 1972; 14:135-141.

44. Nishida T, Tanaka H, Nagagawa S, Sasabe T, Awata T, and Manabe R. Fibronectin synthesis by the rabbit cornea: effects of mouse epidermal growth factor and cyclic AMP analogs. Jpn J Ophthalmol 1984; 28:196-202.

45. Nishida T. Role of fibronectin in corneal epithelial wound healing. In Cavanagh HD, ed. The cornea: transactions of the world congress on the cornea III. New York: Raven, 1988:619-625.

46. Schultz GS, Davis JB, Eiferman RA. Growth factors and corneal epithelium. Cornea 1988; 7:96-101.

47. Hwang DG, Stern WH, Hwang PH, MacGowan-Smith LA. Collagen shield enhancement of topical dexamethasone penetration. Arch Ophthalmol 1989; 107:1375-1380.

48. Ruffini JJ, Aquavella JV, LoCascio JA. Effect of collagen shields on corneal epithelialization following penetrating keratoplasty. Ophthalmic Surg 1989; 20:21-25.

49. Ballen PH. Mucous membrane grafts in chemical (lye) burns. Am J Ophthalmol 1963; 55:302-312.

50. Soong HK, Martin NF, Wagoner MD, et al. Topical retinoid therapy for squamous metaplasia of various ocular surface diseases: a multicenter, placebo-controlled double-masked study. Ophthalmol 1988; 95:1442-1446.

51. Huang AJW, Watson BD, Hernandez E, Tseng SCG. Photothrombosis of corneal neovascularization by intravenous rose bengal and argon laser irradiation. Arch Ophthalmol 1988;106:680-685.

52. Huang AJW, Tseng SCG. Phenotypic alterations of conjunctival flaps on corneal surface by photothrombosis. Invest Ophthalmol Vis Sci 1990; 31:2304.

53. Thoft RA. Conjunctival transplantation as an alternative to keratoplasty. Ophthalmol 1979; 86:1084-1092.

54. Kenyon KR, Tseng SCG. Limbal autograft transplantation for ocular surface disorders. Ophthalmol 1989; 96:709-723.

55. Thoft RA. Indication for conjunctival transplantation. Ophthalmol 1982; 89:335-39.

56. Thoft RA. Keratoepithelioplasty. Am J Ophthalmol 1984; 97:1-6.

57. Turgseon PW, Nauheim RC, Roat MI, Stopak SS, Thoft RA. Indications for keratoepithelioplasty. Arch Ophthalmol 1990; 108:233-236.

58. Kenyon KR. Decision-making in the therapy of external eye disease: non-infected corneal ulcers. Ophthalmol 1982; 89:44-51.

59. Eiferman RA, Snyder JW. Antibacterial effect of cyanoacrylate glue. Arch Ophthalmol 1983; 101:958-960.

60. Kramer SG. Late numerical grading of alkali burns to determine keratoplasty prognosis. Trans Am Ophthalmol Soc 1983; 81:97-106.

61. Brown SI, Bloomfield SE, Pearce DB. A follow-up report on transplantation of the alkali-burned cornea. Am J Ophthalmol 1974; 77:538-542.

62. Cardona H, DeVoe AG. Prosthokeratoplasty. Trans Am Acad Ophthalmol Otolaryngol 1977; 83:271-280.

63. Dohlman CH, Schneider HA, Doane MG. Prosthokeratoplasty. Am J Ophthalmol 1974; 77:694-700.

# 3 Dry Eye Syndromes
## *Current Diagnosis and Management*

**J. Daniel Nelson, MD**

The term "dry eye syndromes" refers to a group of diseases that cause symptoms of dry, irritated, burning, or gritty-feeling eyes. When these diseases affect the conjunctival and corneal surfaces of the eye, they are often termed ocular surface diseases. Although the exact incidence is not known, dry eye syndromes account for many patient visits to the ophthalmologist. Dry eye symptoms are elicited from many older patients whose symptoms can range from very mild to quite debilitating. Many patients "put up" with their symptoms and self-prescribe over-the-counter eye preparations such as boric acid wash or salt water. The box on p. 50 gives the general classification of dry eye syndromes.

## STRUCTURE OF THE TEAR FILM

The precorneal tear film is absolutely necessary for the health of the ocular surface. It provides nutrition, protection and cleansing to the ocular surface. The precorneal tear film is composed of three layers. The outer most lipid (or oily) layer is secreted by the meibomian glands. These glands are located along the posterior aspect of the lid margin and are modified sebaceous-type glands. These glands secrete an oily substance composed of fatty esters onto the surface of the tear film, forming a thin layer that decreases evaporation and provides biomechanical stability to the tear film. The middle layer, and the thickest, is the aqueous layer. The aqueous layer, which comprises over 90% of the tear volume, is secreted by the lacrimal and accessory lacrimal glands. It is the major carrier of dissolved oxygen to the corneal epithelium, stroma, and endothelium. It contains antibodies (IgA), peroxidases, transferrin, and lysozyme which protect the ocular surface from the effects of microbial agents. It also contains electrolytes, trace elements, and proteins. The innermost layer is the mucin layer. Mucin is secreted by goblet cells located on the conjunctival surface. Mucin interacts with the glycocalyx, which is secreted by the corneal epithelial cells, allowing adherence of the hydrophilic aqueous to the hydrophobic epithelium. Tears are spread across the surface of the eye by the movement of the eyelids. This movement (or blink) not only spreads tears across the surface of the eye but also removes debris and desquamated superficial epithelial cells. Tears drain through two slit-like openings, termed the puncta (singular, punctum), at the medial aspect of the upper and lower eyelids, into the canalicular ducts. The inferior and superior canalicular

**General Categories of Frequent Causes
of Dry Eyes**

---

Tear film abnormalities
Eyelid abnormalities
Blink mechanism abnormalities
Ocular surface abnormalities

ducts meet to form a common canaliculus which feeds into the nasal lacrimal sac that exists into the nose. Closure of the eyelid compresses the nasal lacrimal sac, creating a negative pressure in the sac. When the eyelids open, the negative pressure results in tears and debris being aspirated from the eyes into the nasolacrimal system.[1]

## PATHOPHYSIOLOGY OF THE DRY EYE

Because the tear film, ocular surface, lid closure (blink), and lids are critical for maintaining the health of the ocular surface, any dysfunction or disruption of these elements can lead to an abnormality of the ocular surface and to dry eye symptoms. Dry eye signs and symptoms can result from abnormalities of any layer(s) of the tear film.[2] For example, lipid (or oily) layer abnormalities are common in patients with lid margin inflammation (blepharitis). This inflammation may be due to seborrhea, staphylococcal organisms, or dysfunction of the meibomian glands as is seen in ocular rosacea.[3,4] Aqueous-layer abnormalities are seen in patients with lacrimal gland inflammation or degeneration due to Sjögren's syndrome or following radiation therapy to the head. Mucin and glycocalyx abnormalities can be seen in diseases that directly affect the ocular surface— Stevens-Johnson syndrome and ocular pemphigoid. Lid closure (or blink) abnormalities are seen in patients with seventh cranial nerve palsies such as Bell's palsy or after removal of an acoustic neuroma. Many patients also have nocturnal lagophthalmos or inability to close their eyes completely while sleeping. Patients with lid abnormalities, such as ectropion, can develop dry eye signs and symptoms due to the inability to retain enough tears to adequately cover the ocular surface.

Ocular surface disease (OSD) is defined as disease which is noninfectious and involves the conjunctiva *and* cornea. OSD can also cause dry eye due to scarring of the lacrimal gland excretory ducts, loss of goblet cells, or alterations in the epithelium. Examples of OSD include ocular cicatricial pemphigoid, Stevens-Johnson syndrome, vitamin A deficiency, and atopic dermatitis.[5]

## SPECIFIC CAUSES OF DRY EYES
### Environmental Factors

It is well known that patients with dry eye problems, especially those with aqueous tear deficiency (KCS) and blepharitis, are adversely affected by environmental factors that increase evaporation. Cold, dry weather conditions, windy days, car heaters, heat from ovens, and air conditioning are examples of environmental factors that increase evaporation. Patients with KCS are also more susceptible to

**Environmental Factors That Exacerbate
Dry Eye Symptoms**

| | |
|---|---|
| Cold temperatures | Cosmetics |
| Low humidity | Fingernail polish |
| Wind | Hand lotions and soaps |
| Airborne chemicals | Pollen |
| Cigarette smoke | Fabric dyes |
| Fluorescent lights | |

airborne pollutants due to their inability to dilute out the toxic chemicals that dissolve in the tear film. Fabric dyes, newspaper ink, perfumes, and colognes are some examples of airborne chemicals that can irritate the eye with KCS. The box above summarizes other environmental factors that can exacerbate dry eye symptoms.

## Systemic Medications

Many systemic medications, especially those with anticholinergic properties, can cause decreased aqueous tear secretion. Diuretics, psychotropics, and antihistamines are frequent offenders. In addition, dermatological preparations such as topical tretinoin (Retin A) and systemic isoretinoin (Accutane) may cause blepharitis.

## Systemic Diseases

Various systemic conditions can be associated with dry eye syndromes (see box, p. 52). Keratoconjunctivitis sicca associated with Sjögren's syndrome and blepharitis associated with acne rosacea are seen most often. Sjögren's syndrome is classically divided into primary and secondary varieties. Primary Sjögren's syndrome (1° SS) is defined as the presence of KCS *and* xerostomia (dry mouth). 1° SS is often accompanied by decreased vaginal secretions, dry skin, malaise, and occasionally by interstitial pneumonitis and petechial skin rashes. Secondary Sjögren's syndrome (2° SS) is defined as the presence of KCS *and/or* xerostomia *and* a systemic disease such as rheumatoid arthritis, systemic lupus erythematosis, or scleroderma. Patients with 1° SS often have a long, insidious history of increasingly dry mucosal membranes. These patients may have a history of difficulties wearing contact lenses, poor tolerance of dry environments, and conjunctivitis. Patients with 2° SS may present with KCS and/or xerostomia before the onset of systemic disease manifestations, or they may present with systemic symptoms first.[6] KCS is most often found in association with rheumatoid arthritis and systemic lupus. KCS is present in 10% to 25% of patients with rheumatoid arthritis. About 60% of patients who present with KCS and xerostomia have associated connective tissue disease. If a systemic disease is suspected, rheumatological workup, including CBC, antinuclear antibodies, rheumatoid factor, SSA/SSB, and serum protein electrophoresis is indicated. Patients with KCS will complain of a foreign body or of a gritty or sandy sensation (the feeling of sand or gravel) in

### Systemic Conditions Commonly Associated with Dry Eyes

**Blepharitis**

Seborrheic dermatitis
Rosacea
Drug allergy or toxicity

**Ocular surface diseases**

Stevens-Johnson syndrome
Reiter's syndrome
Ocular cicatricial pemphigoid
Sjögren's syndrome
Vitamin A deficiency

**Lid closure abnormalities**

Bells's palsy
Traumatic 7th cranial nerve palsy
Grave's disease

**Decreased or absent lacrimal gland secretion**

Facial nerve lesions between nucleus and geniculate ganglion
Lesions of greater petrosal nerve, sphenopalatine ganglion or lacrimal nerve
Ramsey-Hunt syndrome
Sjögren's syndrome
Rheumatoid arthritis
Systemic Lupus erythematosus
Scleroderma
Polyarteritis nodosa
Amyotrophic lateral sclerosis
Sarcoidosis
Raynaud's phenomenon
Pulmonary fibrosis
Thrombocytopenic purpura
Hashimoto's thyroiditis
Waldenstrom's hyperglobulinemia
Chronic hepatobiliary cirrhosis

After Roy FH. Ocular differential diagnosis, ed 3. Philadelphia: Lea and Febiger, 1984, 74-76.

the eyes. Photophobia (pain with light) and thick, stringy mucus are seen in more severe cases. These symptoms tend to be least upon awakening and more severe as the day progresses. Patients with xerostomia (dry mouth) will have difficulty chewing and swallowing dry foods and meat without accompanying liquids. They will also lack the sensation of saliva in their mouths.

Patients with ocular rosacea blepharitis often have minimal facial findings of rosacea. The major symptoms are of burning (feeling of soap or shampoo) in the eyes and mattering upon awakening. In contradistinction to KCS, symptoms of blepharitis are usually worse upon awakening, improve toward mid-day, and worsen later in the day.

## Acquired Dry Eye Syndromes

The most common acquired causes are those related to age, hormones, blepharitis, lid malposition, or poor blinking. Certain dry eye syndromes are found more frequently in different age groups. KCS is more common in postmenopausal females while rosacea blepharitis is more common in young women (20-40 years old) and older men (> 50 years of age). Although the exact prevalence of KCS in the United States is not known, the prevalence in Sweden is approximately 15%.[7] Lid malposition is more frequent in the elder population due to the increasing laxity of the lids and subcutaneous tissues. Mild lagophthalmos (< 2 mm) is not uncommon and usually is asymptomatic. Severe lagophthalmos is found in patients with seventh cranial nerve abnormalities such as Bell's palsy and among patients following removal of an acoustic neuroma or parotid gland surgery. Poor blinking is common in contact lens wearers, in patients with Parkinsonism, and among those with seventh cranial nerve abnormalities. Severe bacterial or viral conjunctivitis can also result in a chronic dry eye syndrome due to compromise of the ocular surface or scarring of the lacrimal gland excretory ducts.

## Congenital Dry Eye Syndrome

Congenital causes of dry eye syndromes are rare and unlikely to be encountered routinely. They can pose a significant threat to the integrity of the eye. All involve decreased or absent lacrimal gland secretion. These include congenital absence of the lacrimal gland, anhidrotic ectodermal dysplasia, Riley-Day syndrome, and Cri-du-chat syndrome.

## DIAGNOSIS OF THE DRY EYE
### Historical Evaluation

It is incorrect to assume that all dry eyes are due to a lack of aqueous tears. It is imperative that the etiology of the dry eye be determined if at all possible. In other words, the most important aspect in the management of the dry eye is determining the correct etiology of the dry eye.

Unlike other areas of ophthalmology, where clinical examination may be more important than a history, a complete history is of utmost importance in the diagnosis of the dry eye. It is helpful to have a list of standardized questions to ask patients, using defined terms. These include:

1. Do your eyes have the feeling like a foreign body sensation of dust, sand, or gravel in them (mild, moderate, severe)?
2. Do your eyes have a burning sensation similar to water, soap, or shampoo in them (mild, moderate, severe)?
3. Do your eyes itch like a "mosquito bite"?
4. Are bright lights painful or uncomfortable?
5. Are your eyes crusted or mattered shut upon awakening from sleep?

6. Do you have a mucous discharge from the eye during your waking hours?
7. When are your symptoms worse, upon awakening, morning, noontime/ early afternoon, or late afternoon/evening?
8. Can you swallow foods without liquids; is their a sensation of saliva in your mouth?
9. Do you have any systemic diseases?
10. What eye drops are you using?
11. What other medicines (prescribed and over the counter) are you using?

With answers to these questions, a preliminary diagnosis can often be made (Table 3-1). For example, KCS and blepharitis, which are the most common causes of dry eye syndromes that will be seen, usually have differing presentations. Patients with KCS will complain of foreign-body sensation more than of burning. They tend to be more symptomatic as the day progresses due to the effects of evaporation on an already decreased aqueous tear film. Patients with blepharitis commonly complain of burning more than of foreign-body sensation. They also complain of crusting or mattering of the eyes upon awakening from sleep. They tend to be more symptomatic upon awakening (due to crusting and mattering of the eyelids) and better during the morning. Their symptoms worsen later in the day because of the increased effects of evaporation due to a lack of a functional lipid layer of the tear film.

A toxic keratoconjunctivitis due to topical medications or preservatives in artificial tear preparations can "muddy the waters."[8,9] Patients with moderate to

**Table 3-1**   Comparison of Historical Symptoms in Patients with Different Dry Eye Disorders

| Symptom | KCS | Blepharitis | Toxic kerato-conjunctivitis | Allergic kerato-conjunctivitis |
|---|---|---|---|---|
| Foreign-body Sensation | + + + | + | + + + | + |
| Burning | + | + + + | + + + | + |
| Itching | − | − | − | + + + |
| Photophobia | + + | ± | + + | ± |
| Crusting or mat- tering of lids | ± | − | ± | − |
| Symptoms worse | Afternoon, eve- ning | Upon awak- ening, evening | When using eye drops | Seasonal, envi- ronmental |
| Symptoms better | Upon awakening, morning | Mid-day | When not using eye drops | Different envi- ronment |
| Mucous discharge | + + | + + + | ± | + + + |
| Artificial tears | Improve symp- toms | Improve symptoms | Worsen symp- toms | Improve symp- toms |
| Systemic anticho- linergics | Worsen symp- toms | ± | ± | ± |
| Systemic antihis- tamines | Worsen symp- toms | ± | ± | Improve symp- toms |
| Systemic disease | Collagen vascular | Rosacea, seborrheic dermatitis | None | Atopic dermati- tis, hay fever |

severe KCS or blepharitis develop increasing symptoms of burning with the use of the topical preparations. A typical scenario occurs when the patient with KCS is told to use a commercially available preserved artificial tear as "often as you need to." The patient starts using the drops 4-5 times a day and, if symptoms worsen, uses the drops more often. With more frequent usage, patients develop ocular surface toxicity and begin to have stinging and burning on installation of the drop. They then put in more drops to relieve the burning, which leads to a vicious cycle of needing to put in additional drops to relieve the discomfort of the first. It is not uncommon to find patients using preserved artificial tears every five minutes and still not obtaining relief.

Patients must be questioned closely as to what they mean by itching. If the itching is similar to that of a "mosquito bite," allergic conjunctivitis is likely. Symptoms tend to be seasonal or environmentally related and are accompanied by mucous discharge and eye rubbing.

Systemic medications that decrease aqueous tear secretion can aggravate symptoms in patients with KCS. This is especially true of antihistamines, decongestants, and tricyclic antidepressants. It is not uncommon for contact-lens wearers, who are otherwise asymptomatic, to experience dry eye symptoms or contact lens problems on these medications.

Finally, patients with dry eye syndromes (especially KCS) will have worsening of their symptoms when they are exposed to smoky, chemical-laden, or polluted environments. Chemical vapors from clothing dyes, newspaper ink, and cosmetics are particularly irritating in patients with KCS who lack the ability to generate tears to wash or dilute out these substances. Patients with KCS may also develop symptoms of allergic conjunctivitis without a previous history of allergy due to their inability to dilute out airborne or topical allergens.

## Clinical Evaluation

It is important to observe the patient while taking the initial history. Doing so may provide clues to the etiology of the dry eye. Arthritic changes, blink rate, facial skin, and surgical scars, if present, are noted. The mouth is examined with a penlight for evidence of xerostomia (leathery tongue and poor dentition). The skin and scalp are examined for evidence of dermatologic disease such as eczema, acne rosacea, seborrhea, and the skin changes of lupus and scleroderma. The hands are examined for rheumatoid joint disease. The presence of hordeolum, chalazion, ectropion or entropion, decreased blink rate, and lagophthalmos are noted.

The initial slit lamp examination is performed before any topical anesthetics or special stains are used. Both decreased tear film meniscus height and debris are common in KCS. The presence of ectropion, entropion, trichiasis, and lid notching are noted. Lid erythema, telangectasia, poliosis (white eye lashes), loss of lashes, collarettes, and foamy discharge or inspissated material from meibomian glands are seen in blepharitis.

The bulbar and palpebral conjunctiva are examined. Dilated conjunctival vessels and tenacious strings of mucous are common in KCS. Conjunctival filaments and punctate keratitis are seen, with severe KCS, ptosis, and superior limbic keratoconjunctivitis (SLK). Redundant, thickened, and loose superior bulbar conjunctiva is seen with SLK. Conjunctival subepithelial fibrosis, keratinization, symblepharon, generalized foreshortening, and vascularization of the conjunctiva are often seen in cicatrizing diseases such as ocular cicatricial pemphigoid and Stevens-Johnson syndrome.

### Schirmer test

Classically, the Schirmer test has served as the basis for diagnosing the dry eye. The Schirmer test is a measure of the secretion of aqueous tears, and as such it is most useful as an aid in diagnosing KCS. Although the test is relatively specific for KCS (few false positives), it is not very sensitive (many false negatives). That is, if a Schirmer test value is low, it is helpful in the diagnosis of KCS. However, normal or high values do not exclude the diagnosis of KCS. The test is done with or without topical anesthesia. The paper test strip is placed at the juncture of the lateral and middle one-third of the lower lid. The patient is asked to blink normally and the amount of wetting is recorded in five minutes. Because of an initial reflexive tearing component (even when topical anesthesia is used), Schirmer test strips should be left in place for a full five minutes. Removing the test strips at 2.5 minutes and doubling the result is not equivalent to a five-minute test. In patients with severe KCS, one is interested in whether or not the patient still has a functioning lacrimal gland; therefore, a Schirmer test without anesthesia is most useful.

Normal values are ≥ 10 mm wetting/5 minutes. In mild cases or in contact-lens-induced dry eyes, a Schirmer test with anesthesia is most helpful. Normal values with anesthesia are ≥5 mm wetting/5 minutes. Again, it is important to keep in mind that an abnormal Schirmer test does not make the diagnosis of KCS. Supportive history and other clinical and laboratory tests are necessary. The presence of fluorescein and/or rose bengal staining, corneal filaments and/or mucous plaques (Figure 3-1), a decreased marginal tear strip, and blepharitis are also

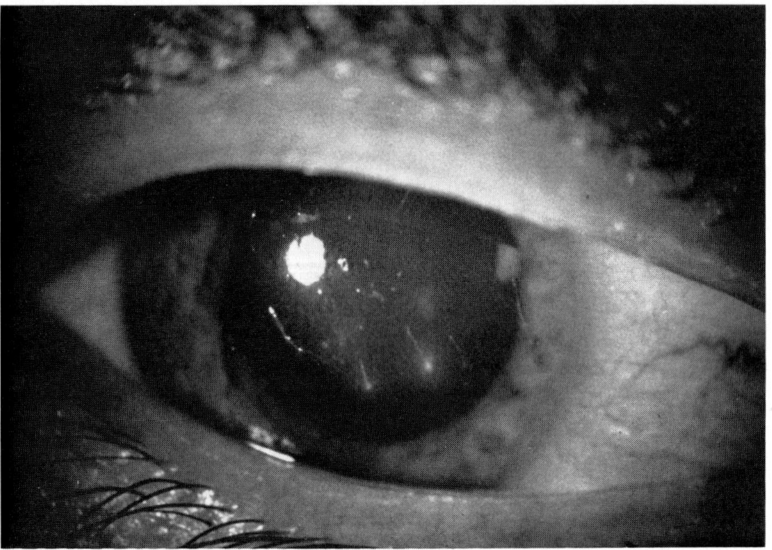

**FIGURE 3-1**    Corneal filaments in a patient with keratoconjunctivitis sicca.

helpful clues as to the etiology of the dry eye. The presence of these findings suggests moderate to severe KCS. In patients with blepharitis due to staphylococcal organisms or seborrhea, scaling and crusting around and on the eyelashes may be seen.

It is not unusual for patients with KCS to have blepharitis, and vise versa. Patients with blepharitis may have low Schirmer test values due to increased evaporation of the tear film. Again, a careful history is helpful in sorting out the etiology of the dry eye.

### Rose bengal staining

Rose bengal, a red aniline dye related to fluorescein, stains devitalized and degenerating corneal and conjunctival cells, mucous, and filaments. The 1% solution is preferable to impregnated sterile paper strips. A grading system where a separate score of 0 to 3 (three being the most severe) is given to the medial and lateral interpalpebral zone and the central cornea for each eye is useful. Examination for staining is best done with the green filter on the slit lamp. There is a total possible score of nine for each eye. A score of three or greater is considered abnormal.[10] Staining with rose bengal has high specificity (few false positives), but low sensitivity (many false negatives) in KCS.[11]

Conjunctival staining in the temporal and nasal interpalpebral zone is seen early in KCS. Staining increases with the severity of the disease. Diffuse corneal staining occurs in more severe disease. The opposite is true in ocular pemphigoid, keratoconjunctivitis medicamentosa, and blepharitis, where the cornea stains more than the bulbar conjunctiva in milder disease. In patients with superior limbic keratoconjunctivitis, the superior bulbar conjunctiva and upper one-third of the cornea stain with rose bengal. Patients with poor blinking and lagophthalmos have characteristic inferior staining.

### Fluorescein staining

Clinically, fluorescein differs from rose bengal because it stains areas of epithelial cell loss and not devitalized epithelium. A moistened sterile fluorescein strip is touched to the inferior tear lake. Conjunctival and corneal staining patterns are similar to those of rose bengal staining.

### Tear breakup time (TBUT)

TBUT is not a useful test in the diagnosis of dry eye since it is almost always abnormal in these patients, i.e., the specificity of TBUT is quite low. It is helpful if TBUT is normal, since this implies a relatively stable tear film. A moistened sterile fluorescein strip is touched to the inferior tear lake. The patient is asked to blink several times, close his or her eyes, then open them. The time from opening of the eyelids to the appearance of the first randomly distributed dry spot on the cornea is the TBUT.

### Impression cytology

Impression cytology (IC) is a technique where surface cells are removed by the direct application of cellulose acetate material onto the conjunctiva. Once the material is removed, it is stained and examined by light microscopy (Figure 3-2). Impression cytology has been used to study the ocular surface in keratoconjunc-

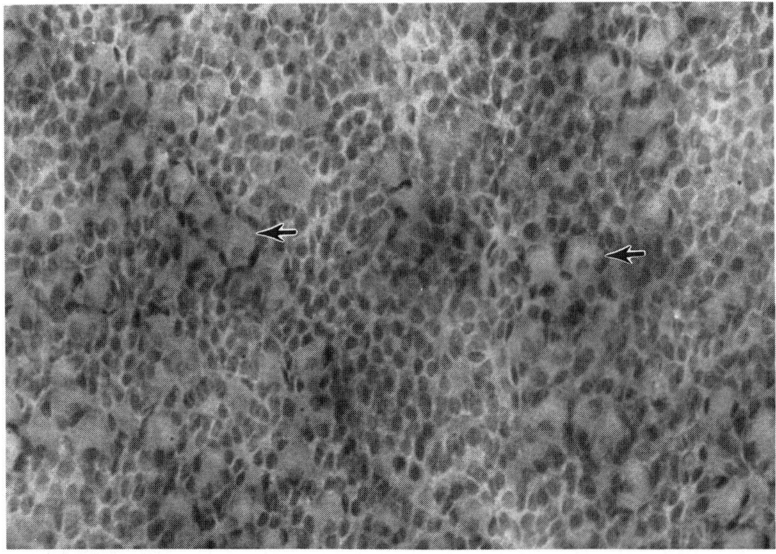

**FIGURE 3-2**     An example of normal conjunctival epithelium and goblet cells (arrows) obtained by impression cytology.

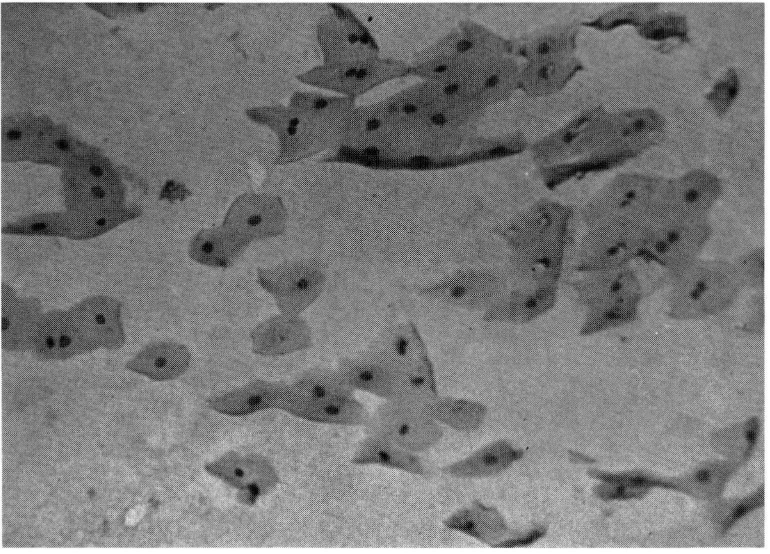

**FIGURE 3-3**     An example of squamous metaplasia of the bulbar conjunctival epithelium obtained by impression cytology.

tivitis sicca, ocular cicatricial pemphigoid, atopic disease, superior limbic keratoconjunctivitis, erythema multiforme, blepharitis, radiation, and chemical-burn-induced dry eye.[12-13]

Impression cytology is useful in differentiating between the etiology of ocular surface disorders. Squamous metaplasia (Figure 3-3) of the bulbar ocular surface with a normal inferior palpebral surface suggests KCS. If there are associated inflammatory cells, then blepharitis, topical drug, or preservative toxicity may be present. Squamous metaplasia of *both* the bulbar and inferior palpebral ocular surfaces suggests an intrinsic corneal and conjunctival disorder such as atopic disease, ocular cicatricial pemphigoid, or Stevens-Johnson syndrome. The presence of inflammatory cells indicates active disease. Impression cytology in patients with superior limbic keratoconjunctivitis (SLK) shows squamous metaplasia of the superior bulbar conjunctiva. In some patients, there is squamous metaplasia of the nasal and temporal bulba conjunctiva, suggesting a more diffuse ocular surface abnormality in SLK.[14]

## Conjunctival biopsy

Conjunctival biopsy allows for full thickness examination of epithelium, basement membrane and substantia propria. Immunofluorescent staining can identify localized deposition of immunoglobulins and complement in epithelial basement membrane. This is helpful in diagnosing disorders such as ocular cicatricial pemphigoid.[15]

## Labial salivary gland biopsy

Labial salivary gland (lip) biopsy provides a relatively simple and safe alternative to lacrimal gland biopsy for diagnosing Sjögren's syndrome (SS). A high correlation between severity of disease and degree of lymphocytic infiltration in the salivary gland is present in patients with SS.[16]

## Laboratory Tests

The following tests are currently used primarily as research tools in the diagnosis of the dry eye. At the present time, they are not in wide use in most clinical ophthalmology practices.

### Lactoferrin

Lactoferrin is an antibacterial glycoprotein secreted by the lacrimal gland. It accounts for about one-fourth of total tear protein. Measurement of tear lactoferrin levels gives an estimate of lacrimal gland output.[16] In KCS, tear lactoferrin levels are decreased. A radial immunodiffusion assay suitable for the office setting is commercially available (Lactoplate).

### Lysozyme

Tear lysozyme is also an antibacterial protein. It comprises 20% to 40% of total tear protein produced by the main and accessory lacrimal glands. Tear lysozyme has been shown to be a sensitive test for the diagnosis of keratoconjunctivitis sicca.[18] As with lactoferrin, tear lysozyme levels are decreased in KCS. There is a commercially available test (Quantiplate) for measuring tear lysozyme activity.

### Tearfilm osmolality

An elevated tear film osmolality is found in dry conditions where tear secretion is decreased or evaporation is increased. It has been shown to be a sensitive and specific test for the diagnosis of KCS.[11,19] Tear samples are obtained by touching a microcapillary pipette to the marginal tear strip. Osmolality is determined by freezing point depression using a commercially available nanoliter, freezing-point depression osmometer.

## TREATMENT OF THE DRY EYE

Treatment of the dry eye is dependent on *its cause or etiology*. Patients with blepharitis often require careful cleansing of the eye lids (lid hygiene), topical antibiotics (drops and ointments), topical steroids, and orally administered tetracycline. Patients with ocular pemphigoid or other immunologic/inflammatory diseases may require systemic steroids and immunosuppressants in addition to topical medications. Patients with KCS require treatments aimed at maximizing tear secretion and flow, including tear supplementation, and minimizing tear drainage. It is helpful to classify KCS as to mild, moderate, or severe disease (Table 3-2).

Managing the dry eye requires a stepwise approach that identifies the minimum amount of therapy required to achieve the desired result. The simpler the treatment regimen, the better the patient compliance. Therapy is directed at providing symptomatic relief and maintenance of the integrity of the ocular surface. Because preservatives are especially toxic to the dry eye, they are to be avoided. Underlying systemic disease, associated blepharitis, inflammation, and allergic conditions are treated. Eyelid abnormalities and disturbances of the normal blink mechanism are corrected. Often the dry eye is a chronic condition that requires continuous therapy and close, consistent followup. The ophthalmologist must be supportive of patients in these situations.

### Treatment of Blepharitis

Lid hygiene at bedtime and upon arising is the mainstay in the management of blepharitis. Patients are carefully instructed on proper technique.[20] Commercially available scrub kits are often helpful.[21,22] Topical erythromycin ointment at bedtime is used in more severe or unresponsive cases. Topical steroids are often required in cases of severe blepharitis to reduce inflammation; and not infrequently they are needed on a chronic basis. Oral tetracycline (250 mg two times a day) taken on an empty stomach is useful, especially when the meibomian glands are involved, as in ocular rosacea. The therapeutic effect of tetracycline may not be seen for as long as two to three months. The dose is tapered according to clinical response, often leading to a maintenance dose of 250 mg daily. It is not unusual to have patients who require nine or more months of daily tetracycline therapy to remain comfortable.

**Table 3-2**    Basic Classification of KCS as to Severity

| Severity | Symptoms | Irritant or emotional tears | Rose bengal staining (0-9) | Schirmer test (mm wetting/5 min)* |
|---|---|---|---|---|
| Mild | Mild | Present | <3 | 5-10 |
| Moderate | Moderate | Absent | 3-5 | 1-5 |
| Severe | Severe | Absent | >5 | <1 |

*Without anesthesia

## Treatment of Allergy

Environmental and seasonal triggers are difficult to identify or avoid. Allergy testing is not helpful in most instances. Cold compresses and systemic antihistamines provide some relief. Sodium cromolyn, which is a mast cell stabilizer, can be given for prophylactic treatment. Some patients can be tapered to as little as one drop a day and remain asymptomatic. Topical steroids on a short-term basis may be required until the therapeutic effect of the cromolyn is achieved. In patients with KCS, allergic symptoms are not uncommon.

## Lid Surgery

Except in ocular cicatricial pemphigoid (OCP), every attempt is made to correct abnormal lid anatomy. Surgical procedures that violate the conjunctiva in patients with OCP can exacerbate or reactivate ocular surface inflammation.

## Surface Lubrication

Artificial tear preparations, ointments, and slow-release polymers (Lacriserts) attempt to provide lubrication of the ocular surface in the face of aqueous, mucin, and lipid deficiencies. Presently available artificial tears should be thought of as lubricants and not as a replacement for normal tears. Most contain a polymeric system to increase and prolong contact time. Preservatives to insure sterility and a buffer to maintain a tolerable pH are also present. Because preservatives are toxic to the dry eye, they should be avoided in moderate to severe disease or when drops are required more than 4 or 5 times daily. Nonpreserved preparations are commercially available. Slow-release pellets of preservative-free hydroxypropyl methylcellulose (Lacriserts) improve symptoms and objective findings in patients with KCS. These work best in younger patients with mild to moderate disease who still have both enough tears to dissolve the pellets and the manual dexterity to place them.

Ointments, best tolerated at bedtime, are useful in patients with KCS and lagophthalmos. Preservative-free, bland ointments are available. Lanolin, which is present in many of these preparations, may cause an allergic dermatitis in sensitized patients.

## Moisture Chambers

Moisture chambers preserve existing tears by providing a mechanical barrier to the environment. They act to decrease evaporation and isolate the eyes from toxic chemicals, smoke, and pollution. Swimmer's goggles, ski goggles, or moisture-chamber spectacles are used.

## Punctal Occlusion

Punctal occlusion is recommended when the patient demonstrates persistent symptoms and ocular surface disease in spite of intensive topical therapy. It is also useful in patients who obtain objective and symptomatic improvement with topical therapy but find the use of frequent drops inconvenient. Interestingly, there is a small group of very symptomatic patients, with normal Schirmer's-test values and no evidence of rose bengal staining, who respond quite favorably to punctal occlusion.

There are both temporary and permanent methods to close puncta. A step-wise approach to punctal occlusion is employed. Temporary methods use silastic plugs or collagen implants. Permanent closure uses cautery, diathermy, or laser coagulation. Collagen implants come in a variety of sizes, to help insure a proper fit. All are 2 mm in length, but they are available in diameters of 0.2, 0.3, and 0.4 mm. They are easier to insert, and better tolerated by the patient with regard to foreign-body sensation, than are silicone plugs. Collagen plugs will hydrolyze over 5 to 10 days. If a patient has noted even minimal improvement in his or her symptoms and does not have epiphora following temporary occlusion, permanent occlusion is indicated.

The technique for argon-laser punctoplasty is as follows: (1) a topical anesthetic is placed in the eye to be treated; (2) a cotton-tipped applicator soaked in topical anesthetic is placed over the puncta and on the palpebral conjunctiva for 10 to 20 seconds; (3) the area around the punctum and canaliculus is infiltrated with lidocaine hydrochloride 2% with epinephrine (from the conjunctival surface for the lower canaliculi and from the skin side for the upper canaliculi); (4) a dot of water-soluble ink from a surgical marking pen is placed on and around the punctum; (5) laser settings are 750 milliwatts, 0.2 seconds, and 100 microns; (6) 25-35 burns are placed around the punctum, and the puncta are ablated with an additional 15-25 burns. Power is adjusted to achieve visible shrinkage of tissue with each burn. Complete occlusion usually results with approximately 50 applications. Well over one-half of the puncta occluded in this manner will reopen. With argon laser, the punta open to 10% to 25% of their original diameter. If the patient continues to have symptoms and ocular surface changes, the upper puncta are treated similarly. If the response is still not adequate, the canaliculi are totally occluded with electrocautery or radiofrequency diathermy. Both diathermy and electrocautery can provide a deep closure. The technique is as follows: (1) topical anesthetic is instilled in the inferior cul de sac; (2) a cotton-tipped applicator soaked in topical anesthetic is placed over the puncta; (3) the area surrounding the punctum is infiltrated with lidocaine hydrochloride 2% with epinephrine; (4) a small burr on a low-speed hand-held drill (used for removing rust rings) is inserted 4-5 mm into the canaliculus and the epithelial lining abraded; (5) a fine epilator wire on the diathermy unit is inserted 8-10 mm into the canaliculus; (6) the very lowest power setting is used; (7) when blanching of the punctum begins, the wire is slowly withdrawn and the pedal is pulsed as the tip approaches the surface to prevent severe burn and laceration of the puncta. A similar technique using a hand-held battery cautery can also be used.

## Tarsorrhaphy

Tarsorrhaphy is very useful, but generally underutilized, in treating ocular surface disorders unresponsive to other forms of therapy. In the dry eye, it provides protection for the ocular surface and reduces tear evaporation by decreasing the amount of exposed ocular surface area. There are many good surgical techniques that work. A lateral tarsorrhaphy is done initially. If the desired improvement does not occur, a medial tarsorrhaphy is done, leaving a central aperture to allow for the placement of artificial tears and medications.

## Agents That Increase Tear Production

If functional lacrimal tissue remains, substances such as bisolvin (Bromhexine) may increase lacrimal gland secretion. Clinical experience is limited to outside the United States as it has not yet been approved by the FDA.

Oil of primrose (Emafol) is thought to be beneficial in treating KCS. Careful, prospective, double-masked, randomized studies have not been done. Neuropeptides and agents that increase cyclic AMP and calcium in the lacrimal gland hold some promise as tear-stimulating agents.

## Anti-inflammatory and Antimetabolite Therapy

Topical and systemic steroids are often required in inflammatory ocular surface diseases. Active, progressive OCP requires systemic immunosuppressive therapy. Azothiaprine (Immuran), cyclophosphamide (Cytoxan), and methotrexate have been used successfully.

## Mucolytic Agents

Acetylcysteine (10% Mucomyst) four times daily is sometimes useful in patients with increased amounts of mucous. Unfortunately, it burns upon instillation, and it is often not well tolerated.

## Therapeutic Contact Lenses and Collagen Shields

Therapeutic contact lenses are useful in a number of ocular surface disorders. Contact lenses provide a protective barrier against mechanical damage from lid scarring and trichiasis, provide symptomatic relief with disrupted epithelium, and promote healing. Caution should nevertheless be exercised in their use in dry eye states. Therapeutic contact lenses are a predisposing factor to serious corneal infection in eyes with cicatricial and dry eye disorders.[23] They can be associated with epithelial, stromal, and endothelial complications.[24]

Collagen shields have been used to promote corneal healing both in patients with acute epithelial defects and after surgery. Use is limited in chronic cicatricial ocular surface and dry eye disorders by the need for frequent replacement. They tend to be quite irritating in patients with severe KCS.

## Cryotherapy

If there are aberrant lashes rubbing on the cornea they must be eliminated. Failure to do so will result in epithelial breakdown and increase the risk of secondary infection. Cryotherapy is the most effective method of treatment. A double-freeze technique ($-80°C$ for 45 seconds, thaw for 60 to 120 seconds and refreeze at $-80°C$ for 30 seconds) with high flow nitrous oxide probes achieves an 85% to 90% success rate.[25] Complications include postoperative pain, lid swelling, pseudomembrane formation, lid scarring and symblepharon, skin depigmentation, and tissue necrosis.

## Conjunctival Resection

Conjunctival resection of the superior conjunctiva is usually curative in patients with SLK. The technique is straightforward and involves the removal of 5 mm of conjunctiva and Tenon's fascia from the 10:00 to 2:00 o'clock positions. As scarring of the conjunctiva to the sclera is the desired result, topical steroids should be used sparingly, if at all.

## EXPERIMENTAL TREATMENTS
### Estrogen Replacement

Systemic and topical estrogens may improve the symptoms associated with KCS.[26] The mechanism of action is uncertain, and may be an effect either on lacrimal or on ocular surface epithelium. Cyclic variation of the conjunctival epithelium with the menstrual cycle does occur in women.[27] Prolactin is also present in human lacrimal glands and in tears.[28] The relationship of hormones both to dry eye and to ocular surface disease requires further study.

## Vitamin A Ointment

Squamous metaplasia of the ocular surface epithelium is seen in many dry eye and ocular surface diseases. Vitamin A is known to reverse squamous metaplasia resulting from vitamin A deficiency. An open-label study of topical vitamin A ointment in patients with various ocular surface disorders, including KCS, noted improvement in symptoms, visual acuity, rose bengal staining, Schirmer testing, and impression cytology after two months of therapy.[29] A later, multicenter, placebo-controlled, double-masked study of vitamin A ointment versus placebo failed to substantiate this earlier report. No significant difference in symptoms or clinical signs was noted in patients receiving four to eight months of treatment with vitamin A ointment. Squamous metaplasia, as demonstrated by impression cytology, did reverse in patients with cicatricial diseases although no significant effect was seen in the patients with KCS.[30] An open-label crossover study of vitamin A ointment in the treatment of keratoconjunctivitis sicca revealed no difference between placebo and topical vitamin A as indicated by Schirmer's testing, rose bengal staining, and tear film osmolality.[31] Adverse reactions associated with vitamin A ointment include conjunctivitis, burning, redness, chemosis and mucous discharge, and corneal calcification. In general, topical tretinoin ointment is useful in patients with severe, noninflammatory ocular surface disease accompanied by squamous metaplasia.

## Topical Cyclosporine A (CsA)

The immunosuppressive agent cyclosporine has been shown to increase tear production and cause marked regression in neovascularization and granulation tissue when used topically in canines with KCS.[32] This study suggested that the effect of CsA was to increase tear production and that this effect was due to its effect on prolactin. It has previously been proposed that prolactin may play an important role in tear secretion.[28] CsA may be useful in the treatment of human patients with KCS, but a randomized, controlled, double-masked clinical trial has not been done.

## Epidermal Growth Factor

Epidermal growth factor is a naturally occurring polypeptide found in tears.[33] EGF appears to enhance epithelial migration by increasing epithelial cell proliferation.[34] However, it had no beneficial therapeutic effect in resurfacing de-epithelialized grafts following penetrating keratoplasty in humans.[35]

## Fibronectin

Fibronectin is a glycoprotein involved in cell-cell and cell-matrix attachment. Fibronectin enhances epithelial wound healing by facilitating epithelial migration.[34] Topical autologous fibronectin has been shown to decrease symptoms and improve fluorescein and rose bengal staining in patients with keratoconjunctivitis sicca of Sjögren's syndrome.[36] Definitive controlled studies have not been reported.

## References


1. Doane MG. Interaction of eyelids and tears in corneal wetting and the dynamics of the normal human eyeblink. Am J Ophthalmol 1980; 89:507-516.
2. Jones DB. Prospects in the management of tear deficient states. Trans Am Acad Ophthalmol & Otol 1971; 83:OP693-OP699.
3. Bowman RW, Dougherty JM, McCulley JP. Chronic blepharitis and dry eye. Internat Ophthalmol Clin 1987; 27:27-35.
4. Lemp MA, Mahmood MA, Weiler HH. Association of rosacea and keratoconjunctivitis sicca. Arch Ophthalmol 1984; 102:556-557.
5. Thoft RA. Relationship of the dry eye to primary ocular surface disease. Trans Ophthalmol Soc UK 1985; 104:452-457.
6. Sjögren H, Bloch KJ. Keratoconjunctivitis sicca and Sjögren's syndrome. Surv Ophthalmol 1972; 16:145-159.
7. Jacobsson LTH, Axell TE, Hansen BU. Dry eyes or mouth: an epidemiological study in Swedish adults, with special reference to primary Sjögren's syndrome. In Talal N, ed. Sjögren's syndrome: a model for understanding autoimmunity. San Diego: Academic Press Ltd, 1989:213-19.
8. Fraunfelder FT, Meter SM. Corneal complications of ocular medications. Cornea 1986; 5:55-59.
9. Wilson FM. Adverse external ocular effects of topical ophthalmic medications. Surv Ophthalmol 1979; 24:57-88.
10. van Bijsterveld OP. Diagnostic tests in the sicca syndrome. Arch Ophthalmol 1969; 82:10-14.
11. Farris RL, Gilbard JP, Stuchell RN, et al. Diagnostic tests in keratoconjunctivitis sicca. 1983; Contact Lenses 9:23-28.
12. Nelson JD, Havener VR, Cameron JD. Cellulose acetate impressions of the ocular surface. Arch Ophthalmol 1983; 101:1869-1872.
13. Nelson JD, Wright JC. Conjunctival goblet cell densities in ocular surface disease. Arch Ophthalmol 1984; 102:1049-1051.
14. Nelson JD. Superior limbic keratoconjunctivitis (SLK). Eye 1989; 3:180-189.
15. Franklin RM, Fitzmorris CT. Antibodies against conjunctival basement membrane zone: occurrence in cicatricial pemphigoid. Arch Ophthalmol 1983; 101:1611-1613.
16. Daniels TE. Labial salivary gland biopsy in Sjögren's syndrome: assessment as a diagnostic criterion in 362 suspected cases. Arthritis and Rheumatism 1984; 26:147-156.
17. Janssen PT, van Bijsterveld OP. A simple test for lacrimal gland function: a tear lactoferrin assay by

radial immunodiffusion. Graefe's Arch Clin Exp Ophthalmol 1983; 220:171-174.

18. van Bijsterveld OP. Diagnostic tests in the sicca syndrome. Arch Ophthalmol 1969; 82:10-14.

19. Gilbard JP, Farris L, Santamaria J. Osmolarity of tear microvolumes in keratoconjunctivitis sicca. Arch Ophthalmol 1978; 96:677-681.

20. Nelson JD. Managing the dry eye: accurate diagnosis is the key. Postgrad Med 1989; 85:38-49.

21. Leibowitz HM, Capino D. Treatment of chronic blepharitis. Arch Ophthalmol 1988; 106:720.

22. Polack FM. Experience with a new detergent lid scrub in the management of chronic blepharitis. Arch Ophthalmol 1988; 106:719-720.

23. Ormerod LD, Fong LP, Foster CS. Corneal infection in mucosal scarring disorders and Sjögren's syndrome. Am J Ophthalmol 1988; 105:512-518.

24. McDermott ML, Chandler JW. Therapeutic uses of contact lenses. Surv Ophthalmol 1989; 33:381-394.

25. Johnson RLC, Collin JRO. Treatment of trichiasis with a lid cryoprobe. Brit J Ophthalmol 1985; 69:267-270.

26. Lemp MA. Recent developments in dry eye management. Ophthalmol 1987; 94:1299-1304.

27. Kramer P, Lubkin V, Potter W, et al. Cyclic changes in conjunctival smears from menstruating females. Ophthalmol 1990; 97:303-307.

28. Frey WH, Nelson JD, Frick ML, et al. Prolactin immunoreactivity in human tears and lacrimal gland: possible implications of tear production. In Holly FJ, ed. The preocular tear film in health, disease and contact lens wear. Lubbock, Tex: The Dry Eye Institute, 1986; 798-807.

29. Tseng SCG, Maumenee AE, Stark WJ, et al. Topical retinoid treatment for various dry-eye disorders. Ophthalmol 1985; 92:717-727.

30. Soong HK, Martin NF, Wagoner MD: Topical retinoid therapy for squamous metaplasia of various ocular surface disorders. Ophthalmol 1988; 95:1442-1446.

31. Gilbard JP, Huang AJW, Belldegrun R, et al. Open-label crossover study of vitamin A ointment as a treatment for keratoconjunctivitis sicca. Ophthalmol 1989; 96:244-246.

32. Kaswan RL, Salisbury MA, Ward DA. Spontaneous canine keratoconjunctivitis sicca: A useful model for human keratoconjunctivitis sicca: treatment with cyclosporine eye drops. Arch Ophthalmol 1989; 107:1210-1216.

33. Ohasi Y, Matakura M, Kinoshito Y. Presence of epidermal growth factor in human tears. Invest Ophthalmol Vis Sci 1989; 30:1879-1882.

34. Watanabe K, Nakagawa S, Nishido T: Stimulatory effects of fibronectin and EGF on migration of corneal epithelial cells. Invest Ophthalmol Vis Sci. 1987; 28:205-211.

35. Kandarakis AS, Page C, Kaufman HE. The effect of epidermal growth factor on epithelial healing after penetrating keratoplasty in human eyes. Am J Ophthalmol 1984; 98:411-415.

36. Kono I, Matsumoto Y, Kono K. Beneficial effect of topical fibronectin in patients with keratoconjunctivitis sicca of Sjögren's syndrome. J Rheum 1985; 12:487-489.

# 4 Chronic Conjunctivitis

**Peter A. Rapoza, MD**

Chronic conjunctivitis, a surprisingly common clinical entity, is a source of frustration to patient and practitioner alike. The term *chronic conjunctivitis* is usually applied to cases of conjunctivitis persisting beyond a minimum of two weeks duration. Burning and irritated eyes, conjunctival injection, and persistent ocular discharge, while seldom sight-threatening, are uncomfortable and unattractive and may interfere with visual function and the ability to wear contact lenses. Diverse etiologies include infections, immune-mediated disorders, irritants, eyelid disorders, and use of ophthalmic medications. Patients with chronic conjunctivitis have often sought assistance from a variety of medical and nonmedical sources, resulting in the application of treatments without identification of a precise etiology and therefore not rendering relief.

This chapter reviews the causes of chronic conjunctivitis, presents a systematic approach to establishing an etiologic diagnosis, and recommends treatment regimens. Careful history taking, performance of appropriate clinical and laboratory examinations, and application of rational treatment strategies will usually allow the clinician to manage patients with chronic conjunctivitis successfully.

## CASE PRESENTATION

A 20-year-old white male student presented with a four-week history of a red left eye associated with ocular discharge and photophobia. The patient was evaluated by an ophthalmologist three days after the onset of symptoms. An examination was performed, but no conjunctival smears were prepared. A topical steroid-sulfa combination was prescribed to treat a presumed bacterial conjunctivitis. Symptoms persisted, and the patient returned to the same ophthalmologist two weeks later. Subepithelial corneal infiltrates were noted. The patient was presumed to have viral conjunctivitis, and the combination topical steroid-sulfa combination discontinued. When the condition persisted, the patient consulted a second ophthalmologist who referred the patient to me for evaluation.

Further history was obtained to reveal that the patient had no exposure to others with conjunctivitis, no identified undue exposure to irritants, and no allergies. The patient was sexually active, but with only one partner for the past few months. He denied any symptoms of urethritis. Examination revealed uncorrected visual acuity of 20/20 OD and 20/50 OS, improving to 20/30 with a pinhole. The right eye was unremarkable. An enlarged, nontender left preauricular lymph node was palpated. Moderately severe conjunctival injection was present. Numerous conjunctival follicles were noted. A moderate amount of white ocular discharge was found. The corneal epithelium was slightly irregular and stained with fluorescein. Several nummular gray subepithelial corneal infiltrates were present, including several within the visual axis. Two-millimeter pannus was detected. The remainder of the ocular examination was unremarkable.

The conjunctiva of the left eye was sampled for bacterial, chlamydial, and viral cultures. Smears were prepared for staining with Gram and Giemsa stain and monoclonal antibody to *Chlamydia trachomatis.* Numerous polymorphonuclear leukocytes, lymphocytes, and epithelial cells were present. No organisms or inclusions were found.

A tentative diagnosis of chlamydial conjunctivitis was entertained. The patient was treated with Doxycycline 100 mg bid po and topical tetracycline ointment qid OS for 10 days. Chlamydial elementary bodies were detected by MicroTrak (Syva Company, Palo Alto, Calif.) and confirmed by isolation of chlamydia in culture. *Staphylococcus epidermidis* was also isolated. The patient reported clinical improvement within two days of beginning treatment. Complete resolution was present one week following the treatment course. The patient was counseled regarding the implications of chlamydial infection, and his partner was referred to her family physician for evaluation.

## ETIOLOGY

*Chronic conjunctivitis* is the term usually applied to inflammation of the conjunctiva of greater than two weeks duration. The causes of the inflammation are myriad. A classic review of the causes of chronic conjunctivitis in over 900 patients in an external disease referral setting was presented by Thygeson and Kimura.[1] Both primary and secondary causes of chronic conjunctivitis have been described. I will attempt to organize an etiologic classification of chronic conjunctivitis based upon primary or direct involvement of the conjunctiva and secondary or indirect mechanisms (see the box, p. 69). The prevalence of the various primary and secondary causes of chronic conjunctivitis is unknown. A recent prospective study of patients with chronic conjunctivitis, excluding those with conjunctivitis secondary to eyelid disease, aqueous tear deficiency, or chronic dacryocystitis, established an etiologic diagnosis in 37 of 55 patients (67%): chlamydia, 11 (20%); virus, 8 (15%); irritant, 6 (11%); allergen, 4 (7%); contact lens associated, 4 (7%); and bacteria, 4 (7%).[2]

## EVALUATION

The evaluation of a patient with chronic conjunctivitis should proceed in a logical fashion to eliminate the secondary causes prior to engaging in the more time- and resource-consuming search for primary etiologies (see the box, top of p. 70).

As in any medical condition, a thorough history must be gathered with particular attention to the characteristics of the chronic conjunctivitis. Potential exposures—including associates with similar symptoms, contact lenses, cosmetics, eyedrops, animals, smoke, industrial or household pollutants, and systemic complaints—should be topics of inquiry.

The physical examination should include a comprehensive ophthalmic examination with particular attention to the external eye and ocular adnexa. Intraocular pressure can and should be measured provided that the tonometer tip is

---

**Etiology of Chronic Conjunctivitis**

I. Primary
  A. Immune-mediated[2]
    Allergic conjunctivitis
    Atopic keratoconjunctivitis
    Contact lens associated conjunctivitis
    Ocular pemphigoid
    Stevens-Johnson Syndrome
    Vernal conjunctivitis
  B. Infection[3]
    Bacteria[1]
      *Actinobacillus mallei**
      *Borrelia burgdorferi*[4]
      *Branhamella catarrhalis*
      Cat-scratch fever*
      *Escherichia coli*
      *Francisella tularensis**
      *Klebsiella pneumoniae*
      *Listeria monocytogenes**
      *Moraxella lacunata*
      Mycobacterium tuberculosis
      *Pasteurella multocida**
      *Proteus mirabilis*
      *Serratia marcesans*
      *Staphylococcus sp.*
      *Streptococcus sp.*
      *Treponema palladium**
      *Yersinia sp.**
    Chlamydia[5,6]
      *Chlamydia psitaci*
      *Chlamydia trachomatis**
    Fungus
      *Actinomyces sp.**
      *Blastomyces dermatidis**
      *Coccidioides immitis**

    Myiasis[7]
    Rickettsia
      *Rickettsia conorii**
    Virus
      Adenovirus[8]
      Epstein-Barr virus*
      *Herpes simplex* virus[9]
      *Herpes zoster* virus
      Mumps virus*
  C. Irritant
    Cosmetics
    Environmental agents[10]
    Foreign bodies[11]
    Medications[12,13]
  D. Neoplasia[14]
    Dysplasia
    Carcinoma in situ
    Squamous cell carcinoma
II. Secondary
  A. Eyelid disorders
    Blepharitis[15]
      Meibomianitis
      Meibomian gland seborrhea
      Meibomian gland obstruction
      Secondary blepharitis (acne rosacea, atopic, fungal, parasitic, psoriatic, viral)
      Staphylococcal
    Floppy eyelid syndrome[16]
    Lagophthalmos[17]
    Neoplasia
      Sebaceous cell carcinoma[18]
  B. Tear deficiency states[19]
  C. Lacrimal duct obstruction[20]

*Causes of Parinaud's oculoglandular conjunctivitis

then sterilized. The posterior segment should at least be evaluated with the direct ophthalmoscope and a dilated examination performed if indicated.

If secondary causes of chronic conjunctivitis have been successfully ruled out, a laboratory evaluation of the condition is usually indicated.[6,21] Conjunctival smears may be prepared for staining with Giemsa and Gram stain. The characteristics of the cellular response may establish a diagnosis or assist in selecting further studies (see the box, bottom of p. 70). Utilizing a dacron swab prewetted with thioglycolate broth, cultures for bacteria (blood agar, chocolate agar, and thioglycolate broth) are obtained. A chlamydial assay (direct immunofluorescence, enzyme-linked immunoassay, or cell culture) is prepared. In comparison to McCoy cell chlamydial culture, direct immunofluorescent monoclonal antibody staining

### Systematic Investigation of Chronic Conjunctivitis

I. History

Demographic data; characteristics of conjunctivitis (symptoms, duration, inciting and relieving factors, previous diagnoses and treatments); allergies; occupational and household exposures; ophthalmic medications; contact lens use and care system; systemic symptoms; past medical history

II. Physical Examination

Lymphadenopathy; eyelid disorders (blepharitis, lagophthalmos, trichiasis); ocular cosmetics; tear meniscus; tear break-up time; Schirmer test; conjunctival alterations (follicles, papillae, foreign bodies including concretions, symblepharon, dysplasia or neoplasia); corneal alterations (epithelial staining with fluorescein and rose bengal; infiltrates, pannus, stromal vascularization, endothelial precipitates); cataract; intraocular pressure measurement; retinal alterations (retinitis, hemorrhages, infarctions); optic neuritis; survey of mucous membranes and skin

III. Laboratory Studies

| | |
|---|---|
| Routine Cytology: | Giemsa stain (or Diff-Quik Wright Geimsa stain) and Gram stain |
| Bacterial Culture: | Reduced blood, chocolate agar, thioglycolate broth |
| Chlamydial assay: | Direct immunofluorescence (DFA), enzyme-linked immunoassay (ELISA), or McCoy cell culture |
| Serology: | For suspected Lyme disease or in cases of Parinaud's oculoglandular conjunctivitis |
| Conjunctival Biopsy: | For suspected dysplasia, malignancy, or ocular pemphigoid |

### Etiology of Chronic Conjunctivitis Based on Cytologic Characteristics of Geimsa-stained Conjunctival Smears

| *Cytologic Characteristics* | *Possible Etiology* |
|---|---|
| Eosinophils, eosinophilic granules | Immune mediated |
| Neutrophils predominate | Bacteria, fungus, |
| Neutrophils, lymphocytes, plasma cells, Leber cells, basophilic intracytoplasmic inclusions | chlamydia |
| Lymphocytes, plasma cells, + multinucleated giant cells or inclusions | Medication, virus |
| Mascara, foreign bodies | Irritant |

resulted in sensitivity of 80%, specificity of 98%, and positive and negative predictive values of 89% and 96% respectively.[6] Due to the relative expense and the low yield, viral cultures are not routinely obtained. The evaluation of patients with Parinaud's oculoglandular conjunctivitis may require fungal cultures or appropriate serologic studies. The latter may be useful in suspected cases of Lyme disease. If the cause of chronic conjunctivitis is not detected by the above studies, or if there is clinical suspicion of ocular pemphigoid or malignancy, a conjunctival biopsy may identify other potentially treatable etiologies.

## TREATMENT

Specific treatment is available for many of the causes of chronic conjunctivitis. Although a comprehensive presentation of therapeutic options is beyond the scope

### Treatment of Common Causes of Chronic Conjunctivitis

| Etiology | Treatment |
| --- | --- |
| Immune-mediated | Curtail exposure to inciting agent; cromolyn sodium 4% 5×/day if exposure control unsuccessful; topical steroids (medrysone or fluoromethalone preferable for longer-term usage); topical immunosuppressives (cyclosporin); or systemic steroids or immunosupressives |
| Bacteria | Broad-spectrum topical antibiotic 4-6×/day for one week, changing to specific coverage upon isolation of organism; appropriate systemic antibiotic for systemic infections (i.e., Lyme disease, Parinaud's oculoglandular conjunctivitis) |
| Chlamydia | Tetracycline 500 mg 4×/day, Doxycycline 100 mg 2×/day, or for 10 days; identification and referral of contacts |
| Virus | No treatment if uncomplicated; cycloplegia and possibly topical steroids for persistent, symptomatic adenoviral keratoconjunctivitis |
| Irritant | Curtailment of exposure to inciting agent; removal of foreign bodies |
| Meibomian gland dysfunction | Warm compresses and Meibomian gland massage 2×/day; Minocycline or Doxycycline 50 mg 2×/day for two weeks, then 1×/day po thereafter; or Tetracycline 250 mg 4×/day for two weeks, then 1-2×/day po thereafter tapered with clinical response |
| Staphylococcal blepharitis | Warm compresses 2×/day with thorough cleansing of lids and lashes; application of broad-spectrum antibiotic or antibiotic/steroid combination to initially establish control |
| Tear deficiency states | Mild: preferred artificial tear 4-8×/day; moderate to severe: nonpreserved artificial tear tiltrated to clinical response while awake and ointment at bedtime, consideration of punctal occlusion |

and intent of this chapter, suggestions for treating more commonly identified conditions are listed (see the box on p. 71). Initial therapy is based upon a synthesis of information gathered from history, physical examination, and the interpretation of routine cytologic stains. If necessary, therapy may be modified when the results of further laboratory studies are known. On occasion, more than one factor may be identified, possibly inciting or contributing to the presence of chronic conjunctivitis. A common example is the cooccurrence of blepharitis and aqueous tear deficiency.

Often, a specific cause of chronic conjunctivitis is not identified. Thygeson and Kimura noted that "an important number of cases . . . resisted all attempts at clinical or etiologic differentiation."[1] My experience, applying the systematic approach to chronic conjunctivitis detailed above, successfully established an etiologic diagnosis in 67% of patients in whom secondary causes of chronic conjunctivitis were ruled out.[6] In my cornea and external disease referral practice, the majority of cases of chronic conjunctivitis are found to be secondary to blepharitis and aqueous tear deficiency, therefore this approach to chronic conjunctivitis of all causes is more successful than implied when only primary causes are examined.

For the patient in whom no specific etiology is identified, reassurance of the patient, reassessment of the case if the conjunctivitis is persistent, and, on occasion, initiation of a therapeutic trial is indicated.

---

## References


1. Thygeson P, Kimura SJ. Chronic conjunctivitis. Trans Am Acad Ophthalmol Oto 1963; 67:494-517.
2. Friedlaender MH. Ocular allergy. J Allergy Clin Immunol 1985; 76:645-657.
3. Chin GN, Hyndiuk RA. Parinaud's oculoglandular conjunctivitis. In Tasman W, Jaeger EA, eds. Duane's clinical ophthalmology. Vol. 4, Chap. 4. Philadelphia: JB Lippincott Co, 1986:1-6.
4. Aaberg TM. The expanding ophthalmologic spectrum of Lyme disease. Am J Ophthalmol 1989; 107:77-80.
5. Bialasiewicz AA, Jahn GJ. Epidemiology of chlamydial eye diseases in a mixed rural/urban population of West Germany. Ophthalmol 1986; 93:757-762.
6. Rapoza PA, Quinn TC, Terry AC, Gottsch JD, Kiessling LA, Taylor HR. A systematic approach to the diagnosis and treatment of chronic conjunctivitis. Am J Ophthalmol 1990; 109:138-142.
7. Reingold WJ, Robin JB, Leipa D, Kondra L, Schanzlin DJ, and Smith RJ. *Oestrus ovis* ophthalmomyiasis externa. Am J Ophthalmol 1984; 97:7-10.
8. Dawson CR, Hanna L, Wood TR, Despain R. Adenovirus type 8 keratoconjunctivitis in the United States III. Epidemiologic, clinical, and microbiologic features. Am J Ophthalmol 1970; 69:473-480.
9. Darougar S, Wishart MS, Viswalingam ND. Epidemiological and clinical features of primary herpes simplex virus ocular infection. Br J Ophthalmol 1985; 69:2-6.
10. Rauzada JK, Dwivedi PC. Chronic ocular lesions in Bhopal gas tragedy. Indian J Ophthalmol 1987; 35:453-454.
11. Chang SW, Hou PK, Chen MS. Conjunctival concretions: polarized microscopic, histopathologic, and ultrastructural studies. Arch Ophthalmol 1990; 108:405-407.
12. Liesegang TJ. Bulbar conjunctival follicles associated with dipivefrin therapy. Ophthalmol 1985; 92:228-233.
13. Wilson LA, McNatt J, Reitschel R. Delayed hypersensitivity to thimerosal in soft contact lens wearers. Ophthalmol 1981; 88:804-809.
14. Crawford JB. Conjunctival tumors. In Tasman W, Jaeger EA, eds. Duane's clinical ophthalmology. Vol. 4, Chap. 10. Philadelphia, 1986, JB Lippincott Co.
15. McCulley JP, Dougherty JM, Deneau DG. Classification of chronic blepharitis. Ophthalmol 1982; 89:1173-1180.
16. Schwartz LK, Gelender H, Forster RK. Chronic conjunctivitis associated with "floppy eyelids." Arch Ophthalmol 1983; 101:1884-1888.

17. Howitt DA, Goldstein JH. Physiologic lagophthalmos. Am J Ophthalmol 1969; 68:355.
18. Doxanas MT, Green WR. Sebaceous cell carcinoma: review of 40 cases. Arch Ophthalmol 1984; 102:245-249.
19. Lemp MA. Recent developments in dry eye management. Ophthalmol 1987; 94:1299-1304.
20. Baker RH, Bartley GB. Lacrimal gland ductule stones. Ophthalmol 1990; 97:531-534.
21. Stenson S, Fedukowicz, Newman R. Laboratory studies in chronic conjunctivitis. Ann Ophthalmol 1983; 15:1160-1164.

# The Argument against Extended-Wear Soft Contact Lenses

**5**


**Jon Walker, MD**
**Matthew E. Dangel, MD**


The evidence against extended-wear contact lenses (EWCLs) comes from two general realms: indirect, inferential data concerning the effect of these lenses on the cornea in "healthy" states and direct epidemiologic evidence that EWCL wearers face an increased risk of ulcerative keratitis. There is a wealth of literature looking at the presumably physiologic changes induced by wearing EWCL compared to daily-wear lenses or no lenses. Because such changes do not appear to damage the cornea directly, they seem to be considered interesting examples of the cornea's adaptive powers and therefore to be physiologically acceptable. Perhaps either further long-term studies or more subtle measures of corneal function will change this perception of harmlessness; nevertheless, our concern is that if another optical option is possible, the patient should not be exposed to the added risk that such "benign" changes may imply.

The breadth of these changes, reviewed by Bruce and Brennan[1] and by Lembach and Stocker,[2] is discussed only briefly here. EWCLs have been shown to cause both corneal epithelial thinning and epithelial microcysts, which are felt to indicate deranged epithelial growth.[3,4] When the lenses that caused microcysts were worn daily, however, no microcysts were formed, indicating that microcysts were the result of extended wear rather than the lenses. Superficial punctate epithelial changes also occur more frequently in EWCL users than in daily-wear lens users.[5] Both these findings are felt to be related to the hypoxic effects of extended wear and to represent an insult to the cornea's primary defense against infection that should be avoided if possible. Nor is it surprising that once some sort of epithelial damage does occur, healing is also retarded by hypoxia, thus prolonging the time that the surface break exists.[6]

Overnight corneal swelling is another observation initially marked in extended wear; and although it eventually decreases, it still represents a significant alteration in corneal function. This edema occurs as a result of the hypoxic accumulation of lactate which increases osmotic pressure and pulls water into the cornea. Decreases in tear osmolarity as part of adaptation to lens wear may also play a role.[1] Finally, this swelling may represent not only an increased osmotic load but also a potentially harmful decrease in the endothelium's ability to deal with the increased load, as discussed later. One possible explanation for the apparent decrease in edema with time has been the observation that stromal thinning occurs with prolonged EWCL use.[3] If this is indeed the case, then the cornea's so-called adaption is really a balance between two clearly abnormal reactions: stromal swelling and stromal thinning.

Of even greater concern are the possible effects on the endothelium. For instance, the stromal edema is associated in some cases with posterior stromal and even Descemet's folds.[7] Actual endothelial edema has also been reported in EWCL use, although it disappears clinically within a week.[8] The simple fact that the cornea does indeed swell beyond the normal range must indicate that the endothelium is pushed beyond maximal capacity, in spite of more reassuring explanations based on osmolarity. All this should be considered evidence of both physiologic and mechanical stress on the endothelium, and we are not quite sure such stresses can really be considered "physiologic." The data on polymegathism are even more disconcerting. Although there is some controversy in the literature about the true significance of the morphologic changes,[1] they must be considered an undesirable side effect, given the crucial, delicate role of the endothelium. Since everyone has only one set of endothelial cells per lifetime, it seems prudent to minimize their discomfort, especially in young individuals such as myopes who insist on extended wear for the sake of convenience.

There are other troubling observations with EWCLs. There is an increased amount of corneal vascularization, felt to be a marker for hypoxia.[9] In a daily wear setting, such vascularization generally represents simply reversible dilation. However, extended wear is associated with real vessel growth; up to four times more often than daily wear in one study of aphakes.[9] Stromal vascularization can also occur, although it is less likely.[9] Because these changes are usually small and stable, they too are considered acceptable. However, we feel this is not completely justified. There are reports of direct deleterious consequences such as hemorrhage and perivascular lipid and cellular infiltrate, primarily seen with the deeper vessels.[1] The fact that damage to these deeper vessels can occur without acute symptoms makes their occurrence even more problematic.[1] Even the relatively benign superficial neovascularization may be more significant than is currently appreciated. The increased blood flow must increase the potential for perilimbal disease processes that are felt to be related to increased immunologic exposure at the border of avascular and vascular cornea. The effect of such vessels in patients who may ultimately be candidates for penetrating keratoplasty or refractive procedures must also be kept in mind.

Extended-wear patients are also essentially the only subset of contact lens patients at risk for the tight lens syndrome because overnight wear is required for the syndrome to develop. Again, because this problem responds so well to removing the lens, it seems to be accepted as part of extended-wear management. The potential, however, for such a marked derangement must be considered yet another reason for avoiding extended-wear use if possible.

We recognize that all these changes are felt to be acceptable because they have not yet been shown to affect the long-term function of the cornea. These changes nevertheless do occur, often as a function of the hypoxia induced by overnight wear, and the fact that they are felt to be "acceptable" at present does not guarantee they will continue to be. Also, even though a minor insult may be well tolerated in isolation, the cumulative effect of continued repeated minor insults may well be serious. As a result, these "acceptable" corneal changes must still be factored into the overall risk–benefit ratio, particularly in cases where alternatives are available. The situation may turn out to be somewhat analogous to the one described in the literature on the effect of long-term ultraviolet exposure on retinal function. Because of the time required, the epidemiologic data demonstrating risk are still equivocal, yet the preponderance of evidence from animal, clinical, and short-term studies makes the association inevitable.

Far more definite evidence against the use of EWCLs comes from the work of the Microbial Keratitis Study Group.[10,11] They found a relative risk of ulcerative keratitis of 3.9 and 4.2 for extended wear versus daily wear users in population and hospital-based samples, respectively. When the subset of extended wear users who wore the lenses overnight was compared to that of daily-wear users, the risk increased to 10 to 15 times. The annual incidence figures reflect a similar increased risk: 20.7 cases per 10,000 EWCL wearers and 4.1 cases per 10,000 daily wearers. It is not clear whether the increased risk from extended wear is secondary to more corneal hypoxia or longer exposure to contaminating microorganisms. It is clear, though, that ulcerative keratitis represents a potentially devastating complication, and the unequivocal evidence of increased risk provides a strong argument against the use of EWCLs unless there are no alternatives.

We do not intend to condemn EWCL use entirely. Instead, we contend it should be acknowledged that like any other therapeutic intervention it has the potential for complications that must be kept in mind. For instance, the myriad "acceptable" alterations induced by EWCLs are certainly more benign than, say, a secondary IOL implantation. Taken together, though, they still make a strong argument for the use of even more benign optical alternatives. The risk of ulcerative keratitis, on top of the so-called physiologic changes, suddenly places EWCLs on an essentially surgical risk–benefit level, with the potential for severe visual loss rather than simple inconvenient side effects.

There are certainly situations where EWCLs are still the only choice, and we do not suggest that they be eliminated entirely from the armamentarium. They should be considered more an alternative of last resort rather than the first choice, particularly in the setting of the healthy young cosmetic-lens wearer. Those patients who require an extended-wear approach must be selected with assiduous care. The ocular surface must be carefully evaluated with attention to tear film, blepharitis, lid function, and preexisting disease. Factors such as access to follow-up and the ability to understand the importance of symptoms must be taken into account. In turn, the dispensing practitioner must be ready to be available 24 hours a day should severe problems develop. It must be acknowledged that among those who are the most justifiable candidates for EWCL use, i.e., aphakes, one or more of the above factors is often suboptimal, which makes extended wear potentially hazardous. However, because the alternatives to EWCL use are surgical, the risk may be tolerable. On the other hand, the ideal candidates in terms of the condition of the ocular surface and comprehension of instructions are usually the young, cosmetic-lens wearers. Because the use of extended wear lenses among these patients is justified primarily by convenience, however, the risks are not tolerable. As progress is made in the development of extended-wear silicone or hard gas-permeable lenses, it is to be hoped that these will prove to be more convenient and less dangerous alternatives to traditional hydrogel lenses.

Finally, some thought should also be given to other, more teleologic contraindications to extended wear. Although there is as yet no definitive literature on the subject, one must wonder why, if the Celestial Design Committee meant us to wear contact lenses, they did not make the delicate architecture of the cornea more compatible with little pieces of plastic. Who knows? Maybe someday we will learn that wearing contact lenses is a sin. Perhaps there is even a special circle of Dante's Inferno set aside for contact lens wearers . . . at least for some of them.

## References


1. Bruce AS, Brennan NA. Corneal pathophysiology with contact lens wear. Surv Ophthalmol 1990; 35:25-58.
2. Lembach RG, Stocker EG. Extended wear contact lenses. Ophthal Clin of North America 1989; 2: 275-289.
3. Holden B, Sweeney D, Vannas A, et al. Effects of long-term extended wear contact lenses on the human cornea. Invest Ophthalmol and Vis Sci 1985; 26:1489-1501.
4. Kenyon E, Pulse K, Seger R: Influence of wearing schedule on extended wear complications. Ophthalmol 1986; 93:231-236.
5. Lebow K, Plishka K: Ocular changes associated with extended wear contact lenses. Int Contact Lens Clinic 1980; 7:49-55.
6. Mauger T, Hill R: Corneal epithelial healing in hypoxic environments. Invest Ophthalmol and Vis Sci 1987; (supp):28(3):2.
7. Holden B, Mertz G, McNalby J: Corneal swelling response to contact lenses worn under extended wear conditions. Invest Ophthalmol and Vis Sci 1983; 24:218-226.
8. Williams L, Holden B. The Bleb response of the endothelium decreases with extended wear of contact lenses. Clin Exp Optom 1986; 69:90-92.
9. Cunha M, Thomassen T, Cohen E, et al. Complications associated with soft contact lens use. Contact Lens Assoc Ophthalmol J 1987; 13:107-111.
10. Schein OD, Glynn RJ, Poggio EC, et al. The relative risk of ulcerative keratitis among users of daily wear and extended wear soft contact lenses. New Eng J Med 1989; 321:773-778.
11. Poggio EC, Ghynn RJ, Schein OD, et al. The incidence of ulcerative keratitis among users of daily wear and extended wear soft contact lenses. New Eng J Med 1989; 321:779-783.

# 6 Therapeutic Uses of Collagen Shields

**Mark R. Sawusch, MD**
**Terrence P. O'Brien, MD**

The collagen corneal shield offers an exciting and important adjunct in the management of several difficult corneal and external disease problems. The composition of the shield provides unique properties of great value not provided by therapeutic contact lenses or other modes of therapy. These properties may have considerable importance in the management of challenging problems involving the ocular surface, including infectious keratitis.

The collagen shield was originally developed by Dr. Svyatoslav Fyodorov to supply the injured cornea with the "building blocks" required for healing. Fyodorov reported that application of collagen shields to animal eyes following keratotomy improved healing rates.[1] Collagen shields, which became commercially available in the United States in 1987, have been FDA approved for use as a corneal bandage in postsurgical, traumatic, and nontraumatic corneal conditions.

Within the last few years, important new applications of collagen shields have been investigated, including use as drug delivery devices. It is in this area that collagen shields potentially have their most useful application.

## PHYSICAL PROPERTIES

Collagen shields are currently manufactured from either porcine or bovine collagen. These collagens are both similar to human collagen and appear to have low allergenicity, although there is a single case report of possible hypersensitivity to a porcine shield.[2]

The shields are similar in size and conformation to soft contact lenses, with a diameter of approximately 14.5 mm and base curve of 9 mm (Figure 6-1). When a shield is hydrated by tear fluids, it softens, conforms to the corneal surface, and forms a pliable, thin film approximately 0.1 mm in thickness. Oxygen permeability (Dk) of porcine collagen shields has been found to be similar to that of hydrogel contact lenses of high water content.[3] Collagen shields may reduce visual acuity up to several lines; and although the bovine-derived shield is claimed by one manufacturer (Chiron Ophthalmics, Inc.) to allow better acuity, there are no published studies to confirm this.

By cross-linking collagen with ultraviolet light, the shields can be manufactured to biodegrade at different rates. Shields with dissolution times of 12, 24, and 72 hours are commercially available, although in practice there may be wide variations in dissolution rates due to differences in lid and tear function and tear-

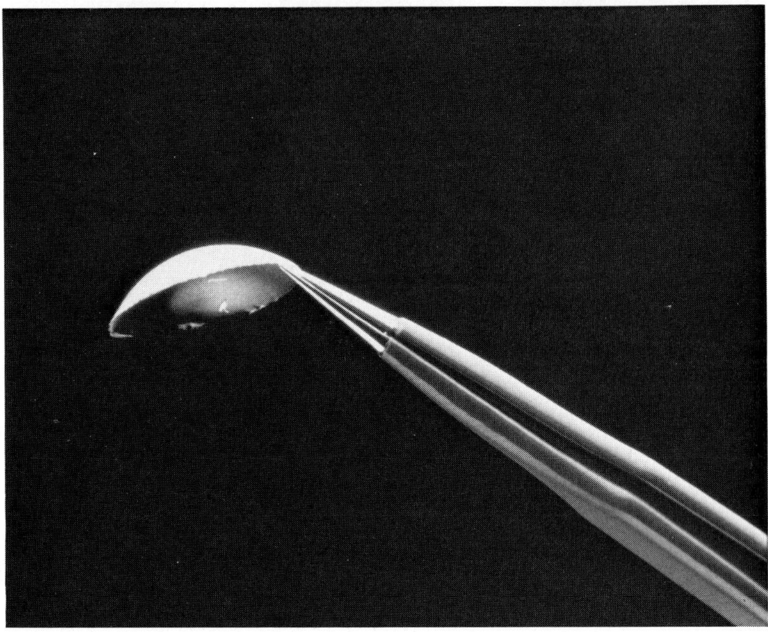

**FIGURE 6-1**    The porcine collagen corneal shield prior to hydration.

film collagenases. In dry eyes, collagen shields may cause irritation and require several days to dissolve.

## APPLICATIONS
### Drug Delivery

The use of collagen shields to enhance delivery of water-soluble drugs was suggested by earlier observations indicating that contact lenses could be used to deliver topical medications, including antibiotics.[4-6] Contact lenses never achieved popularity as drug-delivery devices, possibly because of their cost, fitting requirements, and concern for complications. Collagen shields may also be superior to contact lenses in their ability to enhance penetration and prolong delivery of water-soluble medications, as is suggested by a study that directly compared these methods for topical tobramycin delivery (Figure 6-2).[7] Water-insoluble medications could also be incorporated into a shield in manufacture and then delivered over a sustained period.

The collagen shield may serve as a drug-delivery device by creating a tear reservoir and increasing drug contact time at a steady concentration, or by reversibly binding the drug as it is dosed and then gradually redistributing it into the tear film as the shield itself dissolves.[7-8]

Maintaining concentration and prolonging contact time of drugs are two of the most significant factors affecting penetration of topical medications. Tear production, the lacrimal pump, and conjunctival absorption efficiently remove topically applied ocular medications, limiting corneal penetration. Prolongation of contact time may be achieved by increasing the frequency of administration, or the viscosity of the vehicle, by subconjunctival injection, or by use of a collagen

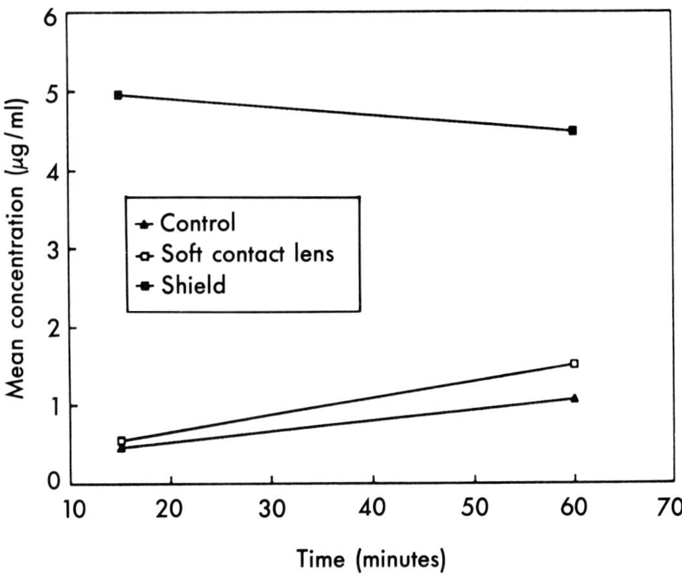



**FIGURE 6-2**    Comparison of the mean aqueous tobramycin concentration in eyes with a collagen shield, with a hydrophilic contact lens, or with no drug delivery device. *(Reprinted with permission from O'Brien TP, Sawusch MR, Dick JD, Hamburg TR, et al. Use of collagen corneal shields to enhance penetration of topical tobramycin. J Cateract Refract Surg 1988; 14:505-507.)*

shield. Drug delivery by collagen shields is potentially more reliable and comfortable than frequent around-the-clock application of drops or painful subconjunctival injection.

Several investigators have found the collagen shield to act as a drug-delivery device to enhance penetration of water soluble medications, including the following:

## Tobramycin

Three studies have found ocular penetration of tobramycin significantly enhanced by collagen shields in comparison to topical dosing alone. O'Brien et al[7] found three-fold higher aqueous concentrations over one hour following topical dosing in rabbit eyes with a shield in place (see Figure 6-2). Sawusch et al[8] found up to 30-fold higher penetration of 3 mg/ml tobramycin over 12 hours in rabbit eyes with shields, with a mean aqueous concentration (6.5 ug/ml) higher than the minimal inhibitory concentrations (M.I.C.s) for commonly encountered organisms. The group without shields had aqueous levels (<0.16 ug/ml) considerably lower than the M.I.C.s for most sensitive strains of *Pseudomonas aeruginosa,* which have been reported to range from 0.25 to 4.00 ug/ml. The collagen shield was not soaked in antibiotic solution prior to application in either of these studies, and tobramycin was dosed at the same frequency in the shield and control groups.

Unterman et al[9] soaked shields in fortified tobramycin (40 or 200 mg/ml) for five minutes prior to application in rabbit eyes. At one, four, and eight hours after application, tobramycin concentrations exceeded the M.I.C.s for most strains of *Pseudomonas.* They were significantly higher than concentrations achieved by subconjunctival injection or topical dosing alone (Figure 6-3).

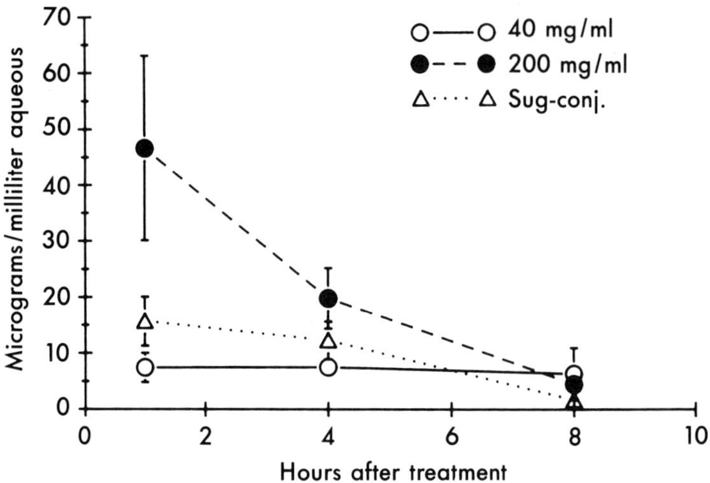


**FIGURE 6-3**    Concentrations of tobramycin in aqueous following application of a collagen shield immersed in 40 mg/ml (open circles) or 200 mg/ml (filled circles) tobramycin, or following a subconjunctival injection of 20 mg tobramycin (triangles). *(Reprinted with permission from Unterman SR, Rootman DS, Hill JM, Parelman JJ, Thompson HW, Kaufman HE. Collagen shield drug delivery: therapeutic concentration of tobramycin in the rabbit cornea and aqueous humor. J Cataract Refract Surg 1988; 14:500-504.)*

Enhanced delivery of tobramycin has been found to enhance treatment of *Pseudomonas* keratitis in animal models. Sawusch et al[8] found a significant decrease in the number of viable *Pseudomonas* organisms in eyes with shields following 12 hours of topical dosing of 3 mg/ml tobramycin compared to those without. The shield was not soaked in antibiotic prior to application.

Hobden et al[10] soaked shields in fortified (40 mg/ml) tobramycin for 10 minutes prior to application in rabbit eyes with *Pseudomonas* keratitis. Drug elution studies showed that soaking for ten minutes was equivalent to soaking for two hours. Following four hours of therapy, the soaked collagen shield was as effective in reducing the number of viable bacteria as was topical dosing every 30 minutes. This study also found that rehydration of a shield with four drops of tobramycin was as effective as exchange with a new shield soaked in tobramycin.

These studies suggest that collagen shields may be a useful adjunct in therapy of bacterial keratitis. Since there may often be a significant delay before a patient with acute microbial keratitis can obtain fortified antibiotic drops, use of a collagen shield may allow high concentrations to be achieved, even with ordinary concentrations of antibiotics, during the critical early period of infection.

Further studies evaluating the precise role of the collagen shield in treatment of corneal infections with particular organisms are indicated. Potential concerns include the shield acting as a nidus for infection or "trapping" virulence factors produced by certain organisms. For example, *Pseudomonas aeruginosa* produces extracellular proteases which contribute to tissue injury, scarring, and ultimate visual loss.[11-16] *Streptococcus pneumoniae* also secretes an ocular toxin highly destructive to the cornea.[17] Collagen shields may theoretically retain these toxins in the preocular tear film, potentially "delivering" higher concentrations to the cornea with possible increased tissue destruction. The shield may also trap polymorphonuclear neutrophils along with their destructive lytic enzymes in the precorneal tear film. Although it has been suggested that shields may act as a nidus for infection, Lucuta et al[18] found that collagen shields did not significantly affect growth of several bacterial species *in vitro* and noted minimal bacterial adherence to the shield.

Further specific investigations addressing these theoretical considerations are necessary to allow specific guidelines for safe usage and to better define the precise role of collagen shields in managing microbial keratitis.

## Gentamicin and Vancomycin

Phinney et al[19] evaluated ocular penetration of gentamicin and vancomycin in rabbit eyes in which a 4 mm corneal epithelial defect was created to simulate ulcerative keratitis. Collagen shields soaked in 40 mg/ml of gentamicin and 50 mg/ml vancomycin were compared to hourly topical dosing. Collagen shields produced significantly higher gentamicin levels in cornea at 30 minutes and 1 hour, but no significant difference in levels between 2 and 6 hours. The collagen shields produced higher earlier levels, but these were not sustained over time compared with the drop regimen.

Phinney found no significant difference in ocular penetration of vancomycin using soaked shields or hourly drops over the 6-hour study period. Vancomycin was released from shields considerably more slowly than gentamicin.

## Amphotericin B

Schwartz et al[20] evaluated ocular penetration of amphotericin B in rabbits with epithelial defects. A single soaked collagen shield provided higher corneal drug levels than hourly topical drops at 1 hour, no difference at 2 or 3 hours, and lower levels at 6 hours.

## Trifluorothymidine

Gussler et al[21] found that collagen shields enhanced penetration of trifluorothymidine in rabbit eyes with epithelial defects created to simulate ulcerative herpetic keratitis. Drug delivery was not enhanced in eyes with intact epithelium. No investigations of possible increased ocular toxicity at these higher concentrations were performed.

## Propamidine

Collagen shields soaked in propamidine isethionate and changed every 24 hours for 5 days were compared to hourly topical dosing in treatment of a rabbit model of Acanthamoeba keratitis by Desai et al.[22] Lower counts of acanthamoeba cysts and trophozoites were found in shield-treated eyes. A comparable reduction in organisms was found for both methods when propamidine was combined with neomycin-polymyxin-gramicidin therapy.

## Antibiotic toxicity

The potential of collagen shields to deliver high concentrations of antibiotics has raised the question of toxicity. Rootman et al[23] noted that high concentrations of gentamicin (400 mg/ml) are toxic to rabbit corneal endothelium when delivered via a collagen shield only when a large epithelial defect is present. Lower concentrations (40 mg/ml) produced minimal endothelial damage. Further studies of the toxicity of antimicrobial agents delivered by collagen shields are indicated.

### Steroids

Rabbit corneal and aqueous penetration of a single drop of prednisolone acetate 1% was enhanced 2-3 fold at 30 minutes in the presence of a collagen shield in a study by Sawusch et al.[24] At 2 hours following administration, prednisolone levels were 4- to 5-fold higher in eyes with a shield. Soaking the shield for 15 minutes prior to application resulted in a further increase of these levels at 30 minutes and 2 hours (Figure 6-4).

Hwang et al[25] found that treatment with a soaked collagen shield plus hourly drops resulted in a 2- to 4-fold increase in rabbit ocular penetration of dexamethasone in comparison to hourly drops alone. A soaked shield by itself yielded equivalent or superior drug delivery in comparison to hourly drops.

### Heparin

Delivery of heparin by soaked collagen shields was found to significantly alter baseline aqueous anticoagulant activity in a rabbit model by Murray et al,[26] whereas a subconjunctival heparin injection did not; no comparison was made to topical therapy with drops. The authors suggest that collagen shield delivery of heparin may prevent postoperative fibrin formation in eyes undergoing vitrectomy or filtering surgery.

### 5-Fluorouracil

Postoperative subconjunctival injections of 5-fluorouracil (5-FU) have been demonstrated to improve success of glaucoma filtering surgery in patients at risk for failure. Sachdev et al[27] investigated the use of collagen shields impregnated with 5-FU and implanted as a subconjunctival drug delivery system to eliminate the need for a regimen of injections. The nonmedicated surgical controls were found to have twice the myofibroblastic cell response of the medicated group. However, no comparison was made to daily subconjunctival 5-FU injections.

---

## Corneal Bandage

Several studies have found the collagen shield to be an effective corneal bandage to enhance healing of epithelial defects. The shield may act in a similar fashion to a bandage contact lens by protecting and lubricating the migrating epithelial cells at the wound margin. Shaker et al[28] found that porcine collagen shields significantly increased wound closure rates of epithelial defects in cats, particularly during the initial few hours following wounding.

Similar results were reported for a rabbit model of superficial keratectomies by Frantz et al,[29] in which collagen shields produced a significant increase in epithelial healing rates.

However, Robin et al[30] noted no significant difference in rabbit corneal reepithelialization rates over 96 hours following chemical debridement, in comparison to treatment with saline or antibiotic ointment.

None of these three studies compared reepithelialization rates to those found with the use of conventional patching, tarsorrhaphy, or soft contact lenses. Thus,

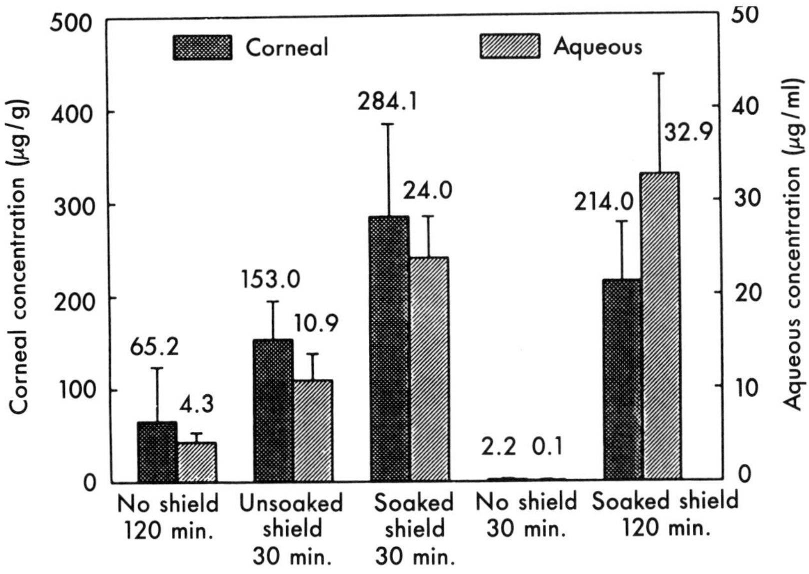


**FIGURE 6-4**    Ocular penetration of prednisolone acetate into rabbit cornea and aqueous. Soaking the shield for 15 minutes prior to application resulted in significantly higher ocular penetration in comparison to application of drops on a dry shield. *(Reprinted with permission from Sawusch et al.[24])*

it is unknown whether collagen shields allow faster reepithelialization than these conventional therapies.

Early clinical data on the use of collagen corneal shields to enhance reepithelialization in humans is not as encouraging as the animal studies suggest. O'Brien and Sawusch[31] noted no significant difference in wound healing rates between collagen shields and patching in a series of 20 patients with acute corneal abrasions. However, the shield was irritating to a few patients and fell out of one, whereas no patients noted discomfort from patching. In a small series of 5 patients with corneal foreign bodies, Moorhead and Jenkins[32] found that collagen shields applied after foreign-body removal were irritating and/or fell out in all 5 cases. Groden and White[33] compared bandage contact lenses to porcine collagen shields in treatment of persistent epithelial defects following penetrating keratoplasty. None of 7 patients treated with collagen shields healed, whereas 16 of 22 patients (73%) treated with bandage lenses healed completely.

There are several anecdotal reports on the use of collagen shields postoperatively, but none of these studies had control groups. Aquavella et al[34] patched over a collagen shield in 44 postoperative patients and noted good tolerance, although no comparison was made to the use of a collagen shield alone.

Although animal studies support the use of collagen shields to enhance rates of reepithelialization, available clinical data do not suggest that shields offer any advantage over conventional therapy such as patching, lubrication, or therapeutic soft contact lenses. Collagen shields may have a role in promoting reepithelialization in one-eyed patients, who would thus retain some vision as they would not with patching, or in patients who require concomitant drug delivery. Some have suggested the use of patching over an antibiotic-soaked shield to provide high antibiotic levels without risk of dislodgement or discomfort. This may be particularly important in patients with contact lens-related abrasions, since these patients occasionally develop bacterial keratitis if treated by a single antibiotic application and patching. Shields are unlikely to replace therapeutic soft contact lenses for treatment of chronic epithelial defects or chronic exposure problems since they do not provide prolonged therapy.

## Filtering Bleb Leaks

Two reports describe the use of collagen corneal shields in the management of leaking blebs following glaucoma filtering surgery. Fourman and Wiley[35] applied a gentamicin-soaked 24-hour shield to a leaking filter bleb and noted sealage within 2 days. Weber and Baker[36] reported sealing a leaking bleb with cyano-acrylate glue, using a collagen shield to cover the glue in a fashion similar to that used with a contact lens. It is unclear from these reports whether collagen shields offer any distinct advantage over conventional therapy in the management of filtering bleb leaks.

## CONCLUSION

The collagen corneal shield offers several exciting new applications for the management of difficult corneal and external disease problems. The most valuable emerging role for collagen shields may be as drug-delivery devices to achieve prolonged, reliably high concentrations of water-soluble medications in the cornea and aqueous humor while avoiding labor intensive frequent instillation or painful subconjunctival injection. Experimental data suggest a role for the shield in enhancing corneal reepithelialization, although no clinical reports have documented advantages over conventional therapies such as patching, lubrication, or bandage contact lenses. Further investigations defining clinical safety and efficacy of collagen shields as adjuncts in the therapy of microbial keratitis are also warranted.

## References

1. Fyodorov SN, Ivashina AI, Bagrov SN, Amstislav-skaya TS, et al. Efficiency of collagen covers: application in cases of keratotomy. In Eye Microsurgery. Moscow: Research Institute of Eye Microsurgery, 1984.

2. Boerner CF. Allergic response to a porcine collagen corneal shield: Case report. Arch Ophthalmol 1988; 106:171.

3. Schwartz SD, Weissman BA, Noel NA, Lee DA, Fatt IF. Oxygen permeability of collagen shields. Invest Ophthalmol Vis Sci 1989; 30(supp):479.

4. Waltman SR, Kaufman HE. Use of hydrophilic contact lenses to increase ocular penetration of topical drugs. Invest Ophthalmol Vis Sci 1970; 9:250-255.

5. Matoba AY, McCulley JP. The effect of therapeutic soft contact lenses on antibiotic delivery to the cornea. Ophthalmol 1985; 92:97-99.

6. Busin M, Goebbels M, Spitznas M. Medicated bandage lenses for sustained gentamicin release. Ophthalmol 1987; 94(supp):124.

7. O'Brien TP, Sawusch MR, Dick JD, Hamburg TR, et al. Use of collagen corneal shields versus soft contact lenses to enhance penetration of topical tobramycin. J Cataract Refract Surg 1988; 14: 505-507.

8. Sawusch MR, O'Brien TP, Dick JD, Gottsch JD. Use of collagen corneal shields in the treatment of bacterial keratitis. Am J Ophthalmol 1988; 106: 279-281.

9. Unterman SR, Rootman DS, Hill JM, Parelman JJ, Thompson HW, Kaufman HE. Collagen shield drug delivery: therapeutic concentrations of tobramycin in the rabbit cornea and aqueous humor. J Cataract Refract Surg 1988; 14:500-504.

10. Hobden JA, Reidy JJ, O'Callaghan RJ, Hill JM, Insler MS, Rootman DS. Treatment of experimental pseudomonas keratitis using collagen shields containing tobramycin. Arch Ophthalmol 1988; 106: 1605-1607.

11. Liu PV. Extracellular toxins of pseudomonas aeruginosa. J Infect Dis 1974; 130(supp):594-599.

12. Morihava K. Pseudomonas aeruginosa proteinase I. Purification and genial properties. Biochem Biophys Acta 1963; 73:113-124.

13. Morihava K, Tsuzuki H, Oka T, et al. Pseudomonas aeruginosa elastase. Isolation, crystallization, and preliminary characterization. J Biol Chem 1965; 240:3295-3304.

14. Kreger AS, Gray LD. Purification of pseudomonas aeruginosa protease and microscopic characterization of pseudomonal protease-induced rabbit corneal damage. Infect Immun 1978; 19:630-648.

15. Kawaharajo K, Abe C, Homma JY, et al. Corneal ulcers caused by protease and elastase from pseudomonas aeruginosa. Jpn J Exp Med 1974; 44: 435-442.

16. Iglewski BH, Bums RP, Cripson IK. Pathogenesis of corneal damage from pseudomonas exotoxin A. Invest Ophth Vis Sci 1977; 16:73-76.

17. Johnson M, Allen J. Ocular toxin of the pneumococcus. Am J Ophthalmol 1971; 72:175-179.

18. Lucuta VL, Kaminsky LA, Witlock DR, Viana MAG, Robin JB. The effect of collagen shields upon microbial growth. Invest Ophthalmol Vis Sci 1990; 31(supp):452.

19. Phinney RB, Schwartz SD, Lee DA, Mondino BA. Collagen shield delivery of gentamicin and vancomycin. Arch Ophthalmol 1988; 106:1599-1604.

20. Schwartz SD, Harrison SA, Engstrom RE, Bawden RE, Lee DA, Mondino BJ. Amphotericin B delivery by collagen shields. Invest Ophthalmol Vis Sci 1990; 31(supp):558.

21. Gussler JR, Ashton P, VanMeter WS, Smith TJ. The effect of collagen shields on the topical delivery of trifluorothymidine into cornea and aqueous. Invest Ophthalmol Vis Sci 1990; 31(supp):485.

22. Desai D, John T, Rockey JH, Sahm D. Use of medicated collagen shields in the treatment of experimental acanthamoeba keratitis. Invest Ophthalmol Vis Sci 1990; 31(supp):421.

23. Rootman DS, Avaria M, Basu PK. Endothelial toxicity of gentamicin delivered by a collagen shield to rabbit eyes. Invest Ophthalmol Vis Sci 1990; 31(supp):558.

24. Sawusch MR, O'Brien TP, Updegraff SA. Collagen corneal shields enhance penetration of topical prednisolone acetate. J Cataract Refract Surg 1989; 15:625-628.

25. Hwang DG, Stern WH, Hwang PH, MacGowan-Smith EA. Collagen shield enhancement of topical dexamethasone penetration. Arch Ophthalmol 1989; 107:1375-1380.

26. Murray TG, Stern WH, Chin DH, MacGowan-Smith EA. Collagen shield heparin delivery for prevention of postoperative fibrin. Arch Ophthalmol 1990; 108:104-106.

27. Sachdev S, Zou X, Higginbotham E. The effect of 5-fluorouracil impregnated collagen shield implants in filtration surgery on rabbits. Invest Ophthalmol Vis Sci 1990; 31(supp):3.

28. Shaker GJ, Ueda S, LoCascio JA, Aquavella JV. Effect of a collagen shield on cat corneal epithelial wound healing. Invest Ophthalmol Vis Sci 1989; 30:1565-1568.

29. Frantz JM, Dupuy BM, Kaufman HE, Beuerman RW. The effect of collagen shields on epithelial wound healing in rabbits. Am J Ophthalmol 1989; 108: 524-528.

30. Robin JB, Keys CL, Kaminshi LA, Viana MAG. The effect of collagen shields on rabbit corneal re-epithelialization after chemical debridement. Invest Ophthalmol Vis Sci 1990; 31:1294-1299.

31. O'Brien TP, Sawusch MR. Collagen corneal shield versus semi-pressure eye patch for treatment of corneal abrasions. Ophthalmology 1989; 96 (supp):119.

32. Moorhead LC, Jenkins DE. Collagen shield management of corneal foreign body injuries in workmen. Ocular Surgery News 1990; 8(10):21-22.

33. Groden LR, White W. Porcine collagen corneal shield treatment of persistent epithelial defects following penetrating keratoplasty. CLAO J 1990; 16:95-97.

34. Aquavella JV, Musco PS, Ueda S, LoCascio JA. Therapeutic applications of a collagen bandage lens: a preliminary report. CLAO J 1988; 14:47-50.

35. Fourman S, Wiley L. Use of a collagen shield to treat a glaucoma filter bleb leak. Am J Ophthalmol 1989; 107:673-674.

36. Weber PA, Baker ND. The use of cyanoacrylate adhesive with a collagen shield in leaking filtering blebs. Ophthalmic Surg 1989; 20:284-285.

# Indications, Techniques, and Results of a Conservative Approach to Radial Keratotomy

**James J. Salz, MD**
**Armand P. Fasano, MS**

## PATIENT SELECTION

As with other refractive surgeries, candidates for radial keratotomy (RK) should have healthy corneas and stable myopia as evidenced by minimal changes in their refractive error on successive yearly eye examinations. Because RK results are not 100% predictable, the procedure should be reserved primarily for patients who are unwilling or unable to wear contact lenses successfully. With proper informed consent, successful contact lens patients are candidates if they have compelling occupational or recreational reasons for the surgery or if they are not satisfied with glasses or contact lenses as their method of vision correction. If the degree of their myopia lies in the range that has a high probability of being significantly improved and if they fully comprehend the risks (and at times unpredictable nature) of the surgery, then RK can be considered. Although we have not operated on patients younger than age 20, we have operated on patients in their sixties for high myopia. On three patients in their seventies who were significantly over-corrected following intraocular lens implantation, we performed 4-incision RKs, the rationale being that a lens exchange would be of greater risk due to previous retinal detachment or high axial myopia.

Our usual patient is between $-2$ to $-8$ D myopic, although we have op-erated on patients with as little as $-1$ D to as much as $-11$ D under special circumstances. The $-1$ D patient was a professional motorcycle racer who was unable to wear contact lenses while racing. The $-11$ D patient was a 60-year-old attorney who was informed he would probably have a significant residual myopia. Fortunately, his response bettered our predictions, and he achieved 11 D of effect from an 8-incision RK with a 3-mm optical zone in one eye and 9 D of effect from a 4-incision, 3-mm optical zone procedure in his other eye.

Patients with 5 D of myopia can usually be corrected independent of their age, but correcting higher amounts of myopia with our surgical technique is age dependent. Patients in their twenties with $-8$ D of myopia are unlikely to achieve satisfactory results, while patients in their fourth or fifth decades, who can usually achieve at least 6 to 7 D of correction, are commonly happy with a residual myopia of 1 to 2 D for reading.

A practical formula for predicting the result from an 8 incision RK with a 3-mm optical zone with our technique is to set the diopters of achieved correction at 2.5 D plus 0.1 times the patient's age in years. Thus a 25-year-old patient can expect 5 D of effect, while a 55-year-old patient might achieve 8 D of correction. There is variability in the results of RK for any patient and this equation yields only an approximation. For example, in female patients in their late thirties, we have observed a range of 3.5 D to 11 D of effect from an 8-incision RK with a 3-mm optical zone.

## INFORMED CONSENT

Pamphlets and videotape presentations are available as aids to obtaining an informed consent. Our present method is to provide patients with a protracted, detailed, written informed-consents at the time of their initial RK consultation. They are urged to take these home and to telephone us regarding any questions about the consent or about RK.

During the initial RK consultation, the surgeon personally discusses the infrequent, but possibly calamitous, complication of infection, both endophthalmitis and keratitis, which can lead to permanent blindness, and the additional risk of rupture along the corneal incisions in the occurrence of severe ocular trauma. The surgeon then discusses and attempts to explain the more usual side effects of RK, which include glare, diurnal fluctuations in vision, increased astigmatism, over- and under-corrections, permanent corneal scars, and temporal instability. Trial lenses are then fitted to patients to demonstrate the most likely amount of myopia reduction for their age in addition to examples of both over- and under-corrections.

We simulate presbyopia by cyclopleging patients and having them attempt to read with their glasses. Mildly myopic patients in their early forties are usually surprised to find that they would need reading glasses if they achieved a complete correction. Periodically we operate unilaterally on presbyopic or prepresbyopic patients with mild myopia to allow them to judge "mono vision" for near with their unoperated eyes. Some find this to be a good compromise and waive surgery on the other eye.

The former chairman of the American Academy of Ophthalmology's Ethics Committee, Dr. Jerome Bettman, counsels not to rely entirely on videotapes, papers, or discussions with assistants when we obtain the patients' informed consent. He feels it is vital for the surgeon personally to discuss with the patient the risks, benefits and possible outcomes of the procedure and to document this by writing a short note in the patient's record, which is then signed and dated, *in his own hand.*[1]

We have examined close to 20 medical legal cases pertaining to RK, and the majority involve issues of informed consent where the surgeon did not fully discuss the possibility of an unforeseen result, usually a significant over- or under-correction. The rest involved unconventional surgical techniques, e.g., 10 reoperations or as many as 78 incisions.

## PATHOPHYSIOLOGY OF RADIAL AND ASTIGMATIC KERATOTOMY INCISION LENGTH

Sato added posterior incisions to his radial keratotomy procedure because he was unable to achieve sufficient effect from the anterior incisions, which began at an optical zone of 6 mm. Unfortunately, a high percentage of Sato's patients developed late bullous keratopathy (Figure 7-1). Fyodorov extended the incisions more centrally and achieved more correction. He also introduced the concept of titrating the effect by adjusting the diameter of the optical clear zone. These were his two greatest contributions to the evolution of RK.

At the University of Southern California, we completed a study on cadaver eyes comparing the keratometric flattening (measured by both the Terry Keratotmeter and corneascopy) following RK incisions with 3-, 4-, 5-, and 6-mm optical zones.[2] This work verified Fyodorov's teaching that smaller optical zones (OZ) produced the maximum effect. A 3-mm OZ, 8-incision RK yielded 9 D of flattening, while the same number of incisions with larger optical zones resulted in the following: 4 mm = 6.5 D; 5 mm = 5.25 D; 6 mm = 2.25 D. A greater change is seen in cadaver eyes than we usually see in the clinical situation. In effect they act as old eyes (which they usually are). If the above values are reduced by 30%, they approach the clinical results one expects in a 30-year-old patient for the 3- and 4-mm optical zones.

Changing the diameter of the optical clear zone by merely 0.5 mm (changing the length of the incisions by only 0.25 mm on each side of the optical zone) is

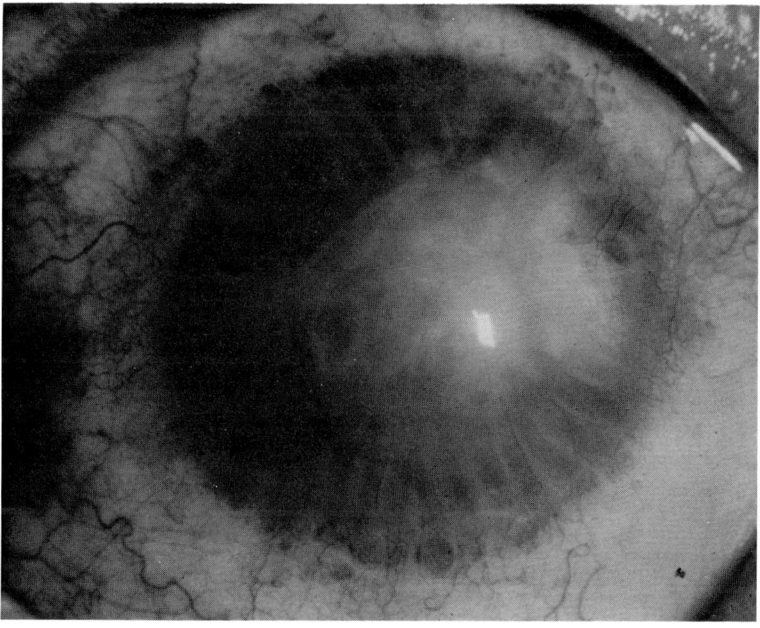

**FIGURE 7-1**    Bullous keratopathy following Sato procedure. *(Reprinted with permission from Thompson FB: Myopia surgery, New York, 1990, Macmillan, p. 32.)*

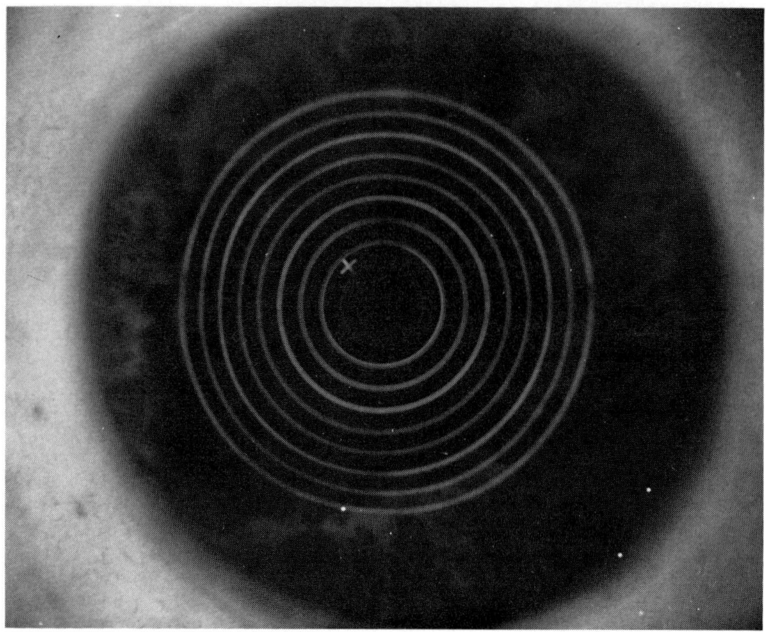

**FIGURE 7-2**    Corneascope photo—cadaver eye, preoperative. *(Reprinted with permission from Thompson FB: Myopia surgery, New York, 1990, Macmillan, p. 36.)*

the most reliable and powerful method of increasing or decreasing the effect of RK incisions.

## NUMBER OF INCISIONS

Fyodorov's first American publication reported his results on 16-incision RK for relatively low amounts of myopia.[3] In our study of 16-incision RK, 4-mm OZ in cadaver eyes, we established that the first 4 incisions produced 60% of the final effect and 8 incisions 90%. Therefore, doubling the number of incisions from 4 to 8 yields only a 30% increase in effect. Doubling the number yet again from 8 to 16 yields only 10% of the final corneal flattening. Preoperative (Figure 7-2) and postoperative (Figure 7-3) corneascope photographs readily demonstrate the significant corneal flattening that occurs after 4-incision RK in cadaver eyes. Increased ring diameter indicates corneal flattening, which is greatest in the meridians of the incisions.

Our cadaver-eye study[2] also compared the effects of 4- and 8-incision RK with three different optical zones. Four incisions produced approximately 85% of the effect with a 3-mm OZ, about 70% with a 4-mm OZ, and about 60% with a 5-mm OZ. Schachar's theoretical model of the cornea predicts that 8-incision RK would produce nearly 90% of the effect of 16 incisions.[4]

## INCISION DEPTH

Jester's statistical analysis of the variables in our cadaver-eye study indicated that incision depth was the most important factor producing significant corneal flat-

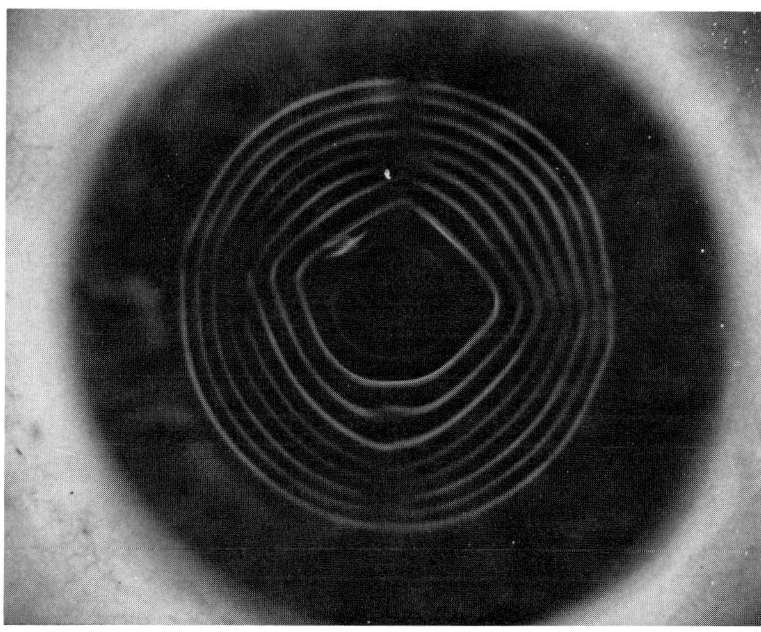

**FIGURE 7-3**    Corneascope photo—cadaver eye following 4-incision RK. *(Reprinted with permission from Thompson FB: Myopia surgery, New York, 1990, Macmillan, p. 37.)*

tening.[5] The significance of proper incision depth has also been stressed in clinical reports by Deitz,[6] Arrowsmith,[7] and the PERK study.[8]

In a cadaver-eye study on RK utilizing ultrasonic pachymetry and micrometer diamond blades, we found histologic verification of uniform incision depth along the entire length of the incisions (Figure 7-4). The histologic incision depths averaged between 80% and 90% in this study.[9]

## SINGLE-PASS INCISIONS, REDEEPENING, AND ZONE CUTTING

We have achieved satisfactory results, with a minimum incidence of complications for the past 10 years, with a single-pass incision technique. This is true even in patients with high myopia.[10] Redeepening and zone-cutting techniques are not necessary in order to correct higher amounts of myopia. The purported purpose of these complicated techniques is to obtain maximum incision depth. There are many reasons to favor the single-pass incision approach.

Cutting the portion of the cornea between 3 mm and 6 mm yields the majority of the flattening of an RK procedure, regardless of the number of incisions. This is evidenced in one of our cadaver-eye studies, which demonstrated that a 4-incision RK with a 3-mm optical zone produced an average flattening of 7.75 D compared to an average flattening of only 1.23 D from 4 incisions with a 6-mm optical zone. It is for this reason that RK surgeons do not ordinarily utilize optical zones larger than 5 mm. We have never used one larger than 5 mm.

Between optical zones of 3 mm and 6 mm, the corneal thickness increases by approximately 10%. Using ultrasonic pachymetry, Hikishima[11] measured a mean central corneal thickness of 0.52 mm, increasing to between 0.57 and 0.60 mm within 2 mm of the limbus on human subjects. For a mean corneal diameter of 12 mm, 2 mm from the limbus is an 8-mm optical zone. The hypothetical average patient might have a corneal profile of 0.52 mm centrally, 0.54 at the edge of a 3-mm OZ, and 0.56 mm at an OZ of 6 mm. An attained incision of 0.50 mm would represent an incision depth of 93% at the 3-mm OZ and 90% at the 6-mm OZ.

This type of an incision, with an achieved depth of 90% or more in the area between 3 mm and 6 mm, will give nearly the full effect for that cornea, even though the incision is only 75% to 80% of corneal thickness perilimbally. Our cadaver-eye study demonstrated histologic evidence of 80% to 90% incision depth along the length of the incisions after single-pass incisions.[9] If these incisions could be accurately recut to 90% in the periphery, this would not significantly increase the effect since optical zones greater than 5 mm produce minimal clinical effects.

We studied peripheral RK incision redeepening in a cadaver-eye study.[2] After performing a single-pass, 8-incision RK with a 3-mm OZ, we recut the 8 incisions from the 6-mm OZ to the limbus with the blade set to 100% of the pachymetry at 6 mm. Although we achieved no meaningful increase in corneal flattening, we perforated a number of the incisions.

There is scant clinical evidence of increased effectiveness for zone cutting or incision redeepening. Deitz performs RK with a single-blade setting, Neumann and Arrowsmith advocate multiple blade settings, with up to 16 incisions and three different blade settings for each incision. In their published results for high myopes, Deitz[12] corrected a higher percentage of patients to 20/40 or better and achieved an average myopia reduction of 6.7 D, compared to 6.2 D for Neumann[13] and 5.7 D for Arrowsmith.[14] Our mean effect from a single-pass, 8-incision RK in high myopes was 6.4 D.[10]

Grandon[15] compared his results from 3-mm OZ, single-pass, 8-incision RK

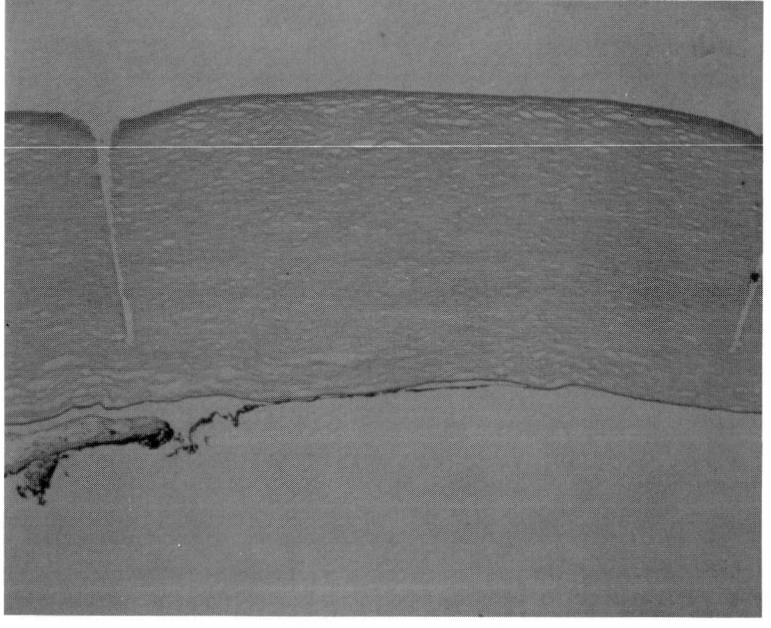

**FIGURE 7-4**     Histologic incision depth of 90~ following RK in cadaver eye. *(Reprinted with permission from Thompson FB: Myopia surgery, New York, 1990, Macmillan, p. 38.)*

in 79 patients with a similar group of 152 patients whose incisions were recut with blade extension from a 5-mm OZ to the limbus. He found merely an additional 0.47 D of effect attributable to the redeepening incisions.

The greater risk of complications, such as increased scarring and perforations, from the more complicated redeepening and zone-cutting techniques of RK are not offset by a demonstrable increase in benefits. For these reasons, our maximum RK procedure consists of 8 single-pass incisions, with a blade setting of 110% of thinnest paracentral pachymetry, and a 3-mm OZ. Patient age is the main determinant of the result with this approach. With suitable patient selection and realistic patient expectations, this comparatively simple approach yields rewarding results.

## RADIAL KERATOTOMY WOUND HEALING

We histologically studied RK incisions in primates and demonstrated that they are healed by avascular wound healing.[16] The epithelium migrates into the incision where it is progressively pushed to the surface by fibroblasts in the first two to three weeks. The fibroblasts are progressively replaced by keratocytes in the subsequent three months.

This repair process can be delayed or remain incomplete. In two normal and two keratoconic corneas (Figure 7-5), epithelial plugs were found in the RK

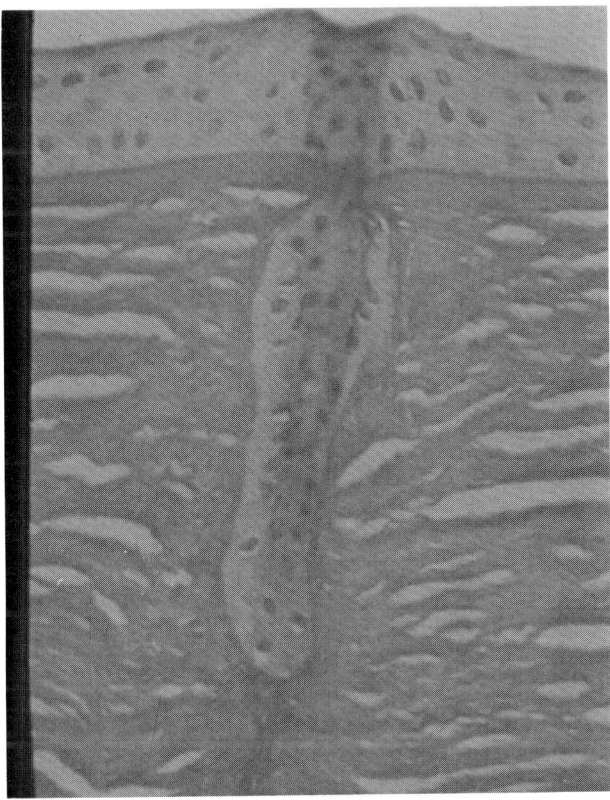

**FIGURE 7-5**     Epithelial plugs in human cornea following RK. *(Courtesy Dr. Perry Binder, reprinted with permission from Thompson FB: Myopia surgery, New York, 1990, Macmillan, p. 41.)*

incisions from 5 to 47 months following the keratotomies.[17] In a patient who died three months following his surgery, Yamaguchi found retained epithelium in the RK incisions in both eyes.[18]

The temporal course of healing is extremely variable. In a case report by Binder[19], a 33-year-old woman had a 16-incision RK in 1980 and 8 additional incisions in 1985. Homoplastic keratomileusis was performed 11 months after the second RK as she remained undercorrected. The button histologically showed incomplete healing of the 11-month-old incisions but evidenced complete healing of the 66-month-old incisions.

## RADIAL KERATOTOMY AND THE ENDOTHELIUM

Hoffer[20] reported endothelial cell loss from 16-incision RK with metal blades as 10% but only 3% after 8-incision RK with diamond blades. In 16 PERK patients at 6 and 12 months, Asbell[21] compared central and mid-peripheral endothelial cell counts between the operated and unoperated eyes. There was no statistically significant difference between the two groups either centrally or paracentrally. Using computer-assisted morphometric analysis, McRae[22] studied the corneas of RK patients. Comparing cell size and cell shape, he found no significant differences between the RK patients and the controls.

## PLANNING THE SURGERY

The novice RK surgeon can choose from an extensive, confusing, and conflicting selection of nomograms, modifiers, and computer programs with procedures for correcting nearly any conceivable myopic refractive error. There are innumerable possibilities—including the number of incisions, optical zones with 0.25 to 0.50 mm steps, cutting directions, single and multiple pass incisions, peripheral re-deepening with two to three zones following a primary incision, or zone cutting with varying blade settings for each of two to three zones of previously uncut cornea, to name a few. The following approach is based on our understanding of the pathophysiology of RK, interpretation of published reports, and clinical observations of both our cases and those of colleagues over the past 8 years.

It is not based on personal experience with the many variations in RK technique. For example, we would not perform deliberate microperforations, even if proof were available that this increases the effect of RK, because this presents an unacceptable risk–benefit ratio. We never perform more than 8 primary incisions, nor do we redeepen incisions, perform zone cutting, or give retrobulbar blocks. Our approach to surgical planning for radial keratotomy is illustrated with specific brief case histories.

## NUMBER OF INCISIONS

Whenever possible, perform a 4-incision RK, usually in the patient's nondominant eye. Start with 4 incisions for myopia less than −4 D, regardless of patient age. This is extended to −7 D for patients in their forties and up to −8 D for patients over fifty years old. The most obvious advantage of a 4-incision RK over an 8-incision is the opportunity to observe the eye's response to the surgery. If undercorrection results one can consider proceeding with an 8-incision RK in the second eye and later adding an additional 4 incisions to the first eye.

## OPTICAL ZONE

If the patient is an appropriate candidate for 4 incisions, the only other decision is the size of the optical clear zone. We usually use optical zones of 3 mm, 3.5 mm, or 4 mm. After 10 years of experience with the procedure, one can as a rule rely on clinical experience, consulting one's own data to see what occurred with patients with conditions similar to the one under consideration. The novice RK surgeon must rely on either a nomogram or computer software to aid the decision. Table 7-1 is a slightly modified nomogram developed by Richard Villasenor, MD. We both feel the patient's age is the major factor influencing the outcome of RK. Keratometry, tonometry, and pachometry values in the normal range do not aid in predicting the results.[23]

For typical patients in their mid-thirties, a 4-incision RK, 3-mm OZ yields around 3.5 D of myopia reduction, 3 D of effect from a 3.5-mm OZ, and about 2.5 D from a 4-mm OZ. For patients in their twenties, predict about 0.5 D less; and for patients in their forties, expect an additional 0.5 D. These figures are approximations, and wide variations in the results are possible. In female patients in their thirties, we have observed from 2 D to 5.5 D of effect from 3-mm OZ, 4-incision RK. In two male patients, ages 55 and 60, the same 4 incisions, 3-mm OZ RK resulted in 3 D of effect in one and 9 D in the other. RK surgeons label these patients as "under or over responders." In any published series of RK results, this can be found under the heading of "range."

As it is impossible to identify these over or under responders before surgery, it behooves us to proceed cautiously. It is especially important to avoid overcorrections because contact lens fitting is particularly difficult in these patients, suturing the RK incisions to reverse the overcorrection is technically demanding, and long-term results of the suturing techniques are not available. Furthermore,

**Table 7-1**   Salz and Villasenor: Four-Incision Radial Keratotomy

| | Optical zone (mm) | | | |
|---|---|---|---|---|
| **Correction (D)** | **Patient age: 30** | **40** | **50** | **60** |
| 4.50 | 3.00* | 3.00* | 3.00* | 3.00 |
| 4.00 | 3.00* | 3.00* | 3.00 | 3.50 |
| 3.50 | 3.00* | 3.50 | 4.00 | 4.25 |
| 3.00 | 3.25 | 4.00 | 4.25 | 4.50 |
| 2.75 | 3.50 | 3.75 | 4.00 | 4.75 |
| 2.50 | 3.50 | 4.00 | 4.25 | 5.00 |
| 2.25 | 3.75 | 4.25 | 4.50 | 5.25 |
| 2.00 | 4.00 | 4.50 | 4.75 | 5.50 |
| 1.50 | 4.50 | 4.75 | 5.00 | 6.00 |

*Probably will result in undercorrection.

NOTE: For myopia greater than $-5.00$, a 3-mm OZ with 8 incisions will average 5.5 D of correction for a patient in their mid-twenties; for a $-5.00$, 40- to 60-year-old patient, start with 4 incisions with a 3-mm OZ. (It is better to undercorrect presbyopes.)

some patients who are initially only slightly overcorrected may become more overcorrected with time ("progressive hyperopia"), as has been reported by Deitz[24] and the PERK study.[25]

Undercorrected myopic patients are usually disappointed but not terribly unhappy with their improvement. Significantly overcorrected myopic patients are quite disappointed about their farsightedness. To reduce the incidence of overcorrection, begin with a 4-incision RK, even if is unlikely to result in full correction. It is always feasible to add 4 incisions. It is not as easy to erase the effects of 4 extra incisions. This should reduce, but not eliminate, the percentage of eyes overcorrected.

A brief discussion of selected individual case histories of patients with low to moderate myopia will demonstrate this approach. The following abbreviations are used in the case histories: SERE—spherical equivalent refractive error; D—diopters; K—keratometry in D; TA—applanation tension; OZ—optical zone; PO—postoperative; VA—visual acuity; sc—without correction; REF—refraction.

## FOUR-INCISION RK CASE HISTORIES FOR LOW TO MODERATE MYOPIA

### Case 1

*A 28-year-old female with a SERE of −3.5 D, K 44.75/46.00, TA 12, underwent 4-incision RK with 3-mm OZ PO VA sc 20/30, REF plano −0.50 × 180. This is expected response from 4-incision RK.*

### Case 2

*A 34-year-old male with a SERE of −2.75 D, K 42.00/42.75, TA 16, underwent 4-incision RK with 3.5-mm OZ PO VA sc 20/30, REF +0.50 -0.75 × 30. Another unexceptional case.*

### Case 3

*A 40-year-old female with a SERE of −2.00 D, K 41.25/41.50. TA 12, underwent 4-incision RK with 3.5-mm OZ. This surgery was performed before we knew to factor in the patient's age. Initially she was overcorrected at +2 D but had 20/30 VA sc. Now she is 4 years PO, and her VA sc is 20/40 and REF is +2.75. On a similar patient today, we would use a 4.5-mm OZ. With this adjustment, this particular patient might still end up overcorrected as she "overresponded," obtaining 4.75 D of effect from 4 incisions with a 3.5-mm OZ.*

### Case 4

*A 25-year-old male, SERE −4.5 D, K 45.00/45.50, TA 16, underwent 4-incision RK, 3-mm OZ. Most RK nomograms or predictive software programs would recommend an 8-incision RK with a 3.5-mm or 3.75-mm OZ for this patient. The problem with this approach becomes evident if the patient is undercorrected by 1.5 to 2 D. Then the surgeon is faced with either adding an additional 4 to 8 incisions or trying to recut the original 8 incisions into a smaller OZ.*

*In this case, the patient was undercorrected by −1.25 D after the first 4 incisions. Now confident that he needed 8 incisions, 3-mm OZ for his other eye, which had a similar refractive error, this was performed in his second eye one month after the 4-incision procedure in his first eye. Two months later, 4 incisions, 3-mm OZ were added to the first eye. His VA sc is 20/25 in both eyes, and his SERE is less than −0.50 D in both eyes. He ended up with 8 incisions, 3-mm OZ in both eyes. Most RK nomograms or predictive software programs would recommend an 8-incision RK with a 3.5-mm or 3.75-mm OZ for this patient, not a 3-mm OZ with 8 incisions as an initial procedure. As a larger OZ would have left him undercorrected, he might have ended up with a 16-incision RK in his first eye.*

### Case 5

*A 47-year-old female with a SERE of −5.25 D, K 45.00/46.25, TA 18, underwent 4-incision RK, 3-mm OZ. In contrast to case 4, this patient had a good chance of obtaining 4 to 5 D of effect from 4 incisions, and this would provide her with satisfactory reading vision if she was undercorrected. She obtained only 3.5 D of effect, a residual myopia of −1.75 D. After observing this result, an 8-incision, 3-mm OZ in her other eye, which had a nearly identical refractive error, yielded a final VA of 20/30 and REF of plano −0.75 × 95. Eight incisions 3-mm OZ in this age group usually average nearly 6.5 D of effect and were not performed initially for fear of overcorrection. After a trial of her "mono vision" (using her undercorrected −1.75 D eye for reading) for a few months, she opted for distance vision in both eyes even if she would require reading glasses. Four more incisions, again 3-mm OZ, in the first eye gave her VA sc of 20/30 and REF −0.50. When adding an additional 4 incisions, generally use the same OZ. This yields only about half the effect that was obtained from the first four incisions.*

### Case 6

*A 34-year-old female, REF −3.50 −1.25 × 180, K45.50/46.25, TA 18 underwent 4-incision RK, 3-mm OZ, plus a single 2-mm transverse incision ("T cut") at a 5-mm OZ in the 90 degree meridian. In this age group, 1 to 2 D of astigmatism can often be corrected by a single "T" cut, preferably superiorly placed where it is partially protected by the upper lid. VA sc is 20/25 and REF is plano −0.50 × 90.*

---

## When to Use 8 Incisions

Although generally preferring 4-incision RK, we find that there are times when it is apparent that a "maximum" response is needed. Some surgeons advocate 16 incisions with "freehand dissection to Descemet's membrane" for a maximum response. Others prefer 16 incisions with "tertiary redeepening," or up to three zones of separate incision depths. These approaches both require 48 individual blade intrusions into the cornea. One surgeon uses 32 single-pass incisions for a maximum effect. Published results of these approaches do not demonstrate clear evidence of increased efficacy over an 8-incision approach with proper incision depth. The increased corneal scarring and increased risk of perforation inherent in these more complicated procedures are not outweighed by a possible small increase in effect.

We feel that an 8-incision, 3-mm OZ, RK performed with a micrometer diamond knife set at 110% of thinnest intraoperative ultrasonic paracentral pachymetry, with the blade setting verified at 100X with the Micronscope, gives the maximum effect with the least risk. The amount of correction obtained, which is essentially related to patient age, varies from 5.5 D in patients in their twenties to nearly 7.5 D for patients in their fifties. Thus patients in their twenties with −5.5 D of myopia will generally receive 8 incisions, but patients in their forties will receive only 4 incisions. In those cases where 4 incisions are initially made in one eye and 4 are added later but 8 simultaneous incisions are made in the other eye, the results have been similar. Eight incisions are appropriate for patients in their thirties with $-6$ to $-8$ D of myopia and for patients over 40 with $-8$ to $-10$ D of myopia. One must inform both groups that they are unlikely to achieve a full correction.

Never perform an 8-incision RK with a larger optical zone than 3 mm. To achieve less effect, the 4-incision RK permits staging of the operation. Only use 8 incisions, 3-mm OZ, when necessary, to achieve the maximum effect possible for a particular patient. If the patient remains undercorrected following 8 incisions of adequate depth (at least 90% near the OZ as estimated with high power slit-lamp biomicroscopy) an additional 8 incisions will give very little effect in most cases and are not warranted. Villasenor[26] reached the same conclusion after reviewing the results of his reoperations.

## SURGICAL TECHNIQUE

**Anesthesia.** Topical 0.5% tetracaine anesthesia is applied (two drops every 5 minutes $\times$ 3). The limbal area is blotted with tetracaine-soaked cellulose sponges or a cellulose ring just before starting the actual surgery.

**Visual axis and optical zone marks and pachymetry.** A sterile 23-gauge needle is used for marking the visual axis, followed by the formerly selected optical zone marker. Once the optical zone is marked, measure the corneal thickness centrally and at the 3, 6, 9, and 12 o'clock positions at the edge of the optical zone mark. Place the rounded edge of the probe at the edge of the optical zone mark (rather than straddling it). You are actually measuring an area of the cornea slightly peripheral to the spot where you will initiate the incision. We use either the Humphrey or portable Biorad Pachpen ultrasonic pachymeter with a velocity of 1640 m/sec. Use an alcohol prep to wipe the tip of the probe prior to touching the cornea. After completing the pachymetry, scrub while the patient is being prepped.

Our technique for marking the visual axis is similar to the PERK method. Instruct the patient to close or cover the nonoperated eye and fixate on the center of the microscope's coaxial light. When marking the patient's operative eye, the RK surgeon closes his or her opposite eye and marks the nasal edge of the light reflex just inferior to it (approximately a 1/2 filament width). Dr. David Guyton[27] has pointed out theoretical optical errors in most of the popular techniques for marking the visual axis, although this technique has served well for several years. He advocates centering the mark over the entrance pupil of the eye.

**Blade setting.** On the day of surgery, the calibration of the diamond knife is verified with the Micronscope by Magnum Diamond (Figure 7-6). This instrument allows you to inspect the blade for chips and debris, assess the alignment and surface of the footplates, and determine the accuracy of the micrometer mechanism at 100X. Because this is a monocular system, parallax is eliminated. The Micronscope has a magnification nearly 10 times that of the operating microscope.

To calibrate the knife on the Micronscope, set the blade to 0.55 mm under the Micronscope and then check the micrometer setting on the knife handle. If the two readings are the same, then the micrometer setting of the knife is accurate for this surgery. If the readings do not coincide, the differences should be noted.

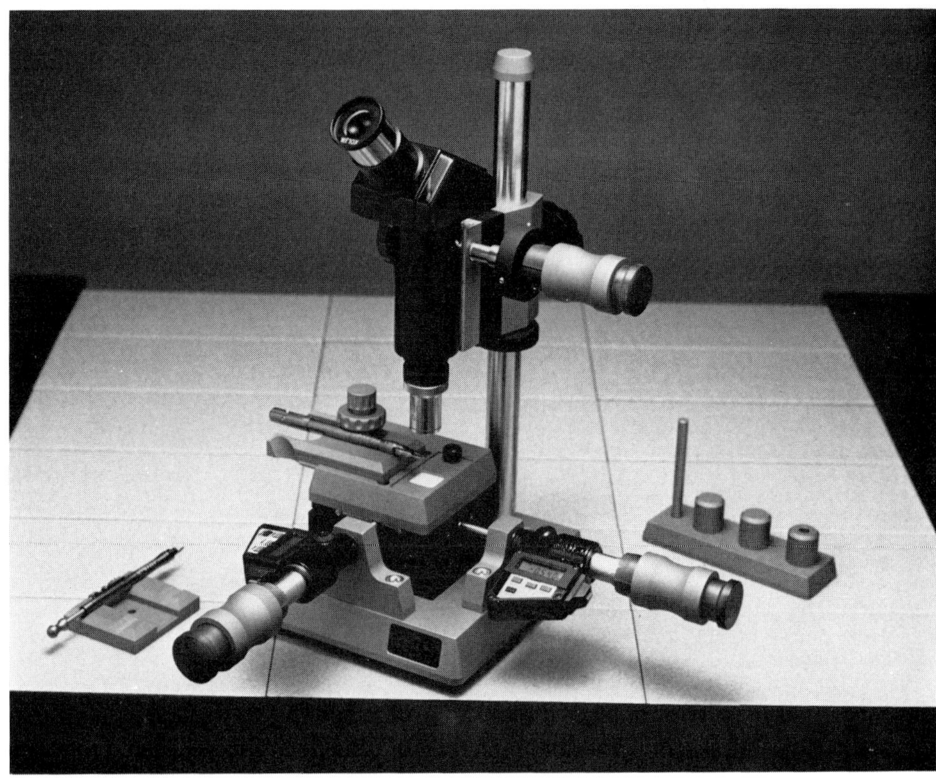

**FIGURE 7-6**    Micronscope. *(Photo courtesy of Doug Mastel.)*

Use the Micronscope's reading as true and set the knife accordingly. At surgery it is a good practice to confirm the setting on the coin gauge, Figure 7-7, merely to insure that there is not a major error in the setting, (e.g., setting the blade at 0.47 mm instead of 0.57 mm but relying on the "corrected" micrometer handle setting as the true reading). This is not a perfect system, but we believe it is the most accurate method presently available.

Generally set the micrometer diamond knife at 110% of the thinnest paracentral ultrasonic corneal thickness and confirm the setting on the coin gauge. The knife is then carefully returned to the coin gauge cradle. You are now finally ready to begin the actual surgery. Note that during the previous maneuvers the patient's eye has not been draped. We now apply the drape, insert the Kratz-Barraquer wire lid speculum, and begin the surgery without delay. The corneal thickness measurements should be unchanged since the eye has not been held open under the operating microscope light.

**Placing the incisions.**  The optical zone mark can be accentuated if necessary by blotting it with a cellulose sponge. For either the right or the left eye, make the 9 o'clock incision first with your right hand. Use a Bores' double-toothed forceps at the 3 o'clock position near the limbus to fixate the eye. Hold the diamond blade like a dart to visualize the tip. The knife can be held at a slightly oblique angle as the tip approaches the OZ mark. When the tip engages the cornea on the OZ mark, the handle is brought up perpendicular to the cornea and the knife is pressed firmly up to the guard (Figure 7-8). Steady the blade without

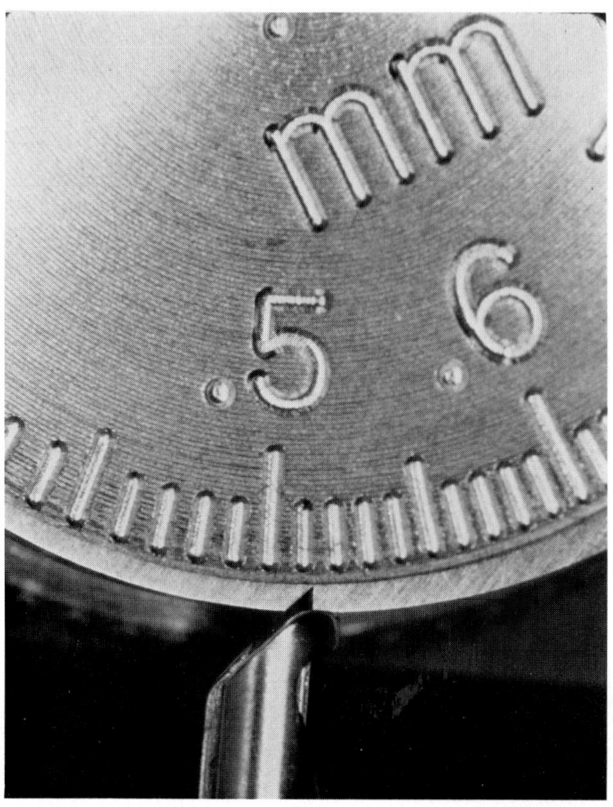

**FIGURE 7-7**     Confirming blade setting with coin gauge. *(Photo courtesy of Doug Mastel, reprinted with permission from Thompson FB: Myopia surgery, New York, 1990, Macmillan, p. 52.)*

cutting for one to two seconds and then incise slowly but smoothly toward the limbus, maintaining equal pressure on each footplate.

After the 9 o'clock incision, the 6 and 12 o'clock incisions should be made with the right hand, followed by the 3, 4:30, and 1:30 o'clock incisions with the left hand, and finally the 7:30 and 10:30 o'clock incisions with the right hand. Always fixate exactly opposite to the incision being made.

Complete all the incisions before inspecting each with the Deitz gauge, and recut any that are not of proper depth. We no longer irrigate the blood free incisions with balanced salt solution. Pressure from a cellulose sponge will control bleeding at the limbal arcade. Apply Garamycin drops, followed by a light pressure dressing. Most patients are more comfortable without it and remove the patch within one to two hours.

**Astigmatic keratotomy.**  If the patient has more than 1.5 D of astigmatism, you can attempt to reduce it with transverse incisions in the steep meridian. Published reports pertaining to the effectiveness of these incisions is minimal. It is widely felt that these incisions should never transect or even intersect the radial incisions because of significant wound-healing problems and epithelial inclusion cysts. This predisposes to irregular astigmatism.

The initial transverse incision ("T-cut") is placed in the steep axis at a 5-mm OZ. Try to make it about 2 mm long. The Deitz gauge, about 2 mm long, can be

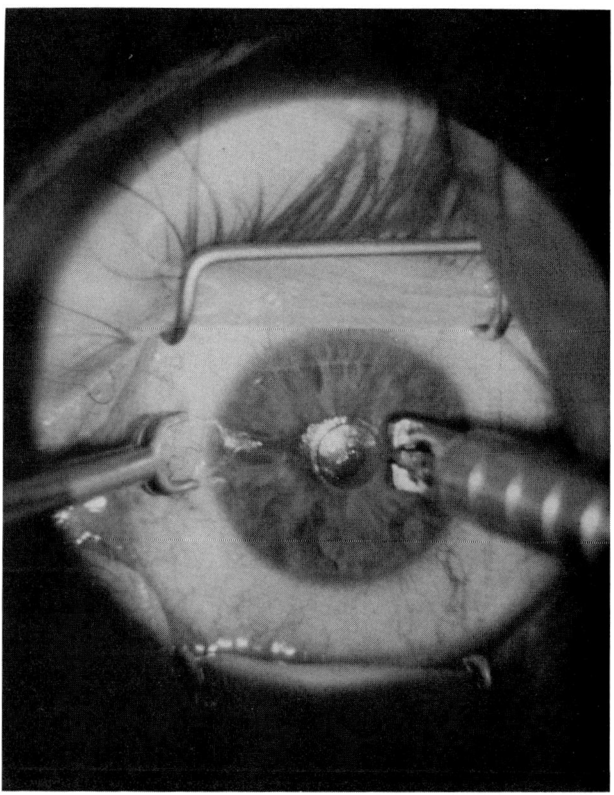

**FIGURE 7-8**    Initiating RK incision at optical zone. *(Reprinted with permission from Thompson FB: Myopia surgery, New York, 1990, Macmillan, p. 53.)*

pressed on the cornea to provide a guide. Start with a single "T" cut for 1 to 2 D of astigmatism for patients in their twenties and thirties. We prefer to place these cuts superiorly where they are partially protected by the patient's lid. Add another "T" cut opposite the first, again at a 5-mm OZ, for 2 to 3 D of astigmatism. A pair of additional "T" cuts are placed at a 7-mm OZ for 3 to 4 D of effect. To produce still more effect (4 to 5 D) place adjacent semiradial incisions to an OZ of 5 mm. For a maximum effect, the semi-radials can extend in to an OZ of 3 mm (5 to 6 D). The Lindstrom modification of the Ruiz trapezoidal keratotomy includes paired "T" cuts at a 5-mm and 7-mm OZ in the steep axis, combined with a pair of nonconnected semiradial incisions from an OZ of 5 mm to 3 mm, depending on the amount of correction desired. Up to 3 to 4 D of effect from a single "T" cut may occur in patients over age 40, so the surgeon and patient must realize that a wide range of effects is possible. Proceed with caution, it is better to undercorrect the astigmatism, leaving the patient with the same axis, than to overcorrect, reversing the cylinder axis.

The sequence of incisions outlined above is the approach to astigmatic keratotomy advocated by Dr. Richard Lindstrom.[28] It is based on quantitative cadaver-eye studies modified by clinical observations. The incisions should never touch each other, and the "T" cuts are never inside a 5-mm OZ, although the adjacent radials can be in to a 3-mm OZ for a "maximum" effect.

The transverse incisions are best performed with a Neumann-style "front-cutting" blade. This provides better visualization to more accurately follow the marks on the cornea. Accurately mark the steep meridian of the cornea, then place the "T" cuts before placing the radial incisions.

**Postoperative care and followup.** The patient should be examined on day one post-op, then at one week, one month, three months, and yearly thereafter. While the epithelium heals in the first three days, treat the operated eye with antibiotic drops only (Garamycin). If the patient is near emmetropia or under-corrected, an antibiotic-corticosteroid combination can be started at 4 to 5 days. Withhold the corticosteroids if the patient is overcorrected by more than 1 D at one week. We believe that the use of corticosteroids for 4 to 6 weeks can increase the effect of RK.

## RADIAL KERATOTOMY RESULTS

Table 7-2 summarizes our results of RK (based on examinations between 3 and 12 months postoperative) categorized according to the degree of preoperative myopia on 225 eyes operated upon over the last 10 years.[29] The relatively small number of patients reflects our conservative approach to this surgery. As previously stated, we do not operate on contented, successful contact-lens wearers unless they have a valid occupational reason (e.g., to qualify for police work). Demonstration of possible results with trial lenses after emphasizing the unpredictability of the surgery discourages many patients from having the surgery. This is the only responsible way to present an elective procedure such as RK, and it reduces the risk of litigation. We have encountered none thus far.

Table 7-2 is based on examinations between 3 months and 1 year. All patients have a minimum 3-month followup exam, and 80% have at least a 1-year follow-up. Many have been followed for 6 to 10 years. Results are not included for 5 patients who were completely lost to followup.

In the low myopia group, all but two patients underwent a single 4-incision RK. The two with 8 incisions had surgery in 1981. Excellent results for this group of patients are reported in most published series. The PERK[8] and Deitz[12] studies achieved uncorrected visual acuities of 20/40 or better in 92% and 95% of their patients respectively and corrected 84% and 90% respectively to within plus or minus one diopter of emmetropia with only 8-incision RK. The 4-incision approach has a significant reduction in the percentage of eyes overcorrected by more than 1 diopter, which was as follows: PERK 11%, Deitz 13%, Salz 3%. Lindstrom,[30] in his low-myopia RK patients, reported no overcorrections greater than 1 diopter with his 4-incision technique.

**Table 7-2**  Summary of Results of RK

|  | Low (> −3.00 D) | Medium (−3.1 to −5.9 D) | High (−6.0 to −12.0 D) |
|---|---|---|---|
| Number of eyes | 34 | 125 | 66 |
| Percentage 20/40 uncorrected | 100 | 73 | 47 |
| Percentage ± 1.0 D | 97 | 81 | 45 |
| Percentage > +1.0 D | 3 | 3 | 3 |
| Percentage 20/80 | 100 | 95 | 80 |

Of the patients with moderate myopia ($-3.1$ to $-5.9$ D), 74% achieved uncorrected 20/40 vision or better, 80% were corrected to within 1 D of emmetropia, and 3% were overcorrected by more than 1 diopter. Deitz[12] reported 88% 20/40 or better, 76% corrected to within 1 diopter of emmetropia, and 13% overcorrected by more than 1 diopter. PERK[8] data at one year (retabulated for moderate myopia to $-3.1$ to $-5.9$ D, courtesy of Mike Lynn and George O. Waring, III, MD) was as follows: 76% 20/40 or better, 55% within 1 diopter of emmetropia, and 11% overcorrected more than 1 diopter. The higher percentage of eyes with uncorrected visual acuity of 20/40 or better reported by Deitz (88%) compared to Salz (74%) is offset by his higher overcorrection rate (13%). Many of his overcorrected patients probably still had active accommodation allowing them relatively good unaided visual acuities. A single 8-incision RK was used for these moderate myopes in the PERK and Deitz studies. In our series, 61% of the moderate myopes underwent 4-incision RK, 7% had additional radial incisions, and 7% had additional transverse incisions. The principal advantage of "staging" the surgery is a reduction in the number of eyes overcorrected, as with the low-myopia group.

Approximately 50% of patients with more than 6 D of myopia achieved 20/40 uncorrected visual acuity or were corrected to within 1 D of emmetropia. These results are competitive with other published reports where the surgeons used more complicated approaches to RK for this group. These approaches include multiple depth incisions, 16 incisions or more, optical zones smaller than 3 mm, and incisions performed from the limbus toward the optical zone. Table 7-3 compares our results for high myopia with those of Neumann,[13] PERK (retabulated to $-6$ to $-8$D courtesy of Mike Lynn and George O. Waring, III, MD),[8] Deitz,[12] Damiano,[31] and Bauerberg.[32] With respect to diopters of mean change and percentage of eyes corrected to 1 diopter of emmetropia, the results are quite similar. Deitz and Damiano achieved a higher percentage of eyes with uncorrected visual acuities of 20/40 or better, with the downside of overcorrections greater than 1 diopter in 16% and 13% of these cases respectively.

The approach to RK discussed in this article has produced results comparable to or better than those of other reported series that have often employed far more complicated techniques. An additional benefit is our much lower incidence of

**Table 7-3**   A Comparison of Results in Six Studies of Eyes with Myopia of $-6.0$ to $-12.0$ D

| | Neumann[13] | PERK[8]* | Deitz[12] | | Damiano[31] | | | | Bauerberg[32] | Current study | | | |
|---|---|---|---|---|---|---|---|---|---|---|---|---|---|
| Year published | 1984 | 1985 | 1987 | | 1989 | | | | 1989 | 1990 | | | |
| Number of Eyes | 50 | 50 | 126 | | 91 | | | | 409 | 65 | | | |
| Number of incisions | 18 | 8 | 8 | 16 | 8 | 12 | 16 | 20 | 8 | 4 | 8 | 4+4 | 8+8 |
| Percentage of Eyes | 100 | 100 | 70 | 30 | 12 | 24 | 60 | 4 | 100 | 9 | 82 | 6 | 3 |
| Multiple Depth Incisions? | Yes | No | No | | Yes | | | | Yes | No | | | |
| Results Include Reoperations? | Yes | No | No | | No | | | | Yes | Yes | | | |
| Percentage 20/40 or Better sc | 68 | 48 | 77 | | 78 | | | | 38 | 47 | | | |
| Percentage PO SE $+1$ to $-1$ D | 62 | 24 | 53 | | 59 | | | | 58 | 45 | | | |
| Mean SE Change | 6.2 | 4.7 | 7.1 | | NR | | | | 6.8 | 6.2 | | | |
| Percentage PO SE $> +1$ D | NR | 4 | 16 | | 13 | | | | 3 | 4 | | | |

*PERK data retabulated $-6.1$ to $-8.0$ D. (Courtesy of Mike Lynn, MS.)
SE = Spherical Equivalent

overcorrections. This is especially noteworthy because a significant percentage of eyes move in a hyperopic direction with time ("progressive hyperopia"). This has been reported by Deitz,[24] Waring,[25] and Sawelson.[33]

What is the definition of a successful RK? Should it be based on percentage of myopia corrected, uncorrected visual acuity of 20/40, closeness to emmetropia, or some combination of these or other measurements? The wide range of postoperative refractions that can produce an uncorrected visual acuity of 20/40 or better makes this definition problematic. In the PERK study, patients with postoperative spherical equivalent refractive errors of $-3$ to $+3$ D were capable of uncorrected visual acuity of 20/40 or better.[34]

Table 7-2 shows that for patients with preoperative myopia greater than $-6$ D the percentage of eyes with uncorrected visual acuity of 20/40 or better corrected to within 1 D of emmetropia falls considerably. However, if these patients are suitably chosen, notably by using patient age as a predictive factor, and if they have realistic expectations, they can be satisfied with the results of RK whether or not they meet these criteria.

The anticipated corrective results should be discussed with the patient. For example, when discussing RK with a 45-year-old, $-8$ D myopic patient, inform him (or her) that he will probably not realize a complete correction of his myopia. The formula presented in surgical planning ($2.5 + 0.1 \times$ patient age) predicts for this patient 7 D of effect from an 8-incision RK, 3-mm OZ. If this patient could read without glasses with residual myopia of $-1$ D, this would be a correction of 87% of his myopia. This result is more striking than correcting a $-2$ D patient to a $-1$ D, even if the latter patient obtains 20/40 vision uncorrected and the former does not. RK in more myopic patients can be gratifying for both patient and surgeon. In our series, 80% of the high myopes attained uncorrected visual acuities of 20/80 or better, a profound improvement for patients with more than 6 D of myopia.

RK is often called an unpredictable operation. For an individual patient, this can be true even though the results for an entire series of patients have been generally satisfactory. The basis for the wide range of possible results of RK surgery is the difference in the biologic responses among corneas, the "over and under responders." Any analysis of RK results will show a wide range. In Table 7-4 it is valuable to look at the mean effects we have seen for 4-incision RK with different optical zones, and for 8-incision RK with 3-mm optical zones, analyzed by patient age.

**Table 7-4**   Mean SE Change by Age, OZ, and Number of Incisions

| | **4 Incisions** | | | | | **8 Incisions** |
|---|---|---|---|---|---|---|
| Optical Zone in mm | 3.0 | 3.5 | 4.0 | 4.5 | 5.0 | 3.0 |
| Number of Eyes | 91 | 25 | 7 | 2 | 1 | 93 |
| Patient Age (yrs) | | | | | | |
| 20-29 | 3.1 | 2.0 | 1.9 | | | 5.3 |
| 30-39 | 3.9 | 2.9 | 2.4 | | | 5.8 |
| 40-49 | 4.5 | 3.5 | | 2.1 | | 6.0 |
| >50 | 5.0 | | | | 1.5 | 7.5 |

**Reoperations.** If an 8-incision RK, 3-mm OZ, has been performed and the patient is undercorrected, do not add incisions if the original 8 are approximately at least 80% to 90% by slit-lamp exam, from the OZ to the mid-periphery. The second 8 incisions rarely add a significant change. Dr. Richard Villasenor concurs with this observation.[26] In fact, both Dr. Villasenor and the PERK study have observed a few patients who became more myopic after reoperation.

The effect of adding a second set of 4 incisions to an original 4-incision RK with the same optical zone, will be approximately 50% of the original result. If a 4-incision RK, 3-mm OZ, gives 4 D of correction, 4 more incisions should add an additional 2 D. This is only a guide, and as with all RK procedures, a wide range of outcomes is still possible.

## COMPLICATIONS

Fortunately, as of yet there have been no vision-threatening complications in either our PERK patients or among our private RK patients. The majority of the complications have been over- and undercorrections and an occasional increase in preoperative astigmatism. There can be more serious complications following RK. These include, but are not limited to, infectious ulcers, endophthalmitis, irregular astigmatism, epithelial downgrowth, corneal perforation, perforation of the globe during retrobulbar injection, optic atrophy, cataract, and traumatic rupture of the globe.

At a special symposium on RK at the American Academy of Ophthalmology meeting in New Orleans discussing the safety issue in radial keratotomy, Dr. Salz pointed out that some of the potentially vision-threatening complications are related to surgical technique. For example, posterior perforation of the globe, optic atrophy, and retinal detachment are possible only if the surgeon injects around the globe. As we use only topical anesthesia, these complications are of no concern.

In order to determine the incidence of complications in a larger series than our own, we combined our private patients with those of Dr. Richard Villasenor, Dr. Richard Lindstrom, and the PERK study (including pilot cases). These radial keratotomies were all performed with topical anesthesia and a micrometer diamond knife. The surgical technique consisted of either 4 or 8 incisions, occasionally with nonconnected transverse astigmatic incisions. This series comprised over 1600 eyes followed from 3 months to 6 years. The only vision-threatening complications were 3 cases of bacterial keratitis, all in the PERK study, of which 2 were affiliated with soft contact lenses. In the combined series, all eyes were correctable to at least 20/40 visual acuity or better following RK.[35]

With the incidence of complications in the combined series mentioned above and the recent studies on the post-RK endothelium, we can state that a properly performed radial keratotomy on properly selected patients is a safe and generally effective operation. The key phrases in this statement are "properly performed" and "properly selected." We have seen unhappy and often litigious patients in consultation. In most cases, the operating surgeon had improperly performed, improperly selected, promised too much, or all three.

**Improper Patient Selection.** The three most common errors in patient selection are operating on presbyopic patients with mild myopia, operating on

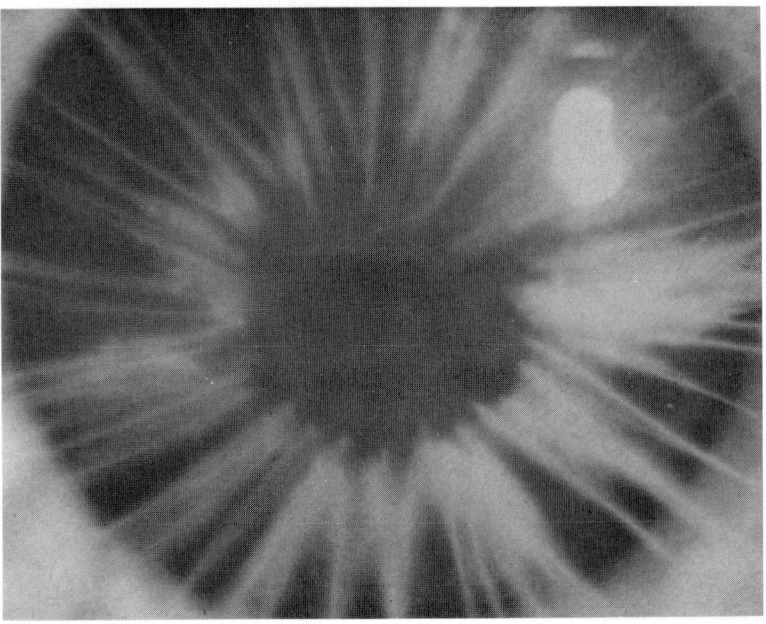

**FIGURE 7-9**    78 RK incisions following 10 operations.

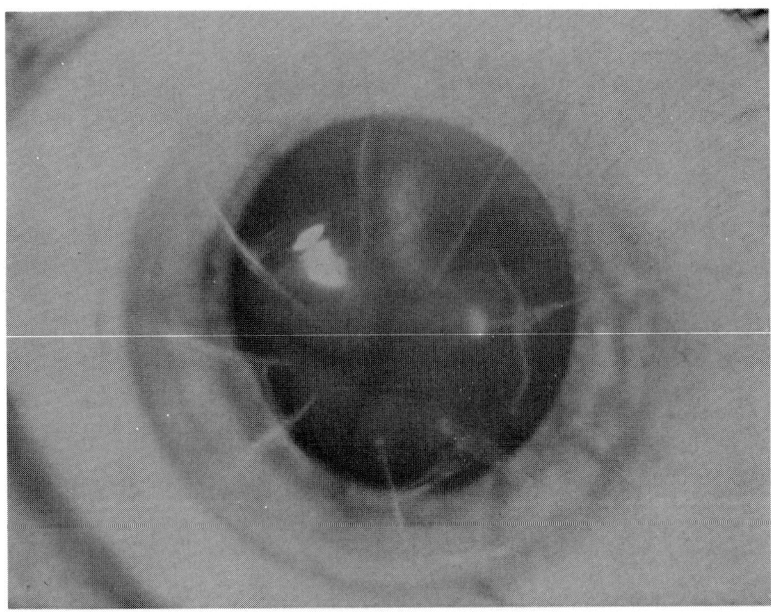

**FIGURE 7-10**    Intersecting radial and astigmatic incisions.

successful contact lens wearers, or operating on patients whose myopia is so high that a good result is extremely unlikely.

When a surgeon advises RK on a successful contact lens wearer, he takes on two extra burdens. Patients want to see as well as they did with their contact lenses, probably 20/20, and published studies show that the majority of RK patients

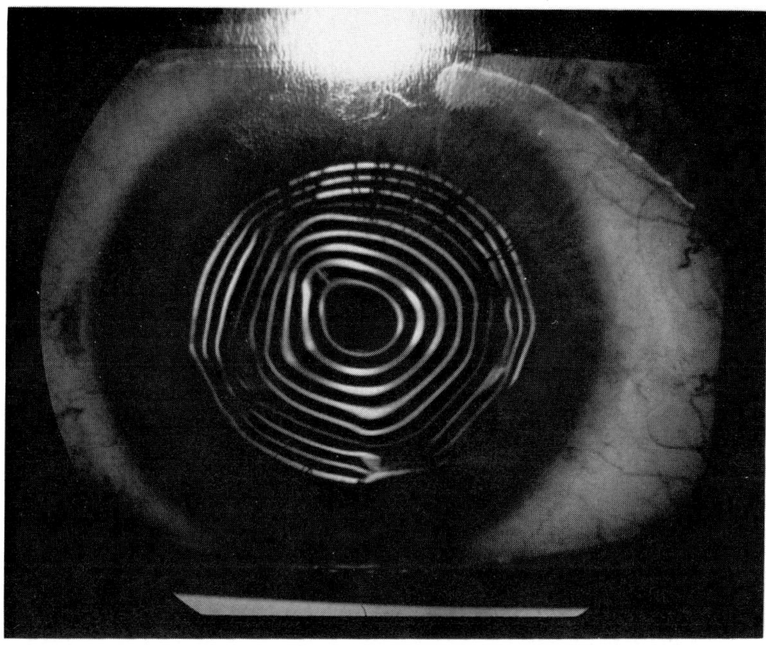

**FIGURE 7-11**    Corneascope photograph of patient in Figure 7-10 demonstrating irregular astigmatism.

do not achieve this level of improvement. Patients will usually not be happy if uncorrected visual acuity is simply improved. If patients do not achieve near 20/20, the surgeon shoulders a second burden, refitting them with contact lenses. Contact lens fitting in post-RK patients is more difficult. Often it is further complicated by the condition of fitting a formerly happy soft lens wearer with gas permeable hard lenses.

Operating on moderately myopic presbyopic patients can also cause patient dissatisfaction. Without RK, a $-2$ D refractive error would allow the patient to read without glasses for many years. Patients do not always understand that RK will force them to use reading glasses that might otherwise be avoided. In discussing presbyopia with these patients, it is helpful to demonstrate presbyopia to them by applying cycloplegic drops and asking them to read with their glasses on, simulating successful bilateral RK. When they find they can read simply by removing their glasses, they frequently lose interest in the surgery. Of the patients who remain interested in RK despite presbyopia, many can adjust to "mono vision" if they have the surgery in only one eye.

**Improper Technique.** Common examples of improper RK technique are numerous reoperations, too many incisions, (Figure 7-9) and transverse incisions that cross or touch radial incisions. As previously discussed in the section on pathophysiology, these predispose to improper wound healing and frequently irregular astigmatism (Figures 7-10 and 7-11).[36]

## FUTURE DIRECTIONS

Refractive surgeons must improve the predictability and reproducibility of the surgery while maintaining a minimal incidence of complications. Two current

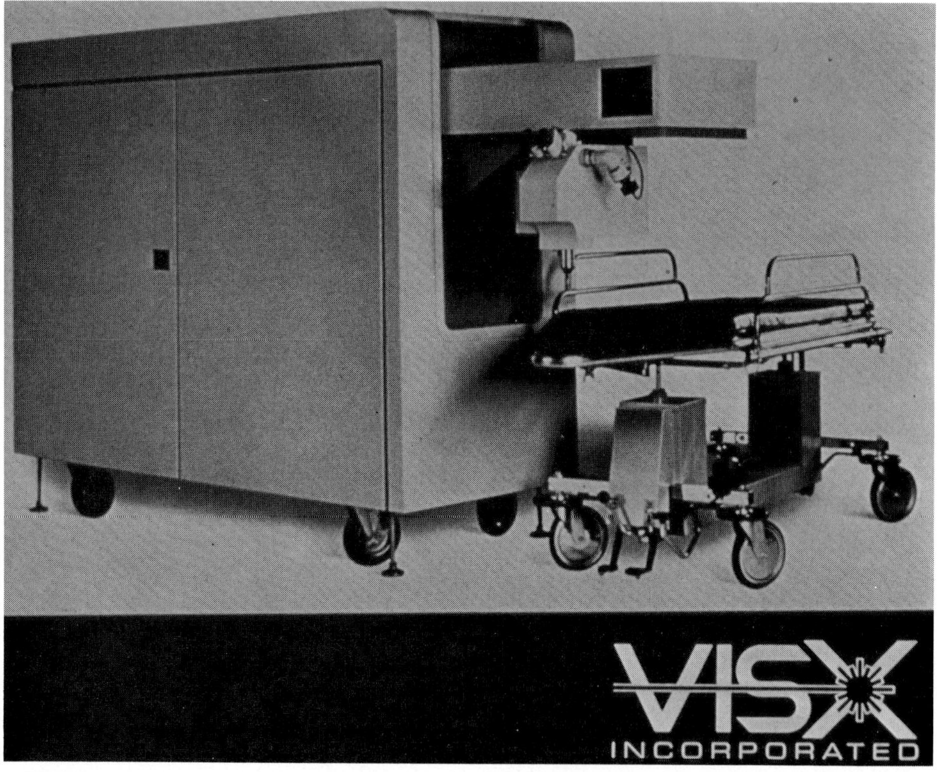


**FIGURE 7-12**   VISX excimer laser.

research areas that should help to achieve this goal are excimer laser photo ablation and synthetic epikeratoplasty. The argon-fluoride excimer (Figure 7-12) laser has the potential to excise corneal tissue accurately and reproducibly, and with minimal long-term loss of corneal clarity. Preliminary reports on sighted eyes are encouraging,[37] but it may not be possible to safely obtain large corrections on the order −10 D. Synthetic collagen lenses are in developmental stages of research. These will be available in almost any power desired and will be placed on the patients own cornea. After complete healing, the excimer laser can be used to refine the correction, if necessary, leaving the central portion of the patients own cornea untouched, except for the removal of the epithelium prior to the placement of the synthetic lens. Waring[38] has coined the term LASE (Laser Adjustable Synthetic Epikeratoplasty) for this procedure. If these research efforts are successful, radial keratotomy may become rare in countries that can afford the luxury of the new technology. Because of the relative safety and simplicity of RK, we expect it to become even more popular in other parts of the world.

## References

1. Bettman JW. Medicolegal considerations in refractive surgery: informed consent. *Refractive Corneal Surgery*. In Sanders DR, Hoffman RF, Salz JJ, eds: Thorofare, N.J., Slack, 1986: 21-32.

2. Salz JJ, Rowsey JJ, Caroline P, Azen SP, Suter M, Monlux R. A study of optical zone size and incision redeepening in experimental radial keratotomy. Arch Ophthalmol 1985; 103:590-594.

3. Fyodorov SN, Durnev VV. Operation of dosaged dissection of corneal circular ligament in cases of myopia of mild degree. Ann Ophthalmol 1979; 11:1885-1890.

4. Schachar RA, Black T, Huang A. A physicist's view of radial keratotomy with practical surgical implication. Denison, Tex.: LAL Publishing, 1980; 195-220.

5. Jester JV, Venet T, Lee J, Schanzlin DJ, Smith RE. A statistical analysis of radial keratotomy in human cadaver eyes. Am J Ophthalmol 1981; 92:172-177.

6. Deitz MR, Sanders DR, Marks RG. Radial keratotomy: an overview of the Kansas City study. Ophthalmol 1984; 91:467-478.

7. Arrowsmith PN, Marks RG. Evaluating the predictability of radial keratotomy. Ophthalmol 1985; 92:331-338.

8. Lynn MJ, Waring GO, Speruto RD, et al. Factors affecting outcome and predictability of radial keratotomy in the PERK study. Arch Ophthalmol 1987; 105:42-51.

9. Salz JJ, Lee TS, Jester JV, Villasenor RA, Steel DL, Bernstein J, Smith RE. Analysis of incision depth following experimental radial keratotomy. Ophthalmol 1983; 90:655-659.

10. Salz JJ, Salz MS. Four and eight incision radial keratotomy for myopia greater than 6.00. J Refrac Surg 1988; 4:45-50.

11. Hikishima H, Nakaisuma H, Takahaski N, Sasaki K. The measurement of the human corneal thickness with corneomap 4500. New Ophthalmol (Jap) 1984; 1:388.

12. Deitz MR, Sanders DR, Raanan MG. A consecutive series (1982-1985) of radial keratotomies performed with the diamond blade. Am J Ophthalmol 1987; 103 (2):417-422.

13. Neumann AC, Ochsner RH, Fenzl RE. Radial keratotomy: a comprehensive evaluation. Doc Ophthalmol 1984; 56:275-301.

14. Arrowsmith PN, Marks RG. Visual, refractive and keratometric results of radial keratotomy: one year follow-up. Arch Ophthalmol 1984; 102:1612-1617.

15. Grandon SC, Grandon GM. Effects of peripheral redeepening on radial keratotomy surgery. J Cataract Refract Surg 1987; 13:268-273.

16. Jester JV, Steel DL, Salz JJ, Miyashiro J, Rife L, Schanzlin DJ, Smith RE. Radial keratotomy in nonhuman primate eyes. Am J Ophthalmol 1981; 92:153-171.

17. Deg JK, Zavala EY, Binder PS. Delayed corneal wound healing following radial keratotomy. Ophthalmol 1985; 92:734-740.

18. Yamaguchi T, Tamaki K, Kaufman HE, Katz J, Shaw EL. Histologic study of a pair of human corneas after anterior radial keratotomy. Am J Ophthalmol 1985; 100:281-292.

19. Binder PS, Nayak SK, Deg JK, Zavala EY, Sugar J. An ultrastructural and histochemical study of long-term wound healing after radial keratotomy. Am J Ophthalmol 1987; 103:432-440.

20. Hoffer KJ, Karin JJ, Pettit TH, Hofbauer JD, Elander R, Levenson JE. Three years experience with radial keratotomy: The UCLA study. Ophthalmol 1983; 90:627-636.

21. Asbell PA, Obstbaum S, Justin N. Peripheral corneal endothelial evaluation post radial keratotomy in PERK patients. Ophthalmology 1984; 91 (Sept Supp 2):122(poster).

22. MacRae SM, Matsuda M, Rich LF. The effect of radial keratotomy on the corneal endothelium. Am J Ophthalmol 1985; 100:538-542.

23. Waring GO. The Lans distinguished refractive surgery lecture. J Refrac Surg 1987; 3:115-116 (editorial).

24. Deitz MR, Sanders DR, Raanan MG. Progressive hyperopia in radial keratotomy. Ophthalmol 1986; 93:1284-1288.

25. Waring GO, Lunn MJ, Fielding B. Results of the prospective evaluation of radial keratotomy (PERK) four years after surgery for myopia. JAMA 1990; 263:1083-1091.

26. Villasenor RA, Cox KO. Radial keratotomy: reoperations. J Refrac Surg 1985; 1:34-37.

27. Uozato H, Guyton DL. Centering corneal surgical procedures. Am J Ophthalmol 1987; 103:264-275.

28. Lindquist TD, Rubenstein JB, Hofmann RF, Lindstrom RL. Astigmatic keratotomy. In Hofmann RF, Lindstrom RL, Neumann AC, Salz JJ, et al, eds: Radial Keratotomy Surgical Techniques. Thorofare, NJ: Slack, 1986: 119-129.

29. Salz JJ, Salz JM, Salz M, Jones DJ. Ten years experience with a conservative approach to radial keratotomy. Refrac and Corneal Surg 1991; 7:12-22.

30. Spigelman AV, Williams PA, Nichols BD, Lindstrom RL. Four incision radial keratotomy. J Cataract Refract Surg 1986; 14:125-128.

31. Shawbitz SD, Damiano RE, Forstot SL. Radial keratotomy in high myopia: an evaluation of one technique. Ann Ophthalmol 1989; 21:375-378.

32. Bauerberg J, Sterzovsky M, Brodsky M. Radial keratotomy in myopia of 6 to 12 diopters using full-length deepening incisions. Refrac Corneal Surg 1989; 5:150-154.

33. Sawelson H, Marks RG. Five year results of radial keratotomy. Refrac Corneal Surg 1989; 5:8-20.

34. Santos VR, Waring GO, Lynn MJ, Holladay JT, Sperduto RD, et al. Relationship between refractive error and visual acuity in the prospective evaluation of radial keratotomy (PERK) study. Arch Ophthalmol 1987; 105:86-92.

35. Salz JJ. How safe is radial keratotomy? J Refrac Surg 1987; 3:188-189.

36. McDonnell P, Caroline P, Salz JJ. Irregular astigmatism after keratotomy. Am J Ophthalmol 1989; 107:42-46.
37. Seiler T, Matallana M, Bende T. Laser thermokeratoplasty by means of a pulsed holmium: YAG laser for hyperopic correction. Refrac Corneal Surg 1990; 6:335-339.
38. Thompson KP, Hanna K, Waring GO. Emerging technologies for refractive surgery: laser adjustable synthetic epikeratoplasty. Refrac Corneal Surg 1989; 5:46-48.

# 8 The Surgical Management of Naturally Occurring and Post-Cataract Surgery Astigmatism

Peter J. Agapitos, MD, FRCSC
Richard L. Lindstrom, MD

Naturally occurring astigmatism is quite common, with up to 95% of eyes having some detectable astigmatic refractive error. The incidence of clinically significant astigmatism has been reported in the literature to be between 7.5% and 75%, depending on the study and the definition of a significant astigmatic refractive error.[1] Between 3% and 15% of the general population may have an astigmatic refractive error of greater than or equal to 2.0 diopters.[2]

Post-cataract surgery astigmatism is a major problem in visual rehabilitation for cataract surgery patients. The incidence of post-cataract astigmatism greater than two diopters is approximately 25% to 30%.[3,4] Corneal astigmatism in cataract surgery patients can continue to change as nylon sutures hydrolyze over the first postoperative year,[5] and more slowly thereafter for up to 5 years. Some studies have documented significant shifts in astigmatism up to 3 years postoperatively.[6]

The major symptom of uncorrected astigmatism is decreased uncorrected visual acuity. Distortion from meridional magnification is present to only a small degree in the uncorrected astigmat (approximately 0.3% per diopter of astigmatism). This is more significant with spectacle correction. Anisometropia, when present, may give rise to aniseikonia. In refractive errors such as simple myopia and simple hyperopia, patients are able to see clearly to some degree at near and at distance, respectively. In contrast, patients with compound astigmatism may not be in focus at any level.

Astigmatism that is corrected by spectacles is prone to the problems of distortion caused by meridional magnification that may give rise to significant difficulties with binocular function. Distortion may be modified by using posterior toric spectacle lenses, minimizing the vertex distance, and altering the astigmatic correction.[7] Contact lenses may improve the correction of these problems; however, not all patients may be successful contact lens wearers.

In this article, we present two case histories to illustrate our approach to the surgical management of post-cataract and naturally occurring astigmatism.

## ASTIGMATISM POST-CATARACT SURGERY

### Case History

*A 19-year-old female patient underwent cataract extraction in the left eye in 1982 subsequent to trauma that occurred in 1979. She underwent secondary intraocular lens implantation in September 1988. One year later, her uncorrected visual acuity was OD: 20/20, Jaeger 1, and OS: 20/80, Jaeger 6. The refractive error was OD: Plano 20/20, OS −3.50 + 5.00 × 70 20/25. Keratometry OS revealed 42.00 D at axis 160 and 48.50 D at axis 70. The ocular examination revealed a well-healed temporal limbal incision without any remaining sutures from the secondary IOL insertion. A well-centered posterior chamber IOL was present. The eye was quiet, and funduscopy was normal. The fellow eye was phakic and normal on examination. This patient had significant symptoms of glare and distortion and could not tolerate spectacles. A trial of contact lenses was unsuccessful. Corneoscopy confirmed the axis of astigmatism.*

*At an optical zone of 6 mm, with a front-cutting diamond knife set at 100% of the thinnest corneal thickness over the 6-mm optical zone in the steep axis, a pair of arcuate keratotomies were performed for 60° total length, each centered on either side of the steep axis. The steep axis was marked intraoperatively at axis 70 using a Terry keratometer. Terry keratometer readings reverted from 39.00 D at axis 160 and 47.00 D at axis 70, to 42.50 D spherical intraoperatively. At 6 weeks postoperatively, the uncorrected visual acuity was 20/20 minus and Jaeger 2, with best corrected visual acuity at 20/20 minus with a refraction of − 1.50 + 1.00 × 95. Keratometry at this visit was 43.75D at axis 160 and 45.75D at axis 70.*

---

## Comment

The result as measured on the operating room table with intraoperative quantitative keratometry indicates that the wound gape present was at that time enough to give approximately 100% correction with spherical readings. Some regression has occurred as postoperatively there were two diopters present on keratometry at the same axis indicating some degree of undercorrection. The achieved shift in astigmatism in this patient was quite large with a delta K of approximately 4.5 diopters. We currently prefer a 7-mm optical zone for most situations, however when larger amounts of correction are necessary, the 6-mm optical zone is reasonable. The patient achieved an improvement in both distance and near uncorrected visual acuity. The final refraction with a spherical equivalent of − 1.00 is not consistent with the uncorrected visual acuity of 20/20, however it is possible that a multifocal effect is present to explain this discrepancy.[8] Alternatively the presence of compound myopic astigmatism in pseudophakic patients may optimize both distance and near uncorrected visual acuity.[9,10]

## NATURALLY OCCURRING ASTIGMATISM

### *Case History*

*A 46-year-old white male underwent cataract extraction and IOL insertion in the right eye in June 1987. He developed a problem with depth perception due to anisometropia and aniseikonia, which he finds particularly troublesome when flying his airplane. Visual acuity is best-corrected to 20/20 in both eyes. Uncorrected visual acuity is OD: 20/40 and OS: 20/200. The refractions are OD: − 0.25 + 1.00 × 180 and OS: −4.00 + 3.50 × 175. Keratometry OS revealed 44.75 D at axis 175 and 41.75 D at axis 85. The ocular examination was within normal limits except for the presence of a posterior-chamber intraocular lens implant in the right eye. The left lens was normal. This patient presents with anisometropia and secondary aniseikonia from myopic astigmatism as a result of contralateral cataract surgery. The difference in spherical equivalent of 2.50 diopters is con-*

*tributing to the problem along with the astigmatism. Spectacle correction and a contact lens trial were not successful.*

*In the left eye, he underwent a 4-incision radial keratotomy (RK) at an optical zone of 4 mm, combined with a 2-incision astigmatic keratotomy (AK) at an optical zone of 6 mm. The AK consisted of a pair of arcuate incisions, each 60° in length, which were performed first at axis 180 with a front-cutting diamond knife (the blade is set in the cornea and pushed away from the starting point along the arc). The blade depth for the AK was set at 100% of the thinnest pachymetry at the 6-mm optical zone in the axis of the astigmatism. The blade depth was set at 100% of the thinnest paracentral pachymetry for the RK, and a back-cutting knife was used (when cutting, the knife blade is pushed towards the limbus, optical zone to limbus). The Terry keratometer was used to determine the steep axis of astigmatism at 175 with readings of 41.25 D at axis 85 and 45.00 D at axis 175. Immediately after surgery, intraoperative Terry keratometry readings were 40.00 spherical. Postoperatively, the patient did well with a refraction of plano and uncorrected visual acuity of 20/20. The keratometry readings were 40.00 D at axis 180 by 41.00 D at axis 90, indicating slight overcorrection.*

---

## Comment

This case of surgery for myopia combined with astigmatic keratotomy demonstrates a relatively large shift in astigmatism with a delta K of approximately 4.0 diopters going from 3 D of astigmatism at axis 175 to 1 D at axis 90. The surgery for myopia is based on the spherical equivalent and not on the spherical component of the refraction in minus cylinder form. Surgery performed at an optical zone of 7 mm may have given less of a shift.

## PREOPERATIVE ASSESSMENT

We always attempt visual rehabilitation with spectacles and contact lenses prior to proceeding with surgery. Patients are informed that the results of surgery are variable and that they may notice daily and/or long-term fluctuation in the resultant refraction. In binocular patients with spectacle-corrected astigmatism, it is important to note that these patients have adapted to the meridional magnification induced by their spectacles. The surgical correction of the astigmatism may induce torsional diplopia caused by meridional aniseikonia and an altered spatial sense.[11] The readaptation to these effects may take many months in some patients. This is a very important point to discuss prior to any surgical intervention. Other potential risks including glare, starbursts, corneal perforation, and infection are also discussed.[12] Only those patients who are truly visually disabled by their astigmatism are candidates for surgery. In addition, patients are advised that a second procedure may be necessary for optimal results.

Prior to surgery, careful refraction, keratometry, and keratoscopy, as well as a complete ophthalmic examination, are performed. Although many patients achieve an improved best-corrected spectacle visual acuity following surgery, most patients do not achieve acuity similar to that which can be obtained with a contact lens. In most cases, the keratometric and refractive cylinder power and axis will be compatible. In case of significant disparity, remeasurement and evaluation with more sophisticated methods of corneal topographical analysis, such as photokeratoscopy, are recommended. Once our diagnostic plan has been formulated and we are comfortable with the patient's diagnosis, optical measures of a conventional nature are initiated, consisting of spectacle correction; and if this is not satisfactory, contact lenses. In the rare instances where patients require uncorrected visual acuity of 20/40 or better for occupational reasons, this could be an indication for surgery.

## Naturally Occurring Astigmatism

In terms of diagnosis, it is necessary to arrive at an accurate etiologic and anatomic diagnosis. Careful clinical examination for findings consistent with keratoconus is absolutely essential, as RK or AK performed in a keratoconus patient is not recommended. This can usually be assessed using slit-lamp biomicroscopy, careful refraction, retinoscopy and corneoscopy. The earliest clinical sign in keratoconus is inferior steepening of the cornea, which is easily discernible on taking regional keratometry readings. The etiology of the astigmatism in most cases is idiopathic. It is important to rule out lenticular astigmatism, and this can usually be done with corneoscopy and keratometry readings. Often a contact lens refraction is useful. Irregular astigmatism, when present, is not an indication for surgery. Patients will probably have an exacerbation of irregular astigmatism after incisional refractive surgery.

## Post-Cataract Surgery Astigmatism

Post-cataract surgery patients should be at least 1 year postoperative. It has been shown that significant shifts in astigmatism can occur up to this point, even when using sutures such as 10-0 nylon which have usually dissolved by this time.[4,5] Careful attention must be paid to concurrent anterior segment abnormalities such as corneal scarring or synechiae which can significantly alter corneal curvature and are likely to be more resistant to modification.

## SURGICAL PLANNING

Surgical planning in post-cataract and naturally occurring astigmatism is based on the refractive cylinder and axis. This is usually a manifest refraction. If there is any doubt, however, a cycloplegic refraction should be performed. The surgical planning for the myopic portion of the surgery is always based on the spherical equivalent and not on the spherical portion of the refraction in minus cylinder form.

The nomograms contained in this article are currently utilized by both the authors, but it should be noted that outcome in astigmatism surgery is quite variable in its efficacy, and no guarantee can be made to the surgeon adopting these guidelines.

The nomogram currently utilized is depicted in Figure 8-1. This nomogram needs to be adjusted to a particular surgeon's technique. The basis for this approach has evolved from laboratory and clinical studies.[13-15] We favor straight or arcuate keratotomies at a 7-mm optical zone, with a blade depth set at 100% of the thinnest pachymetry in the steep axis at the 7-mm optical zone. The 7-mm

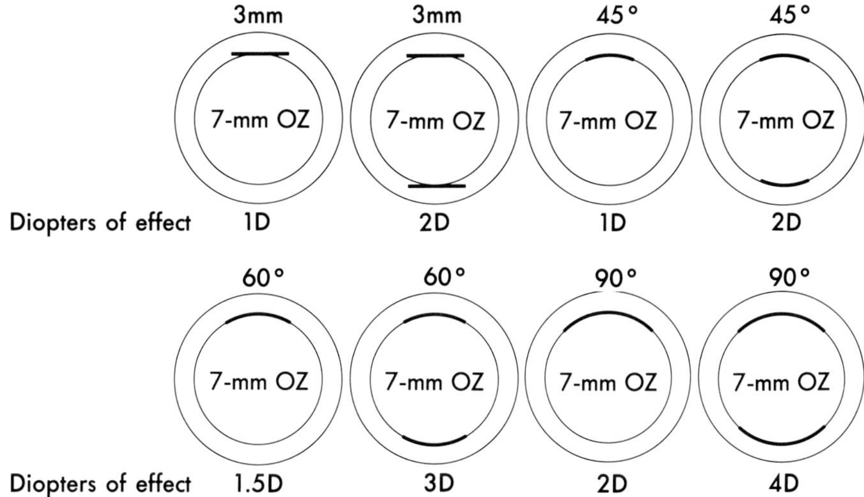



Parameters:
1. Optical zone (OZ): 7 mm
2. Blade depth: 100% of thinnest paracentral pachymetry at 7-mm OZ in the axis of astigmatism
3. Effect of age: Increase/decrease efficacy 2% per year
        Age 20 = 80% of age 30
        Age 55 = 150% of age 30
4. While mild overall flattening may occur, assume a coupling ratio of 1:1.
5. The procedure may be combined with a four-incision radial keratotomy (RK), although radial and tangential incisions should not touch. The RK portion of the procedure is based on the spherical equivalent of the refraction.

**FIGURE 8-1**    Astigmatic keratotomy nomogram.

optical zone is less likely to lead to problems with glare. Although our anatomical studies have shown that the largest shifts occur at optical zones of 5 mm and 6 mm,[14] we prefer a 7-mm optical zone. The age of the patient must also be taken into account since, as with RK, there is an increasing effect with age.[16]

Utilization of the nomogram in surgical planning is illustrated by the following hypothetical cases:

### Hypothetical Case 1

*A 72-year-old post-cataract surgery patient with a refraction of OD: −4.00 + 7.00 × 90, (spherical equivalent −0.50 sphere), OS: −1.00 + 1.00 × 90, (spherical equivalent −0.50 sphere).*

*Considering age, the patient will achieve 100 +(72-30) × 2% or 184% of the effect of a 30-year-old. A paired 90° arcuate keratotomy would achieve 4 × 1.84 diopters, which is equal to 7.36 diopters. A paired 60° arcuate keratotomy would achieve 3 × 1.84, equal to 5.52 diopters. We would favor staying with a pair of 60° arcuates in this case at a 7-mm optical zone performed in the vertical meridian.*

### Hypothetical Case 2

*A 34-year-old male has a refraction of −5.50 + 3.00 × 90, O.U. (spherical equivalent −4.00). He has been unsuccessful at contact lens wear and wishes to enter training as a police officer with a minimum visual requirement of 20/50 without correction. The patient will require combined radial and astigmatic keratotomy. We would favor a 4-incision radial keratotomy with a 3-mm optical zone, basing this on his spherical equivalent. A pair of 45° arcuate incisions could give 108% of the effect on a 30-year-old or 2.16 diopters. A single 60° arcuate incision would give 108% or 1.62 diopters, and a pair of 60° arcuates would give about 3.24 diopters. We find that most patients do best with reduced astigmatism but are not happy if they are converted from "with the rule" to "against the rule." Either a pair of 3-mm straight or 45° arcuate incisions or a single-arcuate incision of 90° is appropriate. Current information is insufficient to recommend one over the other. The astigmatic keratotomy incisions are made prior to the radial incisions in most cases.*

## SURGICAL TECHNIQUE

Recommended equipment includes an operating microscope, Sinskey hook, corneal fixation forceps (we utilize a .12 Colibri forceps), a 3-mm and 7-mm optical zone marker, an 8-, 12-, and 16-cut radial keratotomy incision marker, a skin-marking pencil, a high-quality, front-cutting diamond micrometer knife, an ultrasonic pachymeter, and a bottle of balanced salt solution. An irrigation canula is utilized in wetting the cornea and irrigating the incision. We utilize topical anesthesia with 0.5% proparacaine, though peribulbar anesthesia may also be appropriate. We feel strongly that retrobulbar anesthesia should not be used as this poses additional risk, and fixation by the patient on the microscope light becomes difficult, not permitting accurate centration. Although a surgical keratometer is useful for intraoperative monitoring in complex cases, it is not required.

The patient is centered under the operating microscope and the eye adjusted to be perpendicular to the microscope. The eye is anesthetized with 0.5% proparacaine every 5 minutes beginning at 15 minutes preoperatively. The center of

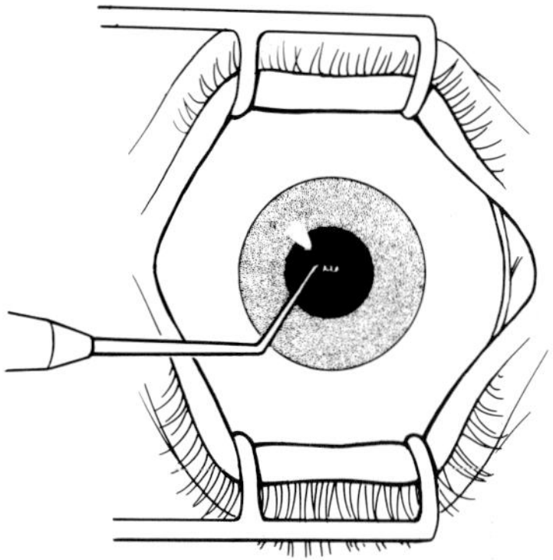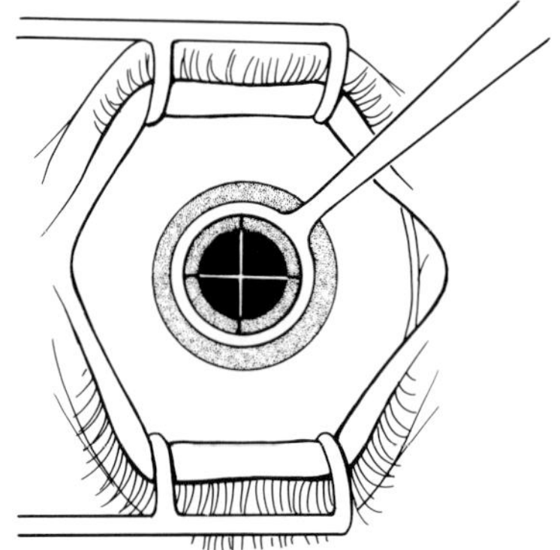

**FIGURE 8-2**    Left, The center of the cornea is marked as the patient fixates on the microscope with a Sinskey hook. Right, A 7-mm optical zone marker is placed onto the cornea.

the pupil is marked with the Sinskey hook by requesting the patient to fixate the operating room microscope light, which is turned down to a low level at this point. The optical zone is then marked with a 7-mm optical zone marker (Figure 8-2). The steeper meridian is marked with a skin marking pen utilizing intra-operative keratometry or preoperative landmarks in the steep axis. If a 3-mm straight incision is selected, a 3-mm optical zone marker is centered over the 7-mm zone mark in the steeper axis to delineate the incision length (Figure 8-3).

If an arcuate keratotomy is preferred, a 16-cut radial keratotomy incision marker is used to delineate an arc of 45° (comprising two segments), a 12-cut RK incision marker is used to delineate an arc of 60° (comprising two segments), and an 8- or 16-cut marker for 90° (2 or 4 segments respectively [Figures 8-4 and 8-5]). When the RK marker is used to delineate the segments of the arcuate incision, an even number of segments must be used so that one of the lines on the marker can be aligned with the steep axis, giving a symmetrical incision in terms of length on either side of the steep axis. An arcuate keratotomy marker designed by

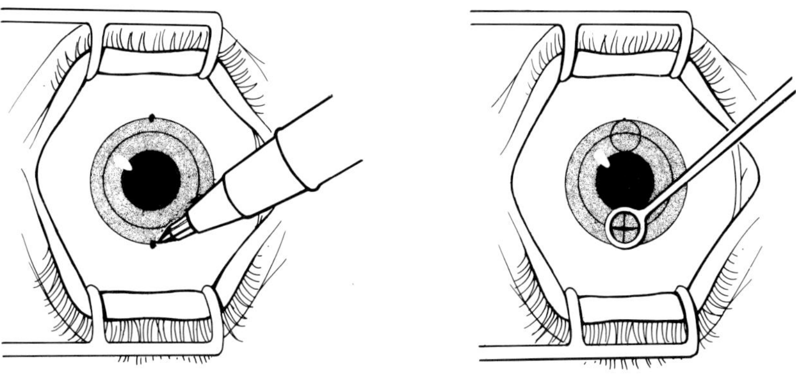

**FIGURE 8-3**    Left, The steep axis of astigmatism is marked with a surgical marker. This is done with the intraoperative quantitative keratometer, but it can also be based on preoperative anatomical landmarks. Right, A 3-mm optical zone marker is centered at the 7-mm optical zone, and these marks can be used to delineate the length of 3-mm straight transverse keratotomies.

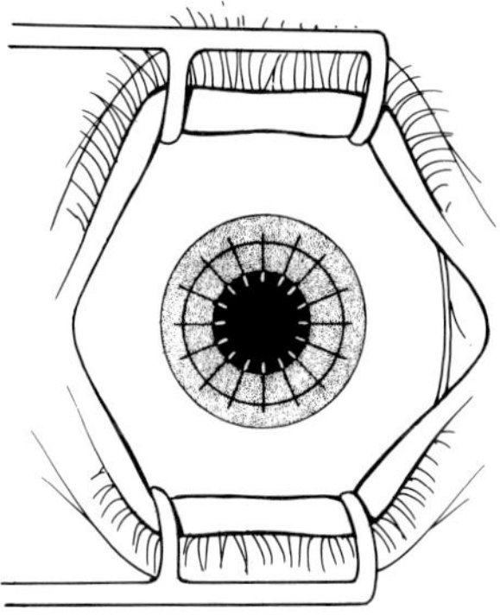

**FIGURE 8-4**    A 16-incision RK incision marker can be used to perform 45° arcuate incisions using two segments for each 45° incision.

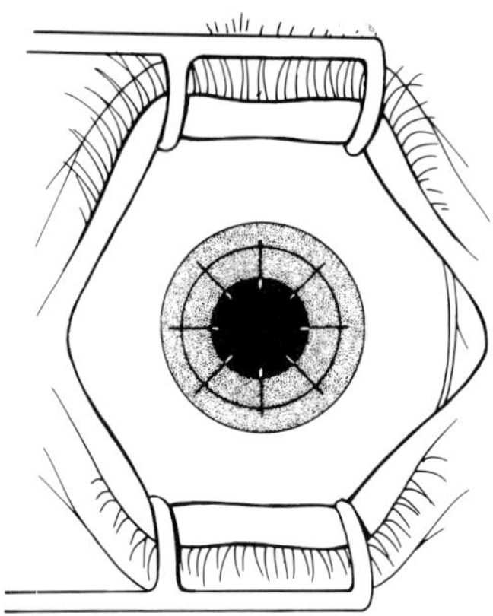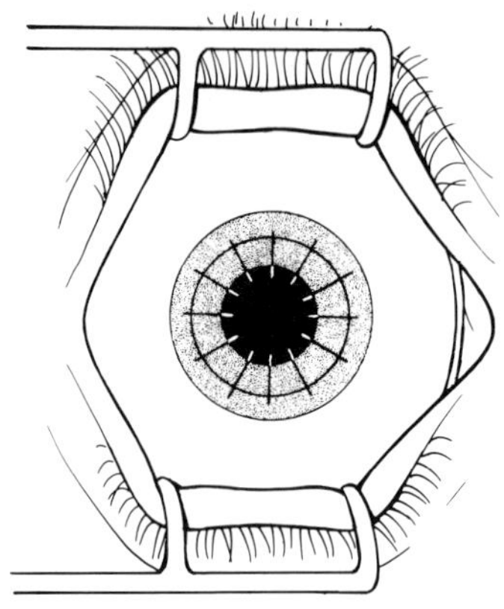

**FIGURE 8-5**     Left, 90° arcuate incisions can be delineated using two segments from an 8-incision RK marker. Right, 60° arcuate incisions can be delineated using two segments from a 12-incision RK marker.

Lindstrom is available from Katena (Figures 8-6 and 8-7). The largest portion of this marker is 90° of arc, followed by 60° and 45° for the two lines closer to the steep axis marker in the center of the instrument. The marker blades may be coated with a skin-marking pencil for better visualization of the radial lines.

The corneal thickness at a 7-mm optical zone is measured on one (for a single incision) or both sides of the cornea either preoperatively or intraoperatively with ultrasonic pachymetry. A high-quality diamond knife is calibrated either preoperatively or intraoperatively with a micronscope. Only extreme care and proper knife selection and maintenance can ensure reproducible cuts. The knife is set at 100% of the thinnest pachymetry. The patient is asked to fixate the operating microscope light, and secondary fixation is achieved with the corneal fixation forcep at the limbus. The knife is set in the cornea, a delay for the count of 1001 is recommended, followed by a slow steady guidance of the knife through the incision. A knife that allows the surgeon good visibility while pushing through the length of the keratotomy improves accuracy. A front-cutting diamond knife is used for all astigmatic incisions, so that the blade is pushed forward through the length of the arcuate or transverse keratotomy. A back-cutting diamond knife is used for the radial keratotomy incisions, so that the blade is inserted at the chosen optical zone and brought towards the limbus. The incision is irrigated with balanced salt solution. Several drops of gentamicin or tobramycin are placed on the eye. We do not routinely patch or use cycloplegics. If a perforation occurs, subconjunctival antibiotic, topical cycloplegia, and a pressure patch are utilized.

## POSTOPERATIVE CARE

The patient is seen at one day, one week and one month, postoperative. Depicted in Figure 8-8 is a patient at three months postoperative. Topical antibiotics are continued for one week. If significant undercorrection is noted on the first postoperative day, we use topical steroid 4 times daily for one to three months in an attempt to delay wound healing and increase incision gape. Incisions may be reopened and extended if significant undercorrection persists after one month. If significant overcorrection is noted early, topical 5% sodium chloride drops are

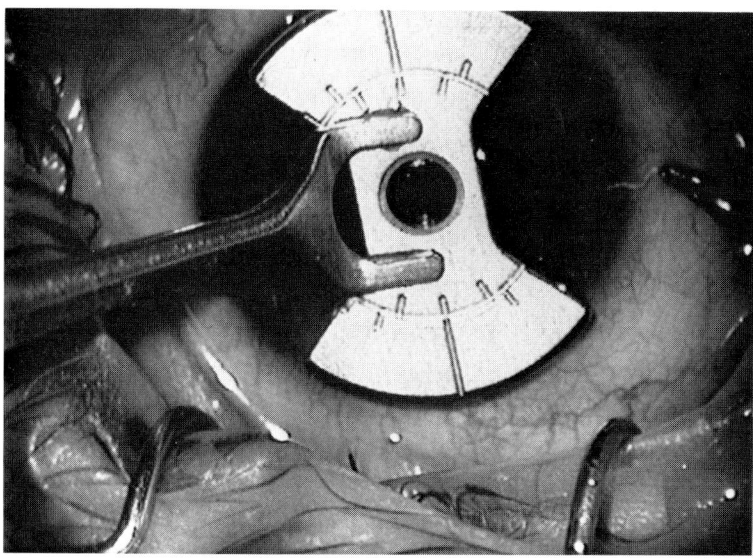

**FIGURE 8-6**    The Lindstrom Astigmatic Keratotomy Marker for a 7-mm optical zone. The center line marks the axis of the incision. The two lines on the interior of the arc delineate 45° of arc. The two lines on the exterior of the arc delineate 60° of arc, and the total length of each arc is 90°.

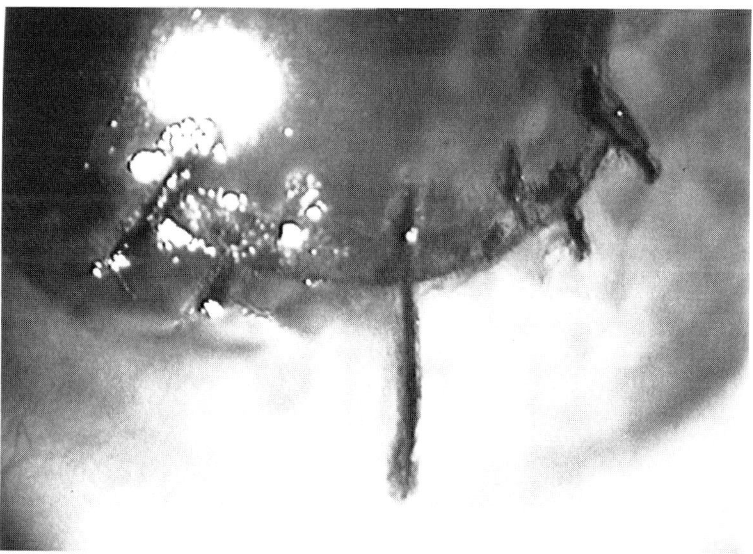

**FIGURE 8-7**    A mark on the cornea using a Lindstrom Astigmatic Keratotomy Marker with a blue surgical marker previously applied to the blades.

started 4 times daily in an attempt to reduce corneal edema and wound gape. If significant overcorrection persists for over one month, we will remove the epithelial plug under topical anesthesia and suture the incision back together with 2 or 3 10-0 nylon or 11-0 mersilene sutures. Intraoperative control of suture tension with a surgical keratometer and the use of slip knots is helpful. We aim for a spherical endpoint or mild overcorrection in the appropriate direction with

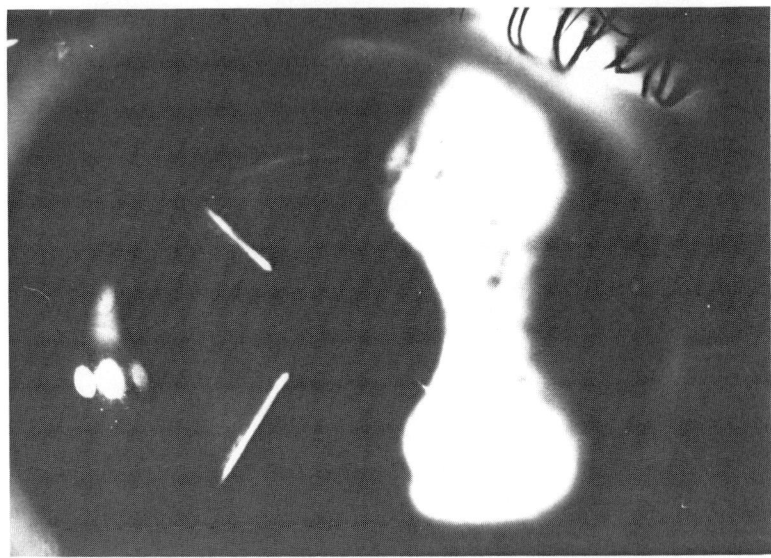

**FIGURE 8-8**  Clinical postoperative photo of a 4-incision radial keratotomy combined with a single-incision arcuate astigmatic keratotomy.

the sutures, and selective suture removal beginning at 8 weeks post-suture placement may be utilized if necessary.

## DISCUSSION

What are the surgical alternatives to our approach as outlined above? With respect to naturally occurring astigmatism, adequate results can be obtained using straight or arcuate keratotomies. We feel that larger shifts can be obtained with arcuate incisions, and this is the experience reported thus far in the literature.[17,18] A single incision or a pair of symmetrical incisions is adequate, and we do not advocate more than two incisions. The optical zone of 6 or 7 millimeters is reasonable, and going any closer to the visual axis than this is not justified and may be fraught with more significant problems with glare. We do not utilize arcuate incisions of over 90° in length, but others have reported success in using incisions of up to 120°.[17] We have abandoned the trapezoidal astigmatic keratotomy or Ruiz procedure because of extreme variability in the results.[15]

Because of the inherent variation in results, it is reasonable in older post-cataract surgery patients to use a single incision, usually under the eyelid, since we have observed large shifts, often unexpectedly, with this approach. A further incision can be added later if necessary. In post-cataract surgery astigmatism, an alternative is wound revision. Since this often involves tissue excision, a longer healing process, and a greater chance of entering the anterior chamber, we usually favor corneal incisional refractive surgery. One exception to this is early postoperative astigmatism associated with wound dehiscence, with or without a fil-

---

The authors have no proprietary interests in any of the instruments or devices mentioned in this article.

tering bleb or iris prolapse. In these cases the wound may be resutured under keratometric control.

When significant astigmatism is present preoperatively in patients with cataract, at the time of cataract surgery we favor performing the cataract incision at the steep axis of preoperative astigmatism, since cataract wounds tend towards against-the-rule astigmatism with time. Intraoperative keratometry can aid us in reducing preoperative astigmatism by titrating the wound to a level of about two diopters of with-the-rule astigmatism. We feel that concurrent astigmatic surgery is rarely indicated. This should be performed later if necessary.

The surgical approach outlined in this chapter has evolved over several years. Much further research is required to delineate the ideal form of surgery. A randomized controlled clinical trial would be ideal. Newer diagnostic techniques, including computer modeling, have permitted us to classify astigmatic patients into heterogenous groups based on their corneal topography. To date we have not been able to suggest accurately variations in surgical technique based on these new diagnostic techniques. This is in progress and will be one of the advances in astigmatism surgery in the coming years.

Although the prognosis for these patients is reasonable, the most common problem with this approach involves the unpredictability which may result in over- or undercorrection of the astigmatism. Although there are medical and surgical options for the management of over- and undercorrection, one cannot overemphasize that thorough and considerable preoperative discussion pertaining to expectations and outcomes is essential.

The key to happy patients is thorough patient education and understanding of what is involved in the surgery. Many patients who cannot be rehabilitated with conventional optical measures benefit significantly from this treatment.

---

## References


1. Duke-Elder SS, Abrams D. Ophthalmic optics and refraction, Vol. 5. System of ophthalmology. St Louis: C.V. Mosby 1970: 274-295.
2. Buzard K, Shearing S, Relyea R. Incidence of astigmatism in a cataract practice. J Refrac Surg 1988; 4:173.
3. Jampel HD, Thompson JR, Baker CC, Stark WJ. A computerized analysis of astigmatism after cataract surgery. Ophthal Surg 1986; 17:786-790.
4. Axt JC. Longitudinal study of postoperative astigmatism. J Cataract Refract Surg 1987; 13:381-388.
5. Richards SC, Brodstein RS, Richards WL, Olson RJ, et al. Longterm course of surgically induced astigmatism. J Cataract Refract Surg 1988; 14:270-276.
6. Parker WT, Clorfeine GS. Longterm evolution of astigmatism following planned extracapsular cataract extraction. Arch Ophthalmol 1989; 107:353-357.
7. Guyton DL. Prescribing cylinders: the problem of distortion, Surv Ophthalmol 1977; 22:177-188.
8. McDonnell PJ, Garbus J, Lopez PF. Topographic analysis and visual acuity after radial keratotomy. Am J Ophthalmol 1988; 106:692-695.
9. Huber C. Planned myopic astigmatism as a substitute for accommodation in pseudophakia. Am Intra-Ocular Implant Soc J 1981; 7:244-249.
10. Sawusch MR, Guyton DL. Myopic astigmatism following cataract surgery: an alternative to multifocal IOLs. Invest Ophthalmol Vis Sci 1990; 31(supp):300.
11. Guyton DL. Prescribing cylinders postoperatively. In Ernest JT, ed, Yearbook of ophthalmology 1985. Chicago: Yearbook Medical Publishers, 1985:63-66.
12. Rashid ER, Waring GO III. Complications of radial and transverse keratotomy. Surv Ophthalmol 1989; 34:73-106.
13. Lindquist TD, Rubenstein JB, Rice SW, Williams PA, Lindstrom RL. Trapezoidal astigmatic keratotomy quantification in human cadaver eyes. Arch Ophthalmol 1986; 104:1534-1539.
14. Duffey RJ, Jain VN, Tchah H, Hofman RF, Lindstrom RL. Paired arcuate keratotomy: a surgical approach

to mixed and myopic astigmatism. Arch Ophthalmol 1988; 106:1130-1135.

15. Agapitos PJ, Lindstrom RL, Williams PA, Sanders DR. Analysis of astigmatic keratotomy. J Cataract Refract Surg 1989; 15:13-18.

16. Agapitos PJ, Williams PA, Sanders DR, Lindstrom RL. Astigmatic keratotomy. CLAO/ISRK Meeting, January 1988 (Poster presentation).

17. Merlin U. Curved keratotomy procedure for congenital astigmatism. J Refractive Surg 1987; 3:92-97.

18. Thornton SP. Astigmatic keratotomy: a review of basic concepts with case reports. J Cataract Refract Surg 1990; 16:430-435.

**Michael E. Sulewski, MD**
**John D. Gottsch, MD**
**Julia A. Haller, MD**
**Walter J. Stark, MD**

# 9 Posterior-Chamber IOL Implantation without Capsular Support

The intraocular lens (IOL) has evolved over the last four decades through many different designs, materials, and manufacturing techniques. The original Ridley lens failed because of poor stability, a result of inadequate fixation and its own heaviness.[1] Attempts to fixate anterior chamber IOLs more securely failed because poor lens design caused progressive and irreparable damage to the corneal endothelium and angle structures.[2-5,6]

With the development of the posterior-chamber lens with J-loop haptics, the modern era of intraocular lens implantation with successful long-term aphakic visual rehabilitation and relatively few complications began. Millions of posterior-chamber lenses have been implanted over the last decade. They have become, by a large margin, the preferred lens for aphakic correction.[7]

The anterior-chamber lens has persisted as an alternative to the posterior-chamber lens for two reasons. First, not all surgeons converted to extracapsular surgery and posterior-chamber lens implantation. Second, in cases of zonular dehiscence or posterior capsular rupture, until recently, the only option for pseudophakic correction was the implantation of an anterior-chamber lens.

Although many anterior-chamber lenses are acceptable, some have been manufactured with serious design flaws such as closed, looped, or rigid haptics. These IOLs, like the original anterior-chamber lenses, have caused endothelial cell loss and pseudophakic bullous edema, frequently with glaucoma, uveitis, and persistent cystoid macular edema.

In response to the real and potential problems with anterior-chamber lenses, alternative techniques for implanting the more successful posterior-chamber lens in the absence of capsular support were sought. In 1985, Hall and Muenzler[8] described techniques for fixating a posterior-chamber lens to the iris during keratoplasty. Several years later, Malbran and coworkers[9] reported a method for implanting a posterior-chamber IOL at the time of keratoplasty using scleral fixation when the posterior capsule was broken or absent. Since then, numerous variations of these techniques have been developed. The practice of IOL implantation without capsular support has now been modified by many surgeons so that a posterior-chamber lens can be sutured during primary extracapsular cataract extraction when there is zonular dehiscence or rupture of the posterior capsule, implanted in combination with an IOL exchange, placed as a secondary lens implantation for aphakic correction, or fixated after repositioning of a subluxated or decentered intraocular lens.

This chapter reviews the various procedures for posterior-chamber lens implantation without capsular support, with their cumulative success rate and potential complications.

## METHODS

The indications for posterior-chamber lens implantation without capsular support include

- Keratoplasty for aphakic bullous keratopathy where an implant is desired, and for pseudophakic bullous keratopathy if an IOL exchange is warranted
- Secondary implantation in aphakic eyes who have undergone a previous intracapsular cataract extraction or suffered capsular rupture during a planned extracapsular cataract extraction
- IOL exchange of an anterior-chamber lens through a limbal approach
- Implantation of a posterior-chamber lens after capsular rupture during a planned extracapsular or phacoemulsification cataract extraction surgery
- The management of dislocated or subluxed intraocular lenses.

These indications are reviewed with regard to the evolution and modification of the surgical techniques developed to manage each problem.

## Keratoplasty

We prefer a modification of the iris-fixation technique first described by Hall and Muenzler[8] for securing posterior-chamber lenses when capsular support is not present during keratoplasty.[10] This allows direct visualization without externalizing sutures through the ciliary body. However, there are situations when iris support is not possible due to absent or inadequate iris tissue. In those cases where there is a large iridodialysis or a large iridectomy, or in an aniridia patient, scleral fixation is preferred.

In the original procedures described for scleral fixation of an IOL, the polypropylene suture-ends on the scleral surface had a tendency to erode through the conjunctiva, thus producing irritation and providing a possible tract for microbial penetration into the eye.[11] To circumvent these problems, a "trap-door" scleral flap was proposed for scleral fixation of anterior[12] and posterior[13] lenses during cataract surgery and was later reintroduced by Hu and associates[14] for transcleral fixation of secondary posterior-chamber lenses. It is likely that sclerally fixated haptics do not become permanently attached to the ciliary sulcus and that the lens can fall back into the vitreous if exposed suture knots are cut.[11,15]

Malbran[9] was the first to report a method of scleral fixation of a posterior-chamber lens in the absence of capsular support during keratoplasty. His technique involved the use of two 28-gauge needles threaded with 10-0 polypropylene sutures that were directed and penetrated the sclera 2 to 3 mm from the limbus at the 3:00 and 9:00 o'clock positions. The needles remained partly in the anterior chamber with the outer end resting on the sclera while the cornea was trephined. The needles were then removed, leaving two loops of suture in the anterior chamber that could be secured to the haptics and fixated externally to the sclera.

## Transcleral fixation during keratoplasty

For transcleral fixation during keratoplasty, a Honan pressure cuff or other controlled ocular pressure-reducing device should be used for 20 minutes prior to surgery to reduce vitreous volume and positive pressure. A 4-0 silk suture is placed beneath the superior and inferior recti for stabilization of the globe. A conjunctival peritomy is performed 3 mm from limbus and dissected 3-4 mm posteriorly. Hemostasis is achieved with wetfield cautery, followed by dissection of a 3-mm half-thickness triangular scleral flap with its base at the limbus, similar to that used in a trabeculectomy. The same flap is created 180 degrees away. Technically, it is easier to make the flap in either the vertical or the horizontal meridians. A large Flieringa ring is then secured that encompasses the dissected partial thickness scleral flaps using either a running or an interrupted 7-0 silk suture. After trephination of the donor corneal button, the recipient cornea is trephined. If a closed loop or unstable anterior-chamber lens is present, causing pseudophakic bullous keratopathy, glaucoma, chronic cystoid macular edema, or uveitis, it should be removed. The techniques for removal of these lenses are described in the section on IOL exchange.

A limited anterior vitrectomy should be performed if there is vitreous in the anterior chamber or around the pupil. A viscoelastic agent is injected into the anterior chamber to keep the vitreous posterior to the pupil and to maintain the anterior chamber. If residual posterior capsule is present and capsular fixation of a haptic is contemplated, the capsular bag can be opened with the viscoelastic substance. If irido-capsular adhesions are present, they should be lysed prior to implantation of the lens. Otherwise these adhesions will result in a displaced or decentered IOL. Placement of the haptics posterior to the capsular remnants will allow proper centration of the lens. Prior to trephining the recipient cornea, a long CIF-4 or CTC-6 Ultima (Ethicon, Inc., Somerville, N.J.) needle with 10-0 polypropylene suture should be tied around each haptic after beading the haptic end with a disposable cautery to prevent slippage of the knot.[14] There are now available 1-piece all-PMMA posterior-chamber lenses which have holes incorporated into the middle of the haptic loops, thereby permitting the polypropylene sutures to be tied around the holes, thus preventing slippage of the fixation suture. A needle holder is used to pass the long curved needle through the pupil, under the iris inferiorly, and out through the ciliary sulcus, exiting the sclera 1 mm posterior to the limbus under the scleral flap. A similar needle pass is made with the other needle through the opposite scleral flap. The inferior haptic loop can be guided into the ciliary sulcus while the polypropylene suture is simultaneously pulled with a tying forceps. The lens optic is then placed through the pupil and into the posterior chamber. This is followed by the placement of the superior haptic into the ciliary sulcus while the superior polypropylene suture, which has already been passed, is gently tugged. The lens can be carefully centered by using a Sinskey hook and pulling lightly on the polypropylene sutures. Adjacent to the site at which the needle exits under the scleral flap, another suture pass is taken into the split thickness scleral tissue, and the suture is tied to itself. The donor corneal button is then sutured in place, after which the Flieringa ring is removed.

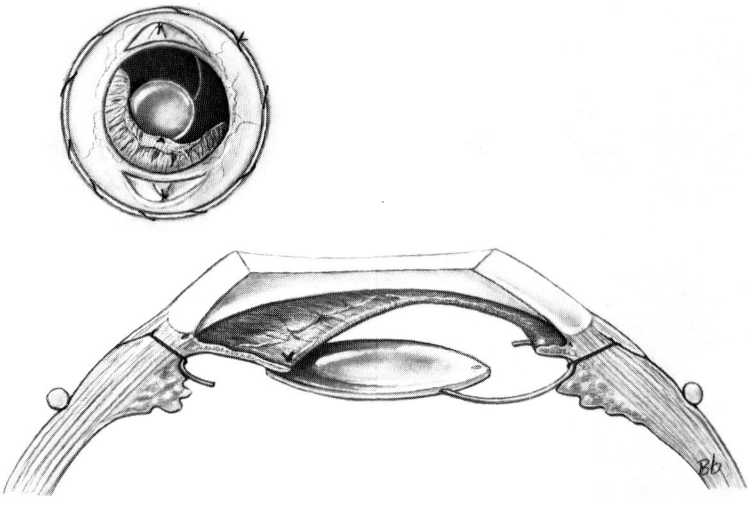

**FIGURE 9-1**     In 3-point fixation of an intraocular lens where large iris defects may exist, 2 sutures are used to fixate one haptic while the other haptic is secured with 1 suture.

The triangular scleral flaps are sutured with a single 10-0 nylon suture at the apex, with the conjunctiva pulled over the flap and closed with an absorbable suture.

Three-point fixation of the IOL may be necessary in some instances to prevent tilting of the lens when there are large iris abnormalities. Two sutures may be used to fixate one haptic while the other haptic is secured with only one suture (Figure 9-1).

## Iris fixation of a posterior-chamber lens during keratoplasty

The technique for iris fixation of a posterior-chamber lens at the time of keratoplasty was first described by Hall and Muenzler.[8] We have modified their technique somewhat as follows: A Flieringa ring is sutured into position approximately 1 mm from the limbus. A 2-holed, 7-mm optic posterior-chamber lens with polypropylene monofilament suture (5 cm) is attached to a double-armed BV100-4 Ethicon needle, which is passed through each hole of the optic (Figure 9-2). The donor button is prepared first, then the recipient corneal button is trephined; and if a problematic IOL is present, it is explanted (see the section on IOL exchange). A limited anterior vitrectomy is performed through the pupil. The optic is then grasped with a pair of McPherson forceps or an intraocular lens forceps, and one haptic is placed behind the iris into the ciliary sulcus at the 3:00 o'clock position (Figure 9-3). Once again, care should be taken not to place the haptic where a capsular remnant with irido-capsular adhesions exists, because a displaced IOL is likely to occur. The suture needles are placed through the iris in the mid periphery, and a single knot is then tied firmly to pull excess suture material so that the IOL will not "hang" from the iris. Bunching of the iris should also be avoided. The other haptic and the optic can be placed in the posterior chamber by gently bending the haptic and manually inserting it into the ciliary sulcus with tying forceps. The other needle secured to the optic is sutured to the iris, taking care that the needle barbs are correctly diagonal and about the same

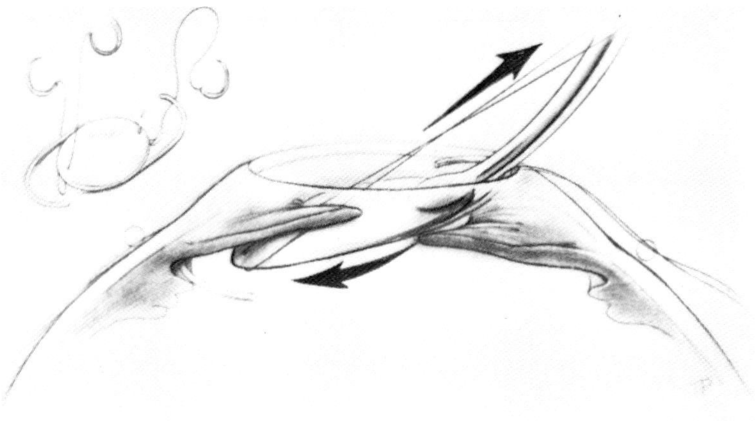

**FIGURE 9-2**    Iris fixation of a posterior-chamber lens during keratoplasty. A 2-holed 7-mm optic posterior-chamber lens with a polypropylene monofilament suture (5 cm) is attached to a double-armed BV100-4 Ethicon needle, which is passed through each hole of the optic.

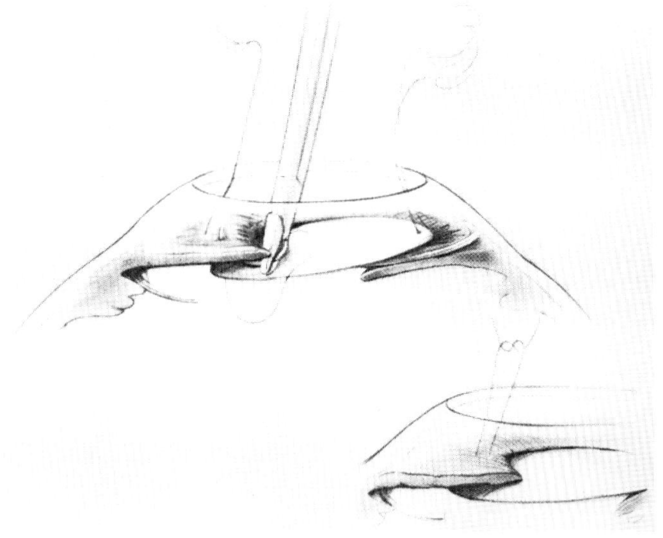

**FIGURE 9-3**    Inferior suture is passed through the iris above the optic hole and tied securely.

distance from the iris root (Figure 9-4). A peripheral iridectomy should be performed, and the corneal graft can then be sutured into position.

There are certain situations where a combination of transcleral and iris fixation of the lens is necessary to ensure long-term lens stability. We have encountered the need for this 3-point fixation technique in a few cases of post-traumatic aphakia where there is partial absence of the iris. A 2-holed posterior-chamber IOL is used with suture-fixation of the optic to the iris remnant, while the two haptics are also transclerally suture-fixated. This method may prevent the lens from tilting. A broad C-loop lens design is also recommended to maximize the area of ciliary sulcus fixation (Figure 9-5).

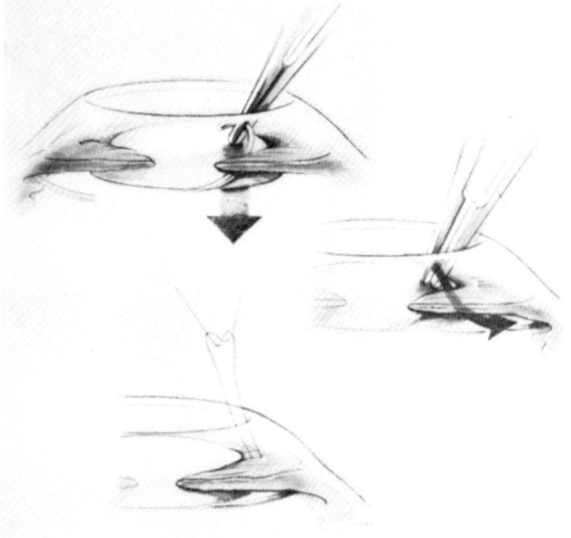

**FIGURE 9-4** Top and middle, Forceps are used to grasp the haptic, and with gentle posterior pressure on the optic, the superior loop is released through the ciliary sulcus. Bottom, Superior suture is passed through the iris and securely tied.

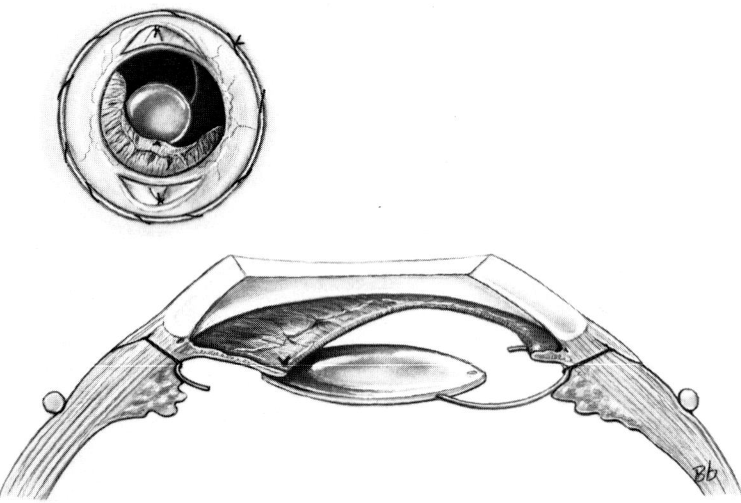

**FIGURE 9-5** A 3-point fixation technique, which is helpful in posttraumatic cases where there is partial absence of the iris. A 2-holed posterior-chamber lens is used with suture fixation of the iris remnant while transscleral fixation sutures are utilized to secure the two haptics. A broad C-loop lens design is recommended for this procedure to maximize the area of ciliary sulcus fixation.

## Secondary Implantation in Aphakia

Many of the techniques outlined in the keratoplasty section are similar to those used for secondary implantation in aphakia, but some modifications are necessary because the surgical approach is not made from an "open sky" but from the limbus.

The technique of secondary posterior-chamber lens implantation in aphakia without capsular support requires transcleral or iris fixation of the lens. These techniques have evolved over the years from several innovative contributors. Choyce[12] described the technique of suturing anterior-chamber lenses to the sclera under a "trap-door" flap in the late 1970s. Mazzacco and coworkers[17] reported their experience with suturing haptics to the iris to stabilize posterior-chamber lenses in eyes without adequate capsular support. Gess[13] reported his technique of suturing the superior haptic to the sclera under a flap to insure proper centration of a posterior-chamber lens at the time of cataract surgery. Procedures using the basic principles of some of these earlier techniques combined with new instrumentation have evolved to permit implantation of a posterior-chamber lens when there is no capsular support.[14,18-20]

After retrobulbar anesthesia, a Honan pressure cuff is used for approximately 20 minutes to reduce vitreous volume and pressure. Inferior and superior rectus 4-0 silk sutures are placed for positioning of the globe. An 8-mm fornix-based conjunctival flap is created at the superior limbus, and a 3-mm inferior peritomy is created. A bipolar cautery is used to achieve hemostasis, and triangular half-thickness scleral flaps are dissected superiorly and inferiorly, with the base positioned at the limbus and the flaps situated 180 degrees apart. A biplanar groove is created superiorly on either side of the flap with a total chord length of 7.5 mm. A 7-mm, no-hole optic with broad spanning haptics (all-PMMA or 3-piece style) is placed in the operative field. A 20-cm double-armed 10-0 polypropylene (Prolene) suture on a CIF-4 or a CTC-6 needle (Ethicon, Inc., Somerville, N.J.) is cut in half, and one end is tied around the inferior haptic. A 5-cm double-armed 10-0 polypropylene suture on a BV100-4 (Ethicon) needle is then tied around the superior haptic. A Ziegler knife is used to enter the anterior chamber. If possible, an anterior vitrectomy is avoided at this stage because of the tendency of the eye to collapse after vitrectomy when the transcleral inferior suture is passed. However, if excessive vitreous is present in the anterior chamber or to the wound, a limited vitrectomy should be performed prior to I$\alpha$ placement. A viscoelastic agent is injected into the anterior chamber to push the vitreous posterior to the pupil and maintain the chamber. If sufficient remnants of the posterior capsule are present, then the capsular bag can support the haptic in the ciliary sulcus, thereby avoiding suture fixation. Iridocapsular adhesions frequently occur, and mechanical lysis to free capsular remnants allows proper posterior-chamber IOL implantation. Freeing capsular remnants inferiorly allows the implantation of a lens in which superior scleral fixation is still necessary but an inferior scleral fixation can be avoided.[21,22] The wound is opened to the full 7.5 mm. A large needle-holder is used to pass the CIF-4 or CTC-6 needle through the corneoscleral incision superiorly, through the pupil and behind the iris inferiorly, and through the ciliary sulcus exiting transclerally 1 mm posterior to the limbus under the scleral flap (Figure 9-6). The inferior haptic loop of the IOL is inserted through the limbal incision, crossing the pupil into the retro-iris space inferiorly, as the external inferior polypropylene suture is gently pulled with a tying forceps. This effectively directs the inferior haptic into the ciliary sulcus. An angled tying forceps can be used to grasp the superior haptic and insert it through the limbal incision. If it is grasped 1 to 1.5 mm distal to its elbow, it can be pronated superiorly and placed directly behind the iris. The double-armed sutures attached to the superior haptic may then be passed through the pupil, under the iris, and through the

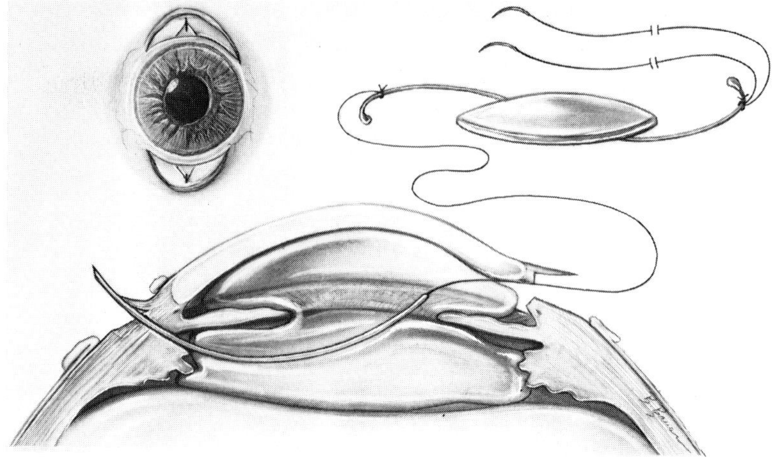

---



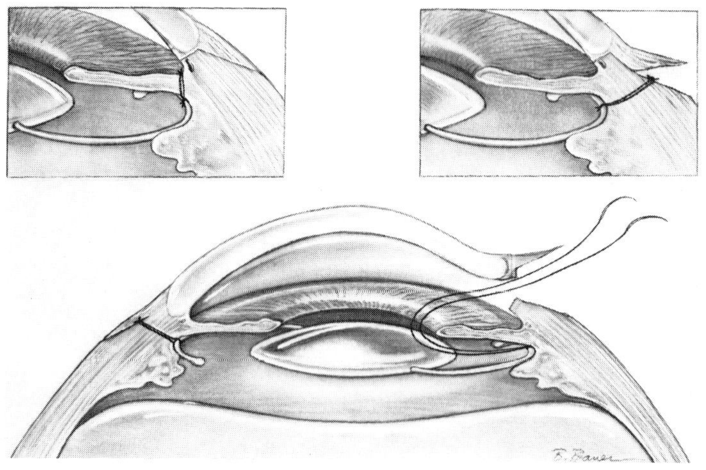

---



ciliary sulcus, exiting from the sclera 1 mm posterior to the limbus within the superior scleral flap. The externalized sutures can then be tied together. Alternatively, if iris fixation of the superior suture is preferred, the needles can be passed through the peripheral superior iris and tied (Figure 9-7). The lens can be gently positioned with a Sinskey hook. The inferior long needle is regrasped, a superficial scleral bite is taken adjacent to the suture bite inferiorly, and the suture is tied to itself and secured under the scleral flap. A miotic is injected into the anterior chamber to constrict the pupil and reform the chamber. The superior wound is closed with interrupted 10-0 nylon sutures, and the scleral flaps may be closed with one 10-0 nylon suture at the apex, with the knots rotated and buried into the sclera. If vitreous is present in the anterior chamber or in front of the lens, a mechanical vitrectomy may be performed prior to placement of the last few sutures, otherwise the viscoelastic substance may be irrigated and aspirated out. An ovoid or peaked pupil may indicate vitreous strands at the pupillary and wound margin, which should be removed with a vitreous cutting instrument. The conjunctiva is closed over the superior wound and the inferior scleral flap with either electrocautery or an 8-0 absorbable suture.

## IOL Exchange

The decision to remove an intraocular lens should be based on several factors. The first consideration is whether the lens in question has a history of causing problems. Closed-loop rigid lenses, such as the Leiske, Surgidev, and Azar 91Z, are well documented to cause progressive pseudophakic bullous keratopathy, chronic uveitis, glaucoma, and cystoid macular edema. In any eye with one of these lenses that has persistent inflammation with early corneal decompensation, chronic uveitis, CME, or glaucoma a lens exchange should be performed.

Second, if other anterior-chamber lens styles are implanted improperly and chronic inflammation and pseudophakic bullous keratopathy develop, an IOL exchange should be performed. Any lens with the foot plate buried into the iris or eroding into the ciliary body, resulting in chronic uveitis or any lens with a foot plate that touches the peripheral cornea, causing chronic endothelial cell loss, should be explanted. Lenses that are too small, that rotate, or that have persistent pseudophakodonesis should be removed before irreversible pseudophakic bullous keratopathy ensues.

If preoperative gonioscopy reveals a closed-loop anterior-chamber IOL that has eroded into the ciliary body, the IOL loops must be cut to create an open loop so the haptic can be rotated out and removed completely (Figures 9-8 and 9-9).[20,23] Much care must be taken in removing embedded haptics. Inadvertent mishandling of the haptics can disinsert the iris, causing severe bleeding into the anterior chamber and vitreous cavity. Leaving an embedded haptic in the angle may allow the plastic to erode through the ciliary body and sclera, causing a wound leak (Figure 9-10). In these cases, the eroded haptic should be removed in the operating room, and the tract should be closed with a partial-thickness scleral autoflap or with a donor scleral patch. Following removal of the anterior-chamber lens, a posterior-chamber lens may be sutured in place as previously described. If uncontrolled glaucoma is present, a trabeculectomy may be performed as well using the already prepared scleral flap.

## IOL Implantation at the Time of a Planned Extracapsular Cataract Extraction or Phacoemulsification

Unfortunately, posterior capsular rupture or dehiscence of zonules may occur during planned extracapsular cataract surgery or phacoemulsification. The capsulorhexis technique provides a platform of stable anterior capsule that can support a posterior-chamber lens in the ciliary sulcus even if the posterior capsule is ruptured. Small posterior capsular ruptures do not preclude the implantation of a posterior-chamber intraocular lens. If vitreous protrudes through the posterior capsular opening, a viscoelastic agent can be used to keep the vitreous back

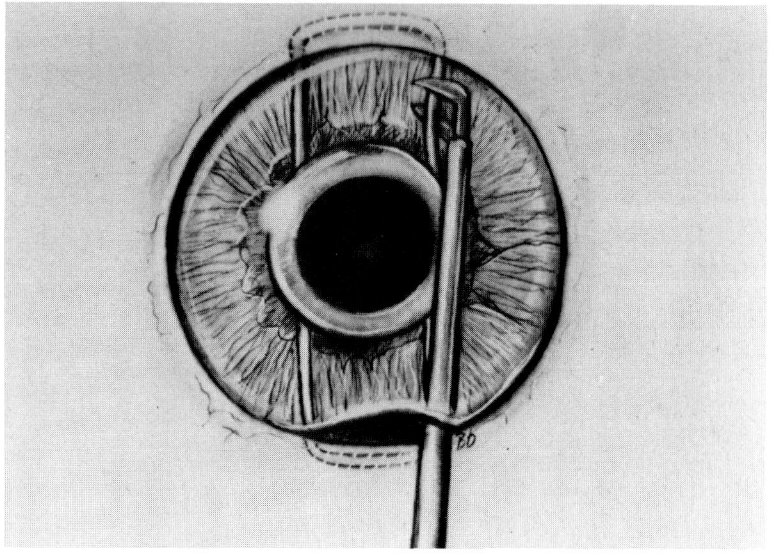

**FIGURE 9-8** IOL removal is performed after first amputating the inferior loop.

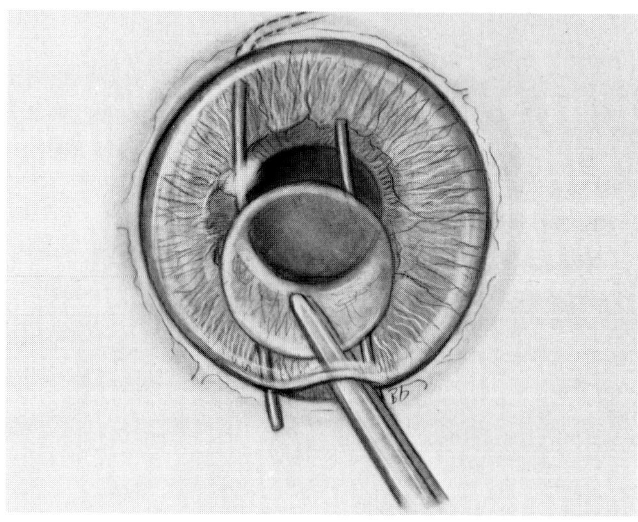

**FIGURE 9-9** In removal of closed-loop anterior-chamber IOLs that have eroded into the ciliary body, the loop must be cut to create an open loop so that the haptic may be removed completely. Once the superior loop is cut in two locations, the lens can be rotated out along with the haptic, thereby avoiding further damage to the iris and ciliary body.

while implantation is performed, or a limited vitrectomy through the rent can be done. If a limited dehiscence of zonules is noted superiorly, superior haptic fixation alone will usually be sufficient to stabilize the lens. Likewise, if a capsular rupture occurs superiorly but there is sufficient capsule inferiorly to implant a posterior-chamber lens, the remaining inferior capsule can be used to stabilize the lens in the ciliary sulcus while superior fixation of the haptic to the iris or sclera may be all that is necessary to stabilize the lens (Figure 9-11).

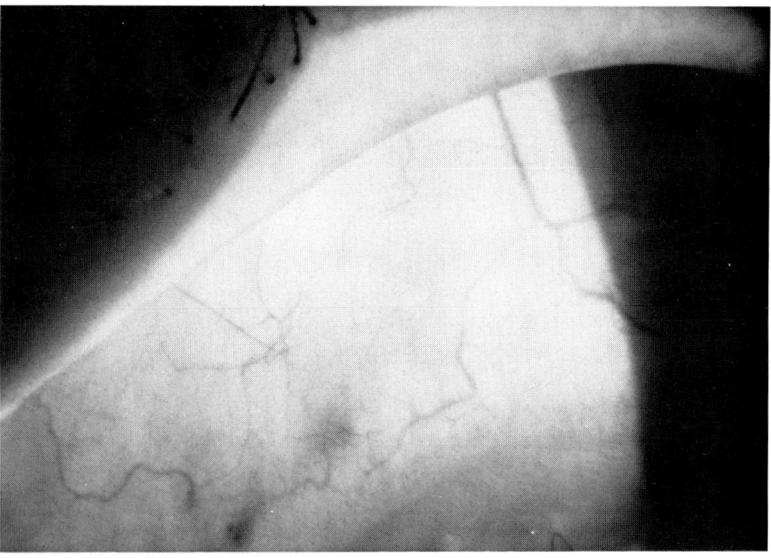

**FIGURE 9-10**    An eroded, amputated, imbedded haptic producing wound leak. Such cases can be closed with a partial-thickness scleral flap.

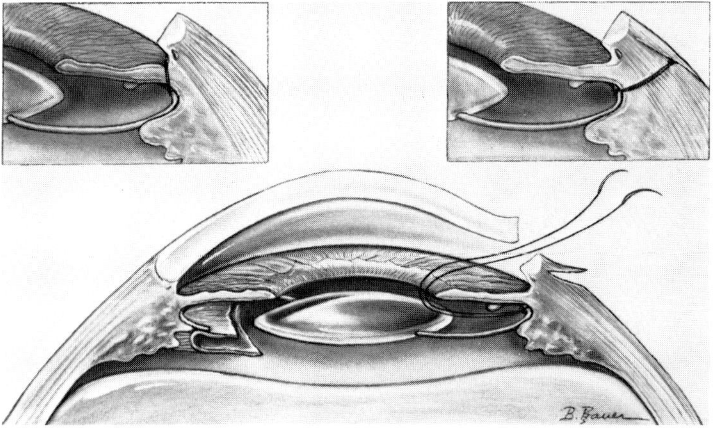

**FIGURE 9-11**    A case of superior dehiscence of zonules or capslar rupture where the lens was stabilized by superior haptic fixation alone. If iris or transscleral fixation of the superior suture is desired, needles can be passed through the peripheral superior iris or under a scleral flap and tied.

In cases of traumatic lens subluxation where there is zonular dehiscence and inadequate capsular integrity, a superior and inferior scleral fixation suturing technique can be utilized to insert a posterior-chamber lens.[24]

## Subluxation or Dislocation of an IOL

Posterior dislocation of an IOL into the vitreous cavity, a more common occurrence when iris-supported IOLs were widely used, is relatively infrequent with current techniques of extracapsular cataract extraction and posterior-chamber intraocular lens implantation. Dislocation is usually secondary to intraoperative iatrogenic rupture of zonular and capsular support. It may also develop postoperatively, after secondary damage to supporting elements, as can occur with further surgery, through an episode of malignant glaucoma, or because of trauma.

Once the IOL is dislocated, several approaches are possible.[25-28] The non-surgical option is to leave the IOL in the vitreous and optically correct the patient with glasses or a contact lens. No known damage has been done to an eye by a free-floating IOL, but certainly the potential exists for hemorrhage or for creating a retinal tear.

Incomplete dislocation of an intraocular lens or a limited dislocation into the anterior vitreous can be approached through the limbus by first grasping the haptic with a tying forceps and then bringing the lens out through the wound where inferior and superior fixation sutures can be secured in place as described in the section on secondary implantation.

A partially subluxed posterior-chamber lens can be secured by a modified McCannel suture through a scleral trap door.[28,49] Alpar has described the use of the Ethicon 1713 suture for placing a McCannel suture to iris-fixate a partially dislocated posterior-chamber lens.[36]

For more posteriorly dislocated IOLs, a pars plana approach permits controlled vitreous excision and precise manipulation of IOLs situated well posteriorly, even on the retinal surface. Preoperative evaluation is crucial to planning a surgical approach. Enough residual capsular shelf may remain to permit at least partial IOL relocation without suturing.

Our initial surgical approach is to excise anterior vitreous and free up the IOL. Some remaining posterior cortical vitreous is ideally left as a cushion for the retina. The IOL is then grasped with intraocular forceps, such as Rappazzo forceps, and carefully reoriented. Several techniques for relocation have been described.[25,26,28,31] In some cases, it is possible to slide the IOL haptics back into their posterior capsular rim of support. When the capsule is absent, stable fixation can occasionally be achieved by placing the haptics in the ciliary sulcus. Gentle testing of stability by pressure on the eye or nudging of the IOL with an intraocular pick may provide reassurance as to the lack of need for sutures.

In most cases, suturing of the IOL is advisable to assure long-term stabilization. One technique is to suture the lens to the iris. In this method, the haptics, once temporarily placed in the sulcus, are sutured to the iris using McCannel sutures. A long curved needle is passed through the limbus and iris, under the IOL haptic and back out the iris and limbus. The suture on either side of the tethered haptic is then grasped through a separate stab incision with a hooked needle, brought out and tied. This can be done with one haptic or both, and has been used with good success.[25] It requires precise suture placement, and can be technically demanding as the haptic capture is not done under direct visualization. There is also the theoretical disadvantage of iris fixation sutures, which may irritate the iris, cause inflammation, or incite CME.

Scleral fixation sutures can also be used with the dislocated IOL. Several approaches are possible. Haptics are externalized through opposite sclerotomies, 9-0 prolene is attached, and the haptics are then sutured to the sclera adjacent to the sclerotomies. One case of endophthalmitis has been reported in a procedure using this technique,[11] suggesting that covering the sutures with a scleral flap may be advisable.

Smiddy[26] has described a method whereby IOL haptics are caught in a loop of 10-0 prolene at 12:00 and 6:00 o'clock. The prolene needle is passed with the left hand through the sclera 1.5 to 2 mm posterior to the limbus and 12:00 o'clock, caught with the right hand, using a Rappazzo forceps, then rotated 180 degrees and handed back to the left hand inside the eye. The right-hand forceps are then passed through the loop of the prolene suture to grasp the superior haptic of the IOL, and it is tied to the sclera externally under a flap. A similar maneuver is used inferiorly. This technique, which requires good visualization of the haptics, is difficult if the lens is quite posterior. Anand and Brown[31] have reported a modification of this technique. They thread a 23-gauge needle with a loop of 9-0 prolene and insert this into the eye at 12:00 o'clock. The loop of suture is then extruded through the needle tip and hooked over the IOL haptic. The authors make 4 such loops, 2 spaced 3 mm apart superiorly and 2 inferiorly, and thread the haptics to provide 4 point fixation for the relocated IOL.

In cases where visualization of intraocular structures is a problem, as occurs with corneal opacities or pupillary membranes resistant to excision, the prolene sutures may be more conveniently attached to the haptics externally. To do this, the haptic is brought out through a superior sclerotomy with Rappazzo forceps, and a 10-0 prolene on a long (CIF-4 or CTC-6) needle is attached. The long needle is then reintroduced into the sclerotomy and across the eye and pushed through the sclera 1 mm posterior to the limbus as the haptic is gently replaced into the vitreous cavity. The opposite haptic is then grasped and brought out through the same sclerotomy, and a 10-0 prolene on a standard cutting needle is affixed. The needle is driven back through the sclerotomy and out the adjacent sclera 1 mm posterior to the limbus, 180° opposite the initial suture. Both sutures are then permanently tied to themselves after an adjacent bite of sclera is taken. A scleral flap can be dissected initially to cover the suture ends.

## Discussion

Many studies have reported that fixation of a posterior-chamber lens to the iris[8,10,16,29,30,32-35] or to the sclera[9,36-38] at the time of penetrating keratoplasty may be more desirable than the implantation of an anterior-chamber lens in eyes where no capsular support exists. Numerous authors have described the complications associated with semiflexible, closed-loop anterior-chamber intraocular lenses and the difficulties of removing the lenses at the time of surgery.[6,10,16,29,30,32-35] Secondary glaucoma with extensive angle damage has been associated with these lenses. Certainly, in eyes with pseudophakic bullous keratopathy with haptics eroded into the angle and iris root, we believe a sutured posterior-chamber lens is preferable to reimplanting an anterior-chamber lens. However, several reports have indicated that the implantation of an open-loop anterior-chamber intraocular lens has results comparable to use of a posterior-chamber lens with sulcus or iris fixation.[29,40,47] The implantation of an anterior-chamber lens, technically easier than suturing a posterior-chamber lens, does not involve externalized sutures, which decreases the potential of a suture abscess and resultant endophthalmitis. Future prospective randomized trials of open-looped anterior-chamber IOLs versus posterior-chamber sutured IOLs may determine which lens is better for a routine case of aphakic or pseudophakic bullous keratopathy.

Most of the published studies prefer iris fixation of the posterior-chamber lens over transcleral fixation. However, there is no convincing evidence to establish one method of fixation as superior to the other. The results and complications of these two methods of posterior-chamber fixation during keratoplasty are summarized in Table 9-1. Concern has been expressed that complications may occur by suturing through the highly vascularized ciliary body. Although no case of intraocular hemorrhage has been reported, we have encountered a referred case of choroidal hemorrhage that occurred upon passing the scleral suture. A systemic medical workup of the patient disclosed a platelet disorder. We now routinely obtain clotting studies on patients undergoing scleral fixation and advise all patients to discontinue aspirin or compounds containing aspirin as well as nonste-

**Table 9-1**   Summary of the Results of Penetrating Keratoplasty with Sutured Posterior-Chamber Lenses in the Absence of Capsular Support

| Study | No. of cases | Avg. followup (months) | Avg. pre-op visual acuity | Avg. post-op visual acuity | Clear grafts (%) | Complications (no.) |
|---|---|---|---|---|---|---|
| **Iris fixation** | | | | | | |
| Wong et al[10] | 20 | 7 | 20/200 | 20/80 | 100 | Retinal detachment 3 weeks post-op in 1 patient which was repaired and achieved visual acuity 1 month later. |
| Soong et al[29] | 133 | 12 (median) | Not given | ≥ 20/40 (45.1%) 20/50-20/100 (30.5%) at 1 year | 97 | Graft rejection (5), retinal detachment (3), glaucoma (16), endophthalmitis (2), CME (44), PAS (28) |
| van der Schaft et al[16] | 29 | 36 | Not given | ≥ 20/40 (45%) 20/50-20/100 (20%) at 1 year | 83 | Bullous keratopathy (7), glaucoma, CME (3), retinal detachment (1) |
| Price and Whitson[35] | 233 | 26 | — | ≥ 20/40 (59.5%) ≥ 20/80 (74%) | 95.5 | Partial iris dialysis (2), IOL dislocation (2), endophthalmitis (10) |
| Hall and Muenzler[8] | 53 | 32 | 90% ≤ 20/200 | ≥ 20/50 (38%) 20/60-20/100 (24.5%) | 88.7 | CME (2), glaucoma (3), graft failure (6), vitreous & AC hemorrhage (1), RD (1) |
| Busin et al[33] | 14 | 7.6 | 20/300-LP | ≥ 20/60 (28.6%) ≥ 20/200 (57%) | 92.8 | Glaucoma (4), goniosynechiae (4), pseudophakodonesis (10), CME (3) |
| **Transcleral** | | | | | | |
| Cowden and Hu[37] | 14 | 6 | HM | 20/400 | 93 | Glaucoma (1), iritis (1), graft failure (1) |
| Spigelman et al[30] | 15 | at least 3 months | — | 20/76 | 100 | Exposed polypropylene suture needed trimming |

roidal, antiinflammatory agents, several weeks prior to surgery. Proper placement of the suture 1 mm posterior to the corneoscleral junction, which avoids the major arterial circle of the iris, should decrease the risk of a significant intra-operative bleeding.[41]

Several cases of endophthalmitis have been reported with iris fixation during keratoplasty.[29,35] It is not clear why endophthalmitis occurred in these series. In over 150 cases of IOL exchange with iris fixation of a posterior-chamber lens with followup to 4 years, however, we have not had a case of endophthalmitis at our institution.

Apple and coworkers[42] studied 4 eyes that had undergone iris fixation in conjunction with keratoplasty and found that 7 of 8 of the haptics were posterior to the sulcus, with the optic secured to the iris. There are no data yet to suggest that the haptics in this position predispose the eye to any complications. However, finding haptics in this position may indicate an improperly secured optic and suggests that the iris fixation sutures are loose,[43] suspending the optic. This could result in a subluxed or tilted IOL and pseudophakodonesis and excessive iris or ciliary-body chafing. In another histopathologic study[44] of 3 eyes that had under-gone penetrating keratoplasty and transcleral suturing of a posterior-chamber lens, only a thin fibrous capsule surrounded the haptics at their attachment site. Lens stability in these cases was not felt to be related to fibrosis of the haptics in the ciliary body. In one case, in which the externalized suture knot was cut, the lens fell back into the vitreous. Thus cutting an exposed suture knot is probably not advisable. Argon-laser melting of an exposed suture (Figure 9-12) can be helpful to promote epithelial closure and decrease chronic irritation, which can result in giant papillary conjunctivitis (Figure 9-13).

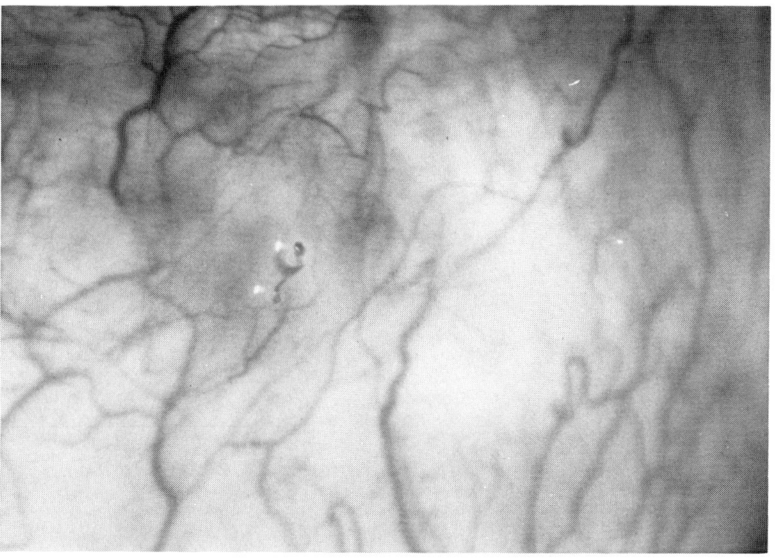

**FIGURE 9-12**    An exposed suture knot causing chronic irritation and giant papillary conjunctivitis. The ends were cauterized with the argon laser, giving the patient symptomatic relief and allowing epi-thelization over the suture.

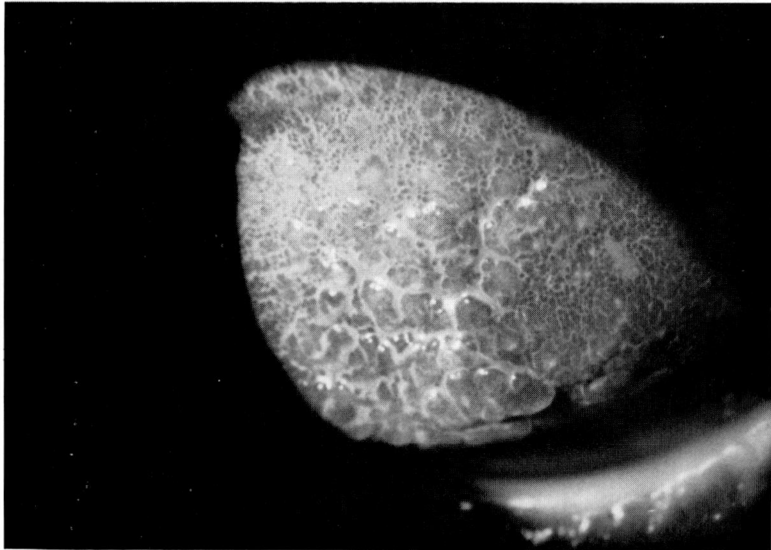

**FIGURE 9-13**    Giant papillary conjunctivitis in a patient with an exposed suture.

Other techniques for secondary implantation of an intraocular lens without capsular support or limited support have been reported. Maas and Sivaligan[45] have used stiff all-PMMA posterior-chamber lenses in the sulcus with only superior transcleral fixation in 6 patients. They have noted no complications with a follow-up of 2 weeks to 17 months. Traykovski[46] has reported his experience with implanting a secondary lens in eyes with an intact anterior hyaloid face but no capsular support. He describes placing a posterior-chamber lens in the ciliary sulcus without suture fixation on a firm vitreous face, lysing iridovitreal adhesions if necessary. The mean follow-up has been 2 years, and all but one of these patients maintained visual acuity comparable to their preoperative acuity. Dahan and coworkers[22] were able to implant secondary all-PMMA IOLs in patients ranging in age from 2 to 67 utilizing the peripheral capsular remnants and placing the haptics in the ciliary sulcus without suture fixation. All eyes had peripheral iridocapsular synechiae which needed lysing prior to implantation of the lenses. The average followup is 13.4 months (range 6 to 24 months), and no long-term complications have been noted thus far.

We have reported a case of a retinal detachment occurring 3 weeks postoperatively.[10] Soong et al[29] reported three cases of retinal detachments for an overall ratio of 2.3%, which was comparable to their rate for all keratoplasties. A meticulous anterior vitrectomy, if needed, and proper handling and placement of the transcleral sutures 1.0 mm posterior to the corneal scleral limbus may decrease the likelihood of a retinal detachment.[41]

Cystoid macular edema was noted in many series, but most cases were felt to have been present preoperatively. Several reports have described cases in which preoperative CME improved after penetrating keratoplasty and IOL exchange.[29,43] Waring et al[9] also report the disappearance of CME following penetrating keratoplasty and reconstructive surgery, suggesting that removing the source of chronic inflammation and restoring anatomic relationships may ameliorate persistent macular edema.

**Table 9-2**   Secondary Posterior-Chamber Intraocular Lens Implantation in the Absence of Capsular Support

| Study | No. cases | Average followup (months) | Post-op visual acuity better than or equal to pre-op acuity | Complications |
|---|---|---|---|---|
| Stark et al[20] | 16 | 9 | 16/16 | Exposed polypropylene suture end causing irritation treated with the argon laser |
| Hu et al[14] | 6 | 8.2 | 5/6 | None |
| Agapitos and Lindstrom[15] | 5 | 2 | 4/5 | Slight decentration of the lens in 1 patient |
| Spigelmen et al[30] | 7 | 3 or greater | 7/7 | Exposed polypropylene sutures |

**Table 9-3**   IOL Exchanges through a Limbal Approach

| Study | No. cases | Average followup (months) | Post-op visual acuity better than or equal to pre-op acuity | Complications |
|---|---|---|---|---|
| Agapitos and Lindstrom[15] | 12 | 5 | 8/12 | Hyphema (2), vitreous hemorrhage (1), exposed polypropylene suture (1), elevated IOP (4), wound leak (1) |
| Stark et al[20] | 8 | 9 | 7/8 | Bleeding from corneoscleral incision (1) |

Results have been good and reported complications few with secondary posterior-chamber implants in either aphakia or with IOL exchange (Tables 9-2 and 9-3). No cases of retinal detachment, new clinically significant CME, or endophthalmitis have been reported to date. These results are encouraging, especially in view of the other series of secondary intraocular lens implantation *with* capsular support that have reported some cases of retinal detachments and CME.[17,21] We have several cases of documented angiographic and visual improvement of CME after secondary IOL exchange. Further followup is necessary to determine if other cases improve and if other complications develop.

Repositioning of posteriorly dislocated IOLs is relatively infrequently performed, and the largest series has recently been reported by Smiddy and Flynn.[48] They describe various techniques for retrieval and refixation of the IOLs in 32 cases. A final visual acuity of 20/40 or better was achieved in 79% of the repositioning cases and in 75% of the IOL-exchange cases. There were 3 cases of new CME and 2 cases of postoperative retinal detachment.

One case of endophthalmitis has been reported,[11] developing 5 months after scleral fixation sutures were used to reposition a traumatically dislocated IOL. In this case, a microabscess was identified at the site of the prolene suture. *Hemophilus influenza* was cultured. Scleral flaps were not used in this case.

The rate of CME after IOL repositioning appears to be relatively low.[48] Theoretically, removal of anterior vitreous connections to the limbal wound and iris at the time of pars plana vitrectomy may reduce the irritative stimulus to the disorder.

Visual prognosis after pars plana repositioning of a dislocated IOL appears to be very good.[48] Results are dependent on associated disorders, and, particularly in cases of trauma, other factors may limit visual return.

## References


1. Ridley H: Intraocular acrylic lenses—past, present and future. Trans Ophthalmol Soc UK 1964; 71:5.
2. Champion R, Green WR. Intraocular lenses: a histopathologic study of eyes, ocular tissue and intraocular lenses obtained surgically. Ophthalamol 1985; 92:1628-1645.
3. Apple DJ, Mamalis N, Loftfield K, et al. Complications of intraocular lenses: a historical and histopathologic review. Surv Ophthalmol 1984; 29:1-54.
4. Apple DJ, Brems RN, Park RB, et al. Anterior chamber lenses. Refract Surg 1987; 13:157-174.
5. Stark WJ, Worthen DM, Holladay JT, et al. The FDA report on intraocular lenses. Ophthalmol 1983; 90:311-317.
6. Kormznehl EW, Steinert RF, Odrich MG, Stevens JB. Penetrating keratoplasty for pseudophakic bullous keratopathy associated with closed-loop anterior chamber intraocular lenses. Ophthalmol 1990; 97:407-414.
7. Stark WJ, Sommer A, Smith RE. Changing trends in intraocular lens implantation. Arch Ophthalmol 1989; 107:1441-1444.
8. Hall JR, Muenzler WS. Intraocular lens replacement in pseudophakic bullous keratopathy. Trans Ophthalmol Soc UK 1985; 5:541-545.
9. Malbran ES, Malbran E Jr, Negri I. Lens guide suture for transport and fixation in secondary IOL implantation after intracapsular extraction. Int Ophthalmol 1986; 9:151-160.
10. Wong SK, Stark WJ, Gottsch JD, Bernitsky DA, McCartney DL. Use of posterior chamber lenses in pseudophakic bullous keratopathy. Arch Ophthalmol 1987; 105:856-858.
11. Heilskov T, Joondeph BC, Olsen KR, Blankenship GW. Late endophthalmitis after transscleral fixation of a posterior chamber intraocular lens. Arch Ophthalmol 1989; 107:1427.
12. Choyce DP. The Choyce Mark VIII and Mark IX anterior chamber implants. J Am Intraocul Implant Soc 1979; 5:217-221.
13. Gess LA. Scleral fixation for intraocular lenses. J Am Intraocul Implant Soc 1983; 9:453-456.
14. Hu BV, Shin DH, Dibbs A, Hong YJ. Implantation of posterior chamber lens in the absence of capsular and zonular support. Arch Ophthalmol 1988; 106:416-429.
15. Agapitos PJ, Lindstrom RL. Transscleral ciliary sulcus fixation of posterior chamber intraocular lens implants. Aust N Z J Ophthalmol 1989; 17:169-172.
16. van der Schaft TL, van Rig G, Renardel de Lavalette JG, Beekhuis WH. Results of penetrating keratoplasty for pseudophakic bullous keratopathy with the exchange of an intraocular lens. Br J Ophthalmol 1989; 73:704-708.
17. Mazzocco TR, Kratz RP, Davidson B, Colvard DM. Secondary posterior chamber intraocular lens implants. J Am Intraocul Implant Soc 1981; 7:341-343.
18. Shin DH, Hu BV, Hong YJ, Gibbs KA. Posterior chamber lens implantation in the absence of posterior capsular support. Ophthalmic Surg 1988; 19:606-607 (letter).
19. Stark WJ, Goodman G, Goodman D, Gottsch J: Posterior chamber intraocular lens implantation in the absence of posterior capsular support. Ophthalmic Surg 1988; 19:240-243.
20. Stark WJ, Gottsch JD, Goodman DF, Goodman GL, Pratzer K. Posterior chamber intraocular lens implantation in the absence of capsular support. Arch Ophthalmol 1989; 107:1078-1083.
21. Lindstrom RL, Harris WS, Lyle WA. Secondary and exchange posterior chamber lens implantation. J Am Intraocul Implant Soc 1982; 8:353-356.
22. Dahan E, Salmenson BD, Levin J. Ciliary sulcus reconstruction for posterior implantation in the absence of an intraocular posterior capsule. J Ophthalmic Surg 1989; 20:776-780.
23. Terry AC, Stark WJ. Removal of closed-loop anterior chamber lens implants. Ophthalmic Surg 1984; 15:575-577.
24. Bleckman H, Hanuschik W, Vogt R. Implantation of posterior chamber lenses in eyes with phacodenesis and lens subluxation. J Cataract Refract Surg 1990; 16:788.
25. Sternberg P Jr, Michels RG. Treatment of dislocated posterior chamber intraocular lenses. Arch Ophthalmol 1986; 104:1391-1393.
26. Smiddy WE. Dislocated posterior chamber intraocular lens. a new technique of management. Arch Ophthalmol 1989; 107:1678-1680.
27. Insler MS, Mani H, Peyman GA. A new surgical technique for dislocated posterior chamber intraocular lenses. Ophthalmic Surg 1988; 19:480-481.
28. Stark WJ, Bruner WE, Martin NF. Management of subluxed posterior chamber intraocular lenses. Ophthalmic Surg 1982; 13:130-133.
29. Soong HK, Musch DC, Kowal V, et al. Implantation of posterior chamber intraocular lenses in the absence of lens capsule during penetrating keratoplasty. Arch Ophthalmol 1989; 107:660-675.

30. Spigelman AV, Lindstrom RL, Nichols BD, Lindquist TD, Lane SS. Implantation of a posterior chamber lens without capsular support during penetrating keratoplasty or as a secondary lens implant. Ophthalmic Surg 1988; 19:396-398.

31. Anand R, Brown RW. Simplified technique for suturing dislocated posterior chamber intraocular lens to the ciliary sulcus. Arch Ophthalmol 1990; 108:1205-1206.

32. Drews RC. Posterior chamber lens implantation during keratoplasty without posterior lens capsule support. Cornea 1987; 6:38-40.

33. Busin M, Branweiler PK, Boker T, Spitznas M. Complications of sulcus-supported intraocular lenses with iris sutures, implanted during penetrating keratoplasty after intracapsular cataract extraction. Ophthalmol 1990; 97:401-406.

34. Koch DD. New optic hole configuration for iris fixation of posterior chamber lenses. Arch Ophthalmol 1988; 106:163-164(letter).

35. Price FW Jr, Whitson WE. Visual results of suture-fixated posterior chamber lenses during penetrating keratoplasty. Ophthalmol 1989; 96:1234-1239, discussion 1239-1240.

36. Alpar JJ. Use of the Ethicon 1713 suture for McCannel suturing. J Am Intraocul Implant Soc 1985; 11:296-298.

37. Cowden JW, Hu BV. A new surgical technique for posterior chamber lens fixation during penetrating keratoplasty in the absence of capsular or zonular support. Cornea 1988; 6:231-235.

38. Insler MS, Kook MS, Kaufman HE. Penetrating keratoplasty for pseudophakic bullous keratopathy associated with semiflexible, closed-loop anterior chamber intraocular lenses. Am J Ophthalmol 1989; 15:252-256.

39. Waring GO III, Stulting RD, Street D: Penetrating keratoplasty for corneal edema with exchange of intraocular lenses. Arch Ophthalmol 1987; 105:58-62.

40. Zaidman GW, Goldman S: A prospective study on the implantation of anterior chamber intraocular lenses during keratoplasty for pseudophakic and aphakic bullous keratopathy. Ophthalmol 1990; 97:757-762.

41. Duffey RJ, Holland EJ, Agapitos PJ, Lindstrom RL. Anatomic study of transclerally sutured intraocular lens implantation. Am J Ophthalmol 1989; 15:300-309.

42. Apple DJ, Price FW, Gwin T, et al. Sutured retropupillary posterior chamber intraocular lenses for exchange or secondary implantation. The 12th annual Binkhorst lecture, 1988. Ophthalmol 1989; 96:1241-1247.

43. Price FW, Whitson WE. Natural history of cystoid macular edema in pseudophakic bullous keratopathy. J Cataract Refract Surg 1990; 16:163-169.

44. Lubniewski AJ, Holland EJ, VanMeter WJ, Gussler D, Pearlman J, Smith ME. Histologic study of eyes with transsclerally sutured posterior chamber intraocular lenses. Am J Ophthalmol 1990; 110: 237-243.

45. Maus M, Sivalingam E: Alternative method for sulcus fixation of posterior chamber lenses in the absence of capsular support. Ophthalmic Surg 1989; 20:476-479.

46. Traykovski A. Secondary lens implantation with sulcus fixation in intracapsular aphakes. J Cataract Refract Surg 1990; 16:367-368.

47. Hassan TS, Soong HK, Sugar A, et al. Implantation of Kelman-style, open-loop anterior chamber lenses during keratoplasty for aphakia and bullous keratopathy (a comparison with iris-sutured posterior chamber lenses). Ophthalmology 1991; 98:875-880.

48. Smiddy WE, Flynn HW. Management of dislocated posterior chamber intraocular lenses. Ophthalmol 1991; 98:889-894.

49. McCannel MA. A retrievable suture idea for anterior uveal problems. Ophthalmic Surg 1976; 7: 98-103.

# 10 Foldable Intraocular Lenses

John S. Parker, MD
Robert W. Panton, MD
Walter J. Stark, MD

Today, more than 20 years since the introduction of phacoemulsification, only a minority of ophthalmologists employ the technique for routine cataract extraction.[1] Despite the slow proliferation of phacoemulsification, it continues to gain in popularity more swiftly than ever.[1,2] Intraocular lens development, while truly remarkable, has been the limiting factor retarding further reduction of cataract wound size and thus inhibiting further benefits from the technique. A Food and Drug Administration (FDA) premarket approved (PMA) lens is available now that allows cataract extraction and lens implantation to be performed through wounds of 4.0 mm. PMA lenses may soon be available that would permit the use of wounds as small as 3.0 mm. Only foldable lenses are in a position to take full advantage of wound sizes in these ranges.

Not surprisingly, controversy surrounds the use of today's foldable lenses. It has been suggested that oval all-polymethylmethacrylate (PMMA) lenses designed for insertion through 5- to 6-mm incisions offer most of the advantages of the foldable lenses with few of their drawbacks.[3] Long-term experience with foldable lenses of any type is minimal in comparison with that available on today's posterior-chamber PMMA lenses.

## Prerequisites

Foldable lenses are not suitable for all surgeons or all patients, but they offer certain advantages when appropriately utilized. At a minimum, the surgeon should be comfortable performing phacoemulsification with continuous-tear anterior capsulotomy. There should be no radial tearing of the anterior capsule, and the capsular opening should be smooth and between 4.5 and 6.0 mm in diameter. The posterior capsule should be intact, and there should not be evidence of significant zonular weakness. Since the optic in currently available foldable lenses is less than 6.5 mm in diameter, we prefer to use these lenses in eyes with relatively miotic pupils. If sphincterotomy is required, we close the pupil with 10-0 polypropylene (Prolene) suture following lens implantation.

## Advantages of Small-Incision Surgery

There are a number of theoretical advantages to be obtained from minimizing cataract wound size. Clinical study supports the common sense notion that visual rehabilitation occurs significantly earlier in patients with a 4-mm wound compared with patients with 6- or 7-mm wounds regardless of wound closure technique.[4,5] Long-term wound slippage, with resulting against-the-rule astigmatism, might be expected to be less of a problem with smaller incisions as well.

A smaller cataract wound means a more resilient globe, should significant trauma be experienced postoperatively. Such resilience is particularly significant in patients whose wound healing might reasonably be expected to be abnormal, as in the elderly patient taking systemic steroids. Cataract wound size and location are likely to be of more critical import in patients with working filtering blebs and in those patients taking anticoagulants.

We have been pleased with the short-term results of foldable silicone intraocular lens use in combined cataract extraction trabeculectomy procedures. Conjunctival closure is less critical and is easily and efficiently managed with a 4-mm scleral wound and a 6-mm peritomy. Since silicone contact is significantly less damaging to corneal endothelium than is PMMA contact,[6] the consequences of a flat anterior chamber postoperatively might well be ameliorated.

## Incision and Closure

Smaller wound size and more posterior-wound location are both associated with less change in corneal curvature following cataract surgery. Recent studies suggest that horizontal "one-stitch" or "no-stitch" wound closure minimizes induced with-the-rule astigmatism associated with small-incision cataract surgery.[7,8] It should be noted, however, that the FDA has not permitted foldable lens manufacturers to claim that a reduced amount of induced corneal astigmatism will result from the use of foldable lenses in cataract surgery with intraocular lens (IOL) implantation. Promotional aspects of "one-stitch" or "no-stitch" techniques may be partially responsible for their increasing popularity in the ophthalmic community.

It is worth noting that the one adverse finding of the CORE study associated with today's FDA-PMA foldable lens was an increased incidence of transient hyphema as compared with the FDA's grid.[9] The hyphemas were not associated with permanent sequela. An increased frequency of transient hyphema is known to be linked with posterior-wound location and it is possible, if not likely, that the finding noted by the CORE study was not related to the lens at all, only to a tendency of surgeons to place small incisions more posteriorly than they would conventional incisions.

A small incision will minimize induced corneal astigmatism for any given wound location. Unless the cataract surgery is to be combined with trabeculectomy, we fashion a scleral tunnel at approximately one-half scleral thickness beginning about 2 mm posterior to the posterior limbus. We prefer not to go more than about 2 mm posterior to the posterior limbus in most patients, simply in order to facilitate the phacoemulsification and to minimize the chance of postoperative hyphema. Since the long-term effect of sutureless surgery is not known, we close all incisions, generally, with 10-0 nylon. Our experience is that induced astigmatism seems to be minimal, regardless of how such small incisions are closed.

## LENS TYPES

There are two fundamental types of foldable intraocular lenses: one-piece lenses and three-piece lenses. This distinction effectively divides lenses into two groups based on both appearance and clinical characteristics.

## Three-Piece Lenses

Three-piece lenses differ from conventional posterior-chamber lenses primarily in optic composition. Most look like conventional PMMA lenses with polypropylene haptics. The optic is typically colorless and 6.0 to 6.5 mm in diameter when unfolded. The characteristics for the following lenses are shown in the box on p. 148.

The only FDA-PMA foldable lens presently available is Allergan Medical Optics' (AMO's) SI-18. The lens costs 50% to 100% more than typical PMMA lenses. Use of the disposable Prodigy insertion device adds up to another $25 to the cost of each case.

The SI-18 can be inserted through a 4.0-mm incision, which means that the original 3- to 3.5-mm phaco incision must be enlarged prior to lens implantation. While not difficult, it requires learning new maneuvers with new equipment.

We do prefer to use AMO's Prodigy device for insertion of the SI-18 although a number of other options are available. The lens can be inserted unfolded through a 5.5- to 6.0-mm wound. Bar-type folders have been largely replaced by specialized lens forceps, such as the Faulkner folder, which are loaded while the lens is secured by a second "holding" forceps prior to folding. We have found foldable-lens insertion with tube-type folders, such as the Prodigy device, to be more controlled than with the various forceps.

Two Prodigy inserters are available for use with the AMO lenses: the Pro-1A and the Pro-1B. The Pro-1A device is useful when inserting lenses of 12 to 21.5 diopter power. Since SI-18 optic-center thickness increases with increasing diopteric strength, a second tube folder is required for use with the thicker lenses (22 to 24 diopter).

We have found the Prodigy device to be quite reliable at placing both haptics in the capsular bag when used as described. It is important to note, however, that considerable stress is placed on the posterior capsule when the SI-18 is extruded from the Prodigy device. Lens placement with such tube-type folders is contraindicated if an opening is present in the posterior capsule.

Although premarket approval of the SI-18 was for both bag and sulcus placement, we would not recommend using any 6-mm lens with polypropylene haptics for bag-sulcus or sulcus-sulcus fixation. Our current minimum prerequisites for SI-18 use include: (1) a continuous smooth anterior capsulotomy, thus minimizing the possibility of a radial tear in the anterior capsule, and (2) zonular strength adequate to maintain a capsular bag position of 360°. Both prerequisites help to insure that the 6.0 mm optic will remain centered.

AMO has two other foldable lenses that have not yet received FDA approval. The first is the SI-20, which, like the SI-18, has a biconvex silicone optic. Another AMO lens, the PC-28, has haptics like the SI-18. The optic of the PC-28, though, contains a rectangular 3-mm × 6-mm PMMA window. On either side of the PMMA

### Three-Piece Foldable Lens Characteristics

| Model | Optic | Haptics |
|---|---|---|
| AMO SI-18 | 6.0-mm biconvex<br>Silicone elastomer<br>UV-blocker | Modified "J" polypropylene<br>Osher tip<br>14-mm overall diameter<br>10° angulation |
| AMO SI-20 | 6.5-mm biconvex<br>Silicone elastomer<br>UV-blocker | Modified "C" polypropylene<br>Notch in superior haptic<br>14-mm overall diameter<br>10° angulation |
| AMO PC-28 | 3-mm × 6-mm plano-<br>convex<br>PMMA<br>UV-blocker | Modified "J" polypropylene<br>Osher tip<br>14-mm overall diameter<br>10° angulation |
| STAAR<br>Elastimide | 6.3-mm biconvex RMX3<br>Silicone elastomer<br>No UV-blocker | Polyimide<br>Modified "C" or "J"<br>No loops or nothces<br>13.5-mm overall diameter<br>Angled or planar |

**Potenital Problems with Foldable Lenses**

- Expense
- Early posterior-capsule opacification
- Difficulty performing YAG capsulotomy
- Dislocation into the vitreous following YAG capsulotomy
- Decentration
- Refolding after implantation
- Accumulation of proteinaceous or cellular deposits
- Lack of a UV filter in some lenses
- Interference with posterior segment visualization following air-fluid exchange

window is an opaque foldable wing such that the shape of the optic, when taken as a whole composed of PMMA and foldable wings, is circular with a 6-mm diameter.

STAAR Surgical Company also offers a number of three-piece lenses that are referred to as "Elastimide" lenses. All of the lenses feature a 6.3-mm biconvex silicone optic capable of being folded before insertion. These lenses are unique in that the haptics are made of polyimide rather than polypropylene as in the AMO lenses. The lenses are available with "J" or "C" type haptic design with each design offering the option of a vaulted or nonvaulted haptic attachment. STAAR offers lens powers ranging from 16 to 25 diopters in 0.5 diopter increments. Lenses of 18 diopter strength and higher have the same center thickness. The RMX3 silicone polymer used in the optic does not contain a UV-blocker.

## One-Piece Lenses

Lens design and size, capsular integrity, and capsulotomy size are of critical importance with one-piece lenses. As a result, one-piece lenses have been associated with problems relating to difficulty maintaining stable lens position. Lenses placed in the ciliary sulcus have had propellering and pigment-dispersion problems. These problems have largely disappeared with capsular bag implantation of appropriately sized lenses, using the continuous-tear anterior-capsulotomy technique to protect the integrity of the peripheral anterior capsule.[10] Early one-piece lenses had problems resisting deformation secondary to capsular contraction when implanted in the capsular bag.

STAAR Surgical has developed a one-piece lens that has been recommended for premarket approval pending receipt of further data by the FDA. FDA approval of the lens was recommended contingent on placement of the lens in a capsular bag with a smooth continuous-tear anterior capsulotomy without radial tearing. Lens implantation is contraindicated if doubt exists about the integrity of the anterior capsulotomy with regard to its susceptibility to radial tearing. An unacceptably high rate of lens decentration has been associated with placement of these lenses in capsular bags with anterior radial tears. The lens is the Model AA-4203 "Elastic" lens, which is made of STAAR's RMX3 silicone polymer. Overall length is 10.5 mm with an integral 6.0-mm diameter biconvex optic. The haptics are solid silicone elastomer with central positioning holes. The lens has been reported to induce minimal capsular fibrosis, and the fibrosis that is induced seems to be relatively isolated to the positioning holes.[11] Early reports suggest that the lens has not experienced significant deformation or decentration problems when implanted in a properly opened capsular bag. Center thickness is constant in lenses of 18.0 diopter and greater power. A prominent advantage of this lens is that it is capable of being inserted through a 3- to 3.2-mm opening, thus eliminating the need to enlarge the wound following phacoemulsification. STAAR offers two reusable tube-type inserters for use with the AA-4203.

No current insertion device is capable of placing both haptics of a one-piece lens inside of a capsular bag. Typically, the inferior haptic is placed inside the capsular bag and a separate two-handed maneuver with hooks is used to place the superior haptic in the bag, while taking care to avoid making a radial tear in the anterior capsule.

## Posterior Capsulotomy and Foldable Lenses

One- and three-piece silicone lenses have been associated with early, extensive capsular fibrosis, and significant difficulty performing posterior YAG capsulotomy has been reported.[3,12,13] Studies have suggested that injection-molded biconvex lenses, whether made of silicone or PMMA, tend to be more easily damaged by a YAG laser than lathe-cut PMMA lenses.[14,15]

Many surgeons, even those quite skilled at performing capsulotomy with conventional lenses, seem to require a learning period in order to perform YAG capsulotomy in eyes with silicone lenses without lens pitting. We prefer to perform YAG capsulotomy on eyes with three-piece silicone lenses earlier than we would on eyes with a PMMA lens, thus making the capsulotomy easier and subjecting the lens to less risk of pitting. We have found deep focus techniques and use of a contact lens to be particularly important in further reducing the likelihood of YAG laser pitting of silicone lenses.

Posterior capsular opacification has been reported to be uncommon following implantation of the one-piece STAAR AA-4203 in the capsular bag.[16,17] The lens has reportedly been associated with dislocation into the vitreous following early posterior capsulotomy.[11] A one-piece hydrogel lens (IOGEL) was recently withdrawn from the market after a persistent problem with dislocation into the vitreous following YAG capsulotomy was demonstrated. There is little capsular-lens fibrosis with either the all hydrogel lenses or the all silicone one-piece lenses. Current recommendations for one-piece silicone lenses are to: 1) minimize the size of the anterior and posterior capsulotomies, and to 2) delay YAG capsulotomy for at least twelve weeks postoperatively in order to minimize the chance for posterior dislocation of the lens following YAG capsulotomy.[11]

## MISCELLANEOUS CONCERNS
### Uveitis and Cellular Accumulation

FDA CORE studies of the AMO SI-18 and the STAAR Elastic and Elastimide lenses have failed to demonstrate an increased frequency of iritis or uveitis with these lenses as compared with the FDA's 1983 grid.[11,19,20] Conflicting data has been published regarding the ability of silicone to activate the alternative complement pathway in human sera.[21,22]

One study has shown that silicone lenses are more likely to accumulate cellular deposits than are all PMMA lenses when both are implanted in the mouse peritoneal space.[23] Studies of lenses implanted in animal eyes, however, have consistently shown equal or less cellular accumulation on silicone lenses as compared to PMMA lenses.[23-28]

### Condensation

Condensation on silicone IOLs following the air-fluid exchange of posterior segment surgery has been reported to result in transient difficulty visualizing the retina.[29] We prefer not to use silicone lenses in eyes at high risk for retinal detachment.

## RESULTS

Visual acuity data from the foldable lenses mentioned in this summary have generally compared favorably with the FDA's 1983 grid of historical data. For example, 513 patients were followed postoperatively for 12 to 14 months in the CORE study of AMO's SI-18. Ninety-two percent of these patients had a final visual acuity of 20/40 or better, compared with only 84% of the patients in the FDA grid.

It can be argued that surgical technique has improved considerably since 1983 and that the population of patients and surgeons in the FDA grid, or even in the FDA Report on Intraocular Lenses,[18] are not directly comparable to those used in CORE studies. Nevertheless, early visual acuity data for today's foldable lenses is in line with expectations.

### The Future

Expansile hydrogels and moisture-sensitive folded acrylics are materials of which future foldable lenses may be composed. Their future, like that of the one-piece

IOGEL lens, involves considerably more uncertainty than the lenses discussed here.

## SUMMARY

Minimization of cataract wound size has been a persistent focus in the refinement of ophthalmic surgical technique. Today, the smallest cataract wounds obtainable, with concomitant lens implantation, are achieved through the use of foldable intraocular lenses. Although only one lens has received FDA premarket approval at the time of this writing, several other fairly similar lenses seem to be close to FDA-PMA. None of the foldable lenses have track records that would permit long-term comparison with conventional posterior-chamber PMMA IOLs. Early findings suggest that foldable silicone lenses can be safe and effective when implanted in stable capsular bags opened anteriorly in a smooth continuous fashion.

## References

1. Leaming DV. Practice styles and preferences of ASCRS members—1989 survey. J Cataract Refract Surg 1989; 16:624-632.
2. Leaming DV. Practice styles and preferences of ASCRS members—1988 survey. J Cataract Refract Surg 1988; 15:689-697.
3. Neumann AC, Cobb B. Advantages and limitations of current soft intraocular lenses. J Cataract Refract Surg 1987; 15:257-263.
4. Brint SF, Ostrick DM, Bryan JE. Keratometruc cylinder and visual performance following phacoemulsification and implantation with silicone small-incision or poly(methylmethacrylate) intraocular lenses. J Cataract Refract Surg 1991; 17:32-36.
5. Steinert RF, Brint SL, Fine IH, White SM. The effect of 4.0 mm vs. 6.5 mm incisions on visual acuity and astigmatism: a prospective, randomized trial. 1990 Annual Meeting, American Academy of Ophthalmol.
6. Herzog WR, Peiffer RL Jr. Comparison of the effect of polymethylmethacrylate and silicone intraocular lenses on rabbit corneal endothelium in vitro. J Cataract Refract Surg 1987; 13:397-400.
7. Sanders DR, Shepherd J, Ernest PH, Fine IH, Maloney WF. Effect of incision size and suture configuration on induced astigmatism and visual rehabilitation. In Gills JP, Sanders DR, eds, Small-Incision Cataract Surgery. Thorofare, NJ: Slack 1990:15-28.
8. Gills JP. Sutureless cataract surgery. In Gills JP, Sanders DR. eds, Small-Incision Cataract Surgery. Thorofare, NJ: Slack, 1990:127-140.
9. Summary of safety and effectiveness data, FDA premarket approval application for the AMO SI-18.
10. Shepherd JR. Continuous-tear capsulotomy and insertion of a silicone bag lens. J Cataract Refract Surg 1989; 15:335-339.
11. Grabow HB, Sanders DR. Implantation of STAAR AA-4203 single-piece silicone lens. In Gills JP, Sanders DR, eds, Small-Incision Cataract Surgery. Thorofare, NJ: Slack 1990:29-56.
12. Milauskas AT. Posterior capsule opacification after silicone lens implantation and its management. J Cataract Refract Surg 1987; 13:644-648.
13. Levy JH, Pisacano AM. Initial clinical studies with silicone intraocular implants. J Cataract Refract Surg 1988; 14:294-298.
14. Bath PE, Romberger AB, Brown P. A comparison of Nd:YAG laser damage thresholds for PMMA and silicone intraocular lenses. Invest Ophthalmol Vis Sci 1986; 27:795-798.
15. Downing JE, Alberhasky MT. Biconvex intraocular lenses and Nd:YAG capsulotomy: experimental comparison of surface damage with different poly(methyl methacrylate) formulations. J Cataract Refract Surg 1990; 16:732-736.
16. Milauskas AT. Capsular bag fixation of one-piece silicone lenses. J Cataract Refract Surg 1990; 16:583-586.
17. Shepherd JR. Capsular opacification associated with silicone implants. J Cataract Refract Surg 1989; 15:448-450.
18. Stark WJ, Worthen DM, et al. The FDA report on intraocular lenses. Ophthalmology 1983; 90:311-317.
19. Lindstrom RL. SI-18 three-piece foldable silicone IOL for small-incision cataract surgery. In Gills JP, Sanders DR, eds, Small-Incision Cataract Surgery. Thorofare, NJ: Slack, 1990:57-88.
20. Utrata PJ. Implantation of STAAR three-piece silicone Elastimide lens. In Gills JP, Sanders DR, eds,

Small-Incision Cataract Surgery. Thorofare, NJ: Slack, 1990:89-101.

21. Mondino BJ, Rajacich GM, Sumner H. Comparison of complement activation by silicone intraocular lenses and polymethylmethacrylate intraocular lenses with polypropylene loops. Arch Ophthalmol 1987; 105:989-990.

22. Gobel RJ, Janatova J, et al. Activation of complement in human serum by some synthetic polymers used for intraocular lenses. Biomaterials 1987; 8:285-288.

23. Uenoyama K, Tamura M, et al. Experimental intraocular lens implantation in the rabbit eye and in the mouse peritoneal space. Part IV. cell adhesion, fibroblast-like cell, and lymphocytic cluster observed on the implanted lens surface. J Cataract Refract Surg 1989; 15:559-566.

24. Cook CS, Peiffer RL Jr, Mazzocco TR. Clinical and pathologic evaluation of a flexible silicone posterior chamber lens design in a rabbit model. J Cataract Refract Surg 1986; 12:130-134.

25. Buchen SY, Richards SC, et al. Evaluation of the biocompatibility and fixation of a new silicone intraocular lens in the feline model. J Cataract Refract Surg 1989; 15:545-553.

26. Kulnig W, Menapace R, et al. Tissue reaction after silicone and poly(methylmethacrylate) intraocular lens implantation: a light and electron microscopy study in a rabbit model. J Cataract Refract Surg 1989; 15:510-518.

27. Menapace R, Skorpik C, et al. Clinicopathologic findings after in-the-bag implantation of open-loop polymethylmethacrylate and silicone lenses in the rabbit eye. J Cataract Refract Surg 1987; 13:630-634.

28. Fogle JA, Blaydes JE, et al. Clinicopathologic observations of a silicone posterior chamber lens in a primate model. J Cataract Refract Surg 1986; 12:281-284.

29. Condensation. Ocular Surgery News Nov 15, 1990:3.

# 11 Clinical Glare Testing

**Gary S. Rubin, PhD**

There has been a surge of interest during the past decade in clinical tests of glare sensitivity. The principal motivation has been the need to document visual disability in cataract patients with mildly reduced Snellen visual acuity. Clinical vision tests are usually administered under controlled illumination conditions that are unrepresentative of real-world situations. Glare-sensitivity tests subject the visual system to some of the demands encountered in everyday life and are now routinely used by many clinicians in the evaluation of visual function.

## Types of Glare

*Glare* can refer to a variety of phenomena. *Discomfort glare* refers to the sensation one experiences when the overall illumination is too bright, for example when the midday sun is reflected from sand or snow. In extreme cases, discomfort glare may result in pain or photophobia. In milder cases, it is sometimes referred to as photoaversion.

*Disability glare* refers to the reduced visibility of a target due to the presence of a light source elsewhere in the visual field. A common example is the reduced visibility of road signs in the presence of oncoming headlights. Disability glare occurs when light from the glare source is scattered by the ocular media. This scattered light forms a veiling luminance which reduces the contrast and thus the visibility of the target. This effect is simulated in Figure 11-1. On the left is a bar pattern (below) with its luminance profile (above). The contrast of the pattern can be defined in several ways, but generally refers to the difference between the luminance of the target and background relative to the average luminance of the scene. The bar pattern on the left of Figure 11-1 has a contrast of 80%. On the right, scattered light raises the luminance of the target and background by the same amount. This reduces the contrast to 50%. Most tests of glare sensitivity are intended to measure disability glare.

*Glare recovery* is a measure of the speed with which the visual system regains function following exposure to a bright light. Any disorder which alters the dynamics of light and dark adaptation may affect glare recovery. Photostress tests are designed to measure glare recovery, but as we shall see, some disability-glare tests may also be affected by glare recovery.

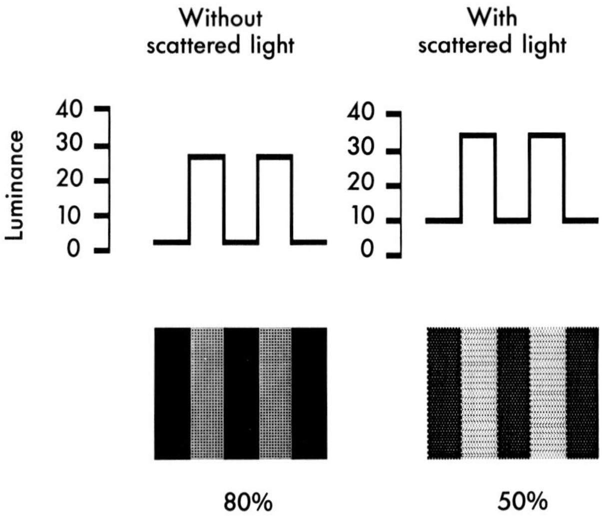


**FIGURE 11-1**    Disability glare is depicted in terms of a veiling luminance. Left panel, The appearance of a bar pattern (below) and its luminance profile (above) in the absence of glare. Right panel, The contrast of the bar pattern is reduced when light scattered from a glare source adds to the target and its background.

## Discomfort Glare

Photophobia and photoaversion are reported in a variety of disorders as diverse as uveitis, ocular albinism, and cone-rod dystrophies. Although there are many anecdotal reports in the literature, there have been few studies of characteristics or causes of the problem. Gawande et al[1] showed that patients with retinitis pigmentosa more often complain of sensitivity to light and trouble seeing in bright sun than patients without ocular pathology. But the patients' problems were not due to supersensitivity to light, per se. Instead, they were traced to reduced-contrast sensitivity in the presence of glare light (disability glare), and slower glare recovery. In the laboratory, discomfort glare is measured by having the patient adjust the brightness of a light source until it reaches an ill-defined threshold of unpleasantness. Even though discomfort glare may figure prominently in the complaints of many patients, there are no practical instruments for clinical assessment of the problem.

## Disability Glare

### Causes of disability glare

Any factor that increases intraocular light scatter may initiate problems caused by disability glare. In normal eyes, glare sensitivity remains fairly constant until about 40 to 45 years of age, after which it begins to increase rapidly.[2] This increase has been attributed to several factors including lens fluorescence which converts incident ultraviolet light into scattered blue light, yellowing of the lens and senile miosis which reduce target illumination at the retina, and "subclinical" lens opacities which scatter light.

Disability glare has been extensively investigated in cataract patients. Hirsch et al[3] compared glare sensitivity, visual acuity, and contrast sensitivity in 186 normal, cataractous, and aphakic eyes. Glare sensitivity was markedly increased in the cataractous eyes, even when adjusted for differences in visual acuity and contrast sensitivity. Glare sensitivity is reported to be correlated with visual acuity in cases of nuclear or cortical opacities, but not in eyes with posterior subcapsular cataracts.[4] Few studies have looked at the improvement in glare sensitivity following cataract extraction. Masket[5] tested 30 eyes of 26 patients before and after phacoemulsifaction with posterior-chamber intraocular lens (PC IOL) implantation. Patients were selected to have 20/20 acuity postsurgically, with clean capsules and no macular abnormalities. Under these best-case conditions, glare-disability scores improved significantly as a result of cataract surgery. Several studies[6,7,8,9] have shown glare sensitivity to be higher in patients with PC IOLs compared to normal controls. However, none of these studies ruled out posterior capsular opacification as the cause of the glare problem. In fact, glare sensitivity is correlated with percent opacification of the capsule,[7] and glare sensitivity is improved following Nd:YAG capsulotomy.[10]

In the normal eye, 70% of intraocular light scatter occurs in the lens, with most of the remaining 30% contributed by the cornea. However, a variety of conditions can cause abnormally high corneal scattering. Keratoconus and corneal edema have been shown to increase glare sensitivity.[11] Experimental studies with induced corneal edema indicate that epithelial edema produces more forward light scatter and is more visually debilitating than stromal edema, even though the latter causes more overall corneal thickening.[12]

The effect of radial keratotomy (RK) on disability glare remains controversial. The PERK study failed to document any significant increase in glare following surgery.[13] But Applegate et al[14] demonstrated a significant increase in glare sensitivity when patients were tested under mesopic light conditions similar to that encountered in nighttime driving. With greater pupil dilation caused by low illumination, areas of the cornea outside the 3-mm clear zone may have contributed more scattered light than in conventional glare testing.

The normal vitreous scatters less than 1% of incident light. But vitreous opacities can significantly increase light scatter and glare sensitivity.[15] Dieter et al[16] reported increased glare sensitivity in patients treated with diathermy for retinal detachment. The increase was correlated with increased vitreous turbidity as visualized during slit-lamp examination.

Another possible source of disability glare is intraocular light scatter at the retinal level caused by macular edema. Unless the edematous tissue is perfectly clear and of the same refractive index as the surrounding fluid and tissue, one might expect it to scatter light. However, since the scattering centers are very close to the image plane, the effect is probably negligible. Verriest and Uvijls[15] reported increased glare sensitivity in diabetic patients with macular edema. However, we found glare sensitivity to be more closely related to lenticular opacities than to the amount of edema.[17]

## Measurement of disability glare

Most disability glare tests are simple in concept. A conventional visual-function test, usually acuity or contrast sensitivity, is administered in the presence of a glare source. The glare source can be a spot, bar, or ring of light, or an extended bright background. The disability-glare score is usually the ratio of performance without glare to performance with glare. This partially factors out differences between patients on the basic visual function being tested (e.g., differences in baseline acuity).

Many glare tests assess the effects of a glare light on contrast sensitivity, either by measuring contrast sensitivity for sinewave gratings or by obtaining a contrast threshold for the detection of optotype targets. Why is a contrast detection task so often used to measure glare sensitivity? The main reason stems from the fact that disability glare can be modelled in terms of a veiling luminance scattered into the test target from the glare source. The veiling luminance effectively reduces image contrast. Since the amount of scattered glare light will determine the magnitude of the contrast reduction, it makes sense to measure contrast sensitivity in order to assess disability glare.

Visual acuity can also be used to measure disability glare because acuity is affected by the contrast of the acuity targets. For a standard letter recognition test, however, acuity is related to contrast by a square-root law. That is, if the contrast is reduced by a factor of 2, acuity will be reduced by the root of 2 or a factor of 1.4.[18] Factors that reduce contrast, such as glare, will have a relatively weak effect on acuity. In a study of glare sensitivity with simulated ocular turbidity, the glare light caused contrast sensitivity to decline rapidly, while visual acuity remained near normal.[19] Therefore, tests based on contrast sensitivity measures should be more sensitive to disability glare than tests based on acuity. The sensitivity of acuity-based glare tests can be improved by either reducing the contrast of the acuity targets or increasing the intensity of the glare source.

In addition to differences in the visual function measured, glare tests vary in the type of glare source used. Most of the early studies used point-source glare. This type of glare source requires simple instrumentation (usually a single light bulb), provides a good simulation of environmental glare sources, such as automobile headlights, and is amenable to simple models of veiling luminance. However, small glare sources require a relatively high luminous intensity to produce the desired effect and tend to draw the observer's fixation away from the target to the glare light.[20] This can result in an afterimage, which may interfere with the visual function measurement. In essence, the disability glare test is turned into a measurement of glare recovery. Extended glare sources, such as a bright annulus produced by a circular fluorescent tube or a bright rectangular background, cause fewer afterimage problems and are said to be better accepted by patients.[18]

Intensities of the glare sources also vary widely from study to study. The Miller-Nadler glare tester,[6] the first such device commercially available in the United States, uses a 1300 cd/m² bright background that the authors compare to the luminance of new snow on a sunny day. At the other extreme, Applegate tested patients with point-source glare that could be as dim as 0.3 cd/m².[13] Two studies have systematically varied glare intensity. Abrahamsson and Sjostrand[20] reported that glare sensitivity in patients with posterior subcapsular (PSC) cataracts increased as luminance of an annular glare source was increased from 2 cd/m² to 200 cd/m². However, Applegate[14] found that lower glare intensities increased glare sensitivity in RK patients. These discrepant findings are probably due to the interaction of pupil size with the pathological cause of light scatter. PSC cataracts are usually centered in the pupil. Bright glare light constricts the pupil, causing a larger proportion of the imaged rays to pass through the cataract. RK produces scars away from the center of the pupil. Under dim illumination the pupil dilates admitting more rays, which have passed through the scars.

Regardless of the visual function test or glare source chosen, there are several basic principles of clinical vision test design that should be followed. First, the test should be "criterion-free." That is, the test results should not be affected by whether the subject is more or less cautious in his or her responses. Tests that allow the patient to decide if the target is visible will produce different results for an individual who is very cautious and demands that the target be clearly discernible before venturing a response, compared to the patient who is willing to guess at anything. Forced-choice procedures circumvent this problem. A standard eye chart uses a forced-choice procedure when the patient is asked to identify the letters (to make a "forced choice") and the examiner determines whether the answers are correct or incorrect. If the patient is allowed to answer that he or she cannot see the letter, then the test is not forced-choice. Forced-choice tests yield more reliable results than criterion-dependent tests, especially with unpracticed observers.[21,22]

Second, the test targets should follow a uniform progression. For acuity targets this means that letter size should decrease in equal logarithmic steps. For contrast sensitivity, target contrast should decline in equal logarithmic steps. Uniform step size is important for making quantitative comparisons, such as comparing glare sensitivity before and after cataract surgery across patients who may have different baseline sensitivities. Surprisingly, many Snellen acuity charts do not follow a uniform progression of letter sizes although the ETDRS acuity chart,[23] which is quickly becoming a clinical standard, adheres to this principle.

Finally, to ensure high test-retest reliability, it is necessary to have several trials at each level of difficulty, and an appropriate scoring procedure must be used. If the test is to be scored by the line (e.g., 20/20 vs. 20/40) then requiring two correct responses out of three trials provides an optimal compromise between test efficiency and reliability.[24] However, the sensitivity of the test is improved by giving partial credit for each correct answer (e.g., counting the number of correctly identified letters on an acuity test). In order to make sense of the score, the test must follow a uniform progression with a constant number of trials at each level of difficulty. The ETDRS acuity chart and the Pelli-Robson letter sensitivity chart[23] meet both of these criteria.

## Clinical utility of disability glare tests

Glare tests have been promoted for a variety of clinical purposes. As a diagnostic tool, its utility is limited. Obviously, the clinician does not need a glare test in order to diagnose a cataract or corneal disorder. However, it is not always clear whether the patient's visual impairment can be accounted for entirely by the anterior segment pathology or is caused in part by retinal or neural disease. Glare testing might help in these ambiguous situations, but there have not been any clinical studies to address this issue. Instead, most clinicians rely on various potential acuity tests to "bypass" the eye's cloudy optics. (See Odom et al[25] and Rubin[26] for reviews of potential acuity tests.)

Disability glare tests show promise for large-scale screening to detect early lens changes. As I noted above, glare tests are more *sensitive* to these changes than other clinical tests of visual function, including visual acuity and contrast sensitivity. In addition, glare tests are more *specific* to anterior segment disease than other tests. Although the contrast sensitivity function (CSF) has been promoted for detecting early lens changes, there is no pattern of CSF loss that is unique to any particular vision disorder. Contrast sensitivity may be reduced by retinal or neurological disorders in which the ocular media are entirely clear. In fact, a study of CSFs in diabetics with retinopathy and cataracts[27] could not distinguish between CSF losses encountered in patients with cataracts and no retinopathy and patients with retinopathy and clear lenses. Glare sensitivity, on the other hand, has been shown to correlate with the extent of posterior subcapsular opacification in cataract patients[19] and subclinical lens opacification in normal elderly patients.[2]

The principal utility of disability glare testing (and the driving force behind commercialization of the test) has been the objective documentation of visual disability in patients with mild cataracts. Glare testing has been applied to two types of vision problems: 1) reduction of visual acuity out-of-doors in bright sunlight and 2) visual disability related to nighttime driving. Several studies have evaluated the ability of commercial glare testers to predict outdoor visual acuity. The Miller-Nadler glare tester[6] measures contrast sensitivity for identification of a Landolt C in the presence of a bright, square, glare source. Hirsch et al[28] found the test to be a good predictor of visual acuity measured while the patient was facing the sun, accounting for 64% of the variance in a sample of 84 cataractous eyes. The Brightness Acuity Tester, or BAT, is a brightly illuminated hemispherical cup held in front of the eye through which a conventional eye chart is viewed. Holladay et al[29] also found it to be a good predictor of outdoor acuity, accounting for 71% of the variance in a sample of 64 normal and cataract patients. However, studies comparing several glare testers using the same group of patients have been inconclusive. Prager et al[30] compared the BAT with the Miller-Nadler test and reported that neither instrument was very good at predicting acuity facing the sun (each accounting for less than 25% of the variance in a sample of 47 eyes). The BAT overpredicted outdoor acuity and the Miller-Nadler test underpredicted. Finally, Neumann et al[31] compared five of the most popular commercial glare testers. Unfortunately, the results are difficult to interpret. Different vision tests were used for various devices, and in some cases, the authors based their predictions on tables provided by the manufacturer, rather than determining the predictive accuracy from their own data.

Many of the commercial glare testers provide a glare source that simulates the headlight of an oncoming automobile. In a laboratory study of drivers with normal visual acuity, it was shown that glare sensitivity correlates with simulated nighttime driving performance and with subjective complaints about glare from oncoming headlights.[32] However there are no quantitative data comparing how well these tests predict visual disability during actual nighttime driving. It is important to remember that pupil dilation under dim ambient illumination may change the amount of intraocular light scatter, depending on the size and location of opacities in the lens.

### Disability glare in low vision

Glare can be particularly disabling to patients with severe visual impairment ("low vision"). Most of these individuals have reduced contrast sensitivity. Glare further reduces the contrast of the retinal image, making it more difficult to read or recognize faces and objects. It is often thought that glare is wavelength dependent. According to the Rayleigh scattering formula, light scatter is inversely related to wavelength—short wavelength light is scattered more than long wavelength light. This has led to the use of tinted lenses that filter out short wavelength light to control glare problems. While the tinted lenses may have a beneficial effect for some patients, the benefit is probably not related to glare reduction in most cases. Rayleigh scattering only applies when the scattering particles are small, compared to the wavelength of light. Lenticular scattering is caused by relatively large structures and has a weak dependence on wavelength.[33] However, corneal scattering is more strongly wavelength dependent, and colored filters may have the desired effect.[34]

Regardless of the source of the scattered light, there is a solution that benefits many patients with low vision. We have demonstrated[35] that low-vision observers with cloudy ocular media have superior near acuity and read better when the contrast of the text is reversed (white letters on a black background). With normal black-on-white text, the white background is a large source of light for scattering. With reversed-contrast text the light available for scattering is reduced, while the contrast of the text remains high. These effects are illustrated in Figure 11-2. The graph plots reading as a function of letter size (magnification) for a low-vision subject with corneal opacification secondary to Stevens-Johnson syndrome. His near acuities, measured with the Sloan continuous-text reading cards were 20M at 40 cm for normal black-on-white text, and 14M at 40 cm for white-on-black text. His peak reading rate was higher with reversed-contrast text (100 words per minute compared to 66 words per minute) and he required less magnification for optimal reading performance 15× compared to 60×).

Unfortunately, the only low-vision devices that can reverse contrast are computer-assisted or closed-circuit television readers.

---

## Glare Recovery

### Causes of delayed glare recovery

Glare recovery has received much less attention in clinical literature than disability glare. Most of the published studies have concentrated on the relation of glare recovery, or photostress, to retinal disease. Exposure to a bright light bleaches photopigments in the outer segments of the photoreceptors, making them less sensitive to light and reducing visual function. The speed with which visual function returns to its prestress level is an indirect measure of the rate of photopigment resynthesis. Resynthesis depends on the integrity of the photoreceptors, retinal pigment epithelium, and choroid. Diseases that disrupt these structures, or their juxtaposition, are expected to prolong glare recovery. On the other hand, diseases that affect the anterior segment or neural pathway may impair visual function, but should not affect glare recovery.

Glare recovery has been studied over the lifespan of normal subjects with

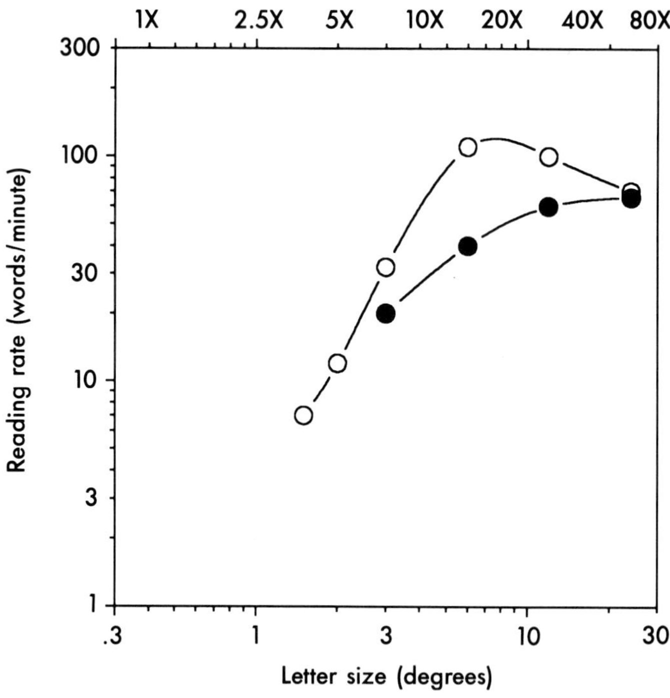



**FIGURE 11-2**   Reading rate is graphed as a function of letter size (lower x-axis) or magnification (upper x-axis) for a subject with corneal vascularization secondary to Stevens-Johnson syndrome. Filled symbols plot reading performance for conventional black letters on a white background. Open symbols plot reading performance for reversed-contrast text.

mixed results. Most studies have shown that recovery times increase by about 10% past 40 years of age,[36,37,38] but Smiddy and Fine[39] found no correlation with age in elderly patients with drusen and no other ocular pathology. Glare recovery is significantly delayed in a variety of retinal diseases, including active central serous chorioretinopathy,[36] diabetic retinopathy,[40] and macular edema (diabetic and aphakic cystoid).[36] Glaser et al[37] also reported increased glare-recovery times in most patients with submacular drusen and no detectable serous detachment, but Smiddy and Fine[39] found no correlation with severity of drusen.

Normal glare recovery times are reported for patients with optic nerve disease, even in the presence of reduced visual acuity. Glare recovery times were within the normal limits for 19 of 20 patients with various optic nerve diseases and visual acuities from 20/20 to 20/70.[36]

## Measurement of glare recovery time

Unlike disability glare, there has been very little commercial interest in clinical photostress testing. Perhaps the reason is that the test can be administered with equipment already available in every ophthalmologist's office. Typically, glare recovery is evaluated by recording visual acuity under normal conditions, exposing the patient to a bright light, and measuring the time to return to the same or one-line-worse acuity. As in disability glare testing, there is no *a priori* reason why visual acuity should be used. In laboratory studies of photoreceptor kinetics, investigators typically use a contrast discrimination task where the observer must detect a small increase or decrease in the brightness of a test target. Theoretically, it is much simpler to relate the resynthesis of photopigment to contrast detection than to visual resolution (visual acuity), and some clinical studies have measured glare recovery times for the detection of a small flashing disk. (See, e.g., Severin et al.[36]) But visual acuity tests are much more widely available, and until someone shows that a contrast test provides better information for the clinician, acuity will continue to be the clinical test of choice. Whichever vision test is used, it should conform to the standards of test design described above.

Various types of light sources are used for photostress testing: ophthalmoscopes, xenon flash-tubes, and penlights. For reliable and repeatable testing it is necessary to use a standardized light source. Penlights do not fulfill this requirement. Light intensity varies with the age of the batteries and the optical characteristics of the bulb. Ophthalmoscope lights could be calibrated by the user, but seldom are. Flash-tubes have several advantages. They deliver a standard amount of light and the exposure is too brief to be affected by pupillary constriction or eye movements (provided that the patient properly fixates prior to the flash). The Brightness Acuity Tester (see above) can also be used for photostress testing. It has a calibrated light source and the hemispherical field minimizes the effects of small eye movements during exposure.

Little attention has been paid to the intensity of the glare light. Many of the clinical papers do not even report light levels, and those that do vary as to whether the glare is measured in units of luminous intensity, illuminance, or retinal illuminance. Clearly, further work needs to be done to determine whether the intensity of the glare source affects the sensitivity and specificity of the test.

## Clinical utility of glare recovery tests

Since glare recovery depends on the integrity of the photoreceptors, retinal pigment epithelium, and choroid, several investigators have proposed that the test could be used to differentiate retinal disease from optic nerve disease in patients with unexplained vision loss. The work reviewed above supports this proposition. However, in a recent paper by Sherman and Henkind,[38] significantly longer glare recovery times were reported for patients with chronic open angle glaucoma. The authors did not control pupil size, but discount the possibility that the effect was caused by meiosis, resulting from glaucoma therapy. No explanation is offered for this paradoxical finding.

It has also been suggested that glare recovery could be used to monitor patients who are at risk for developing retinal disease. Zingirian et al[40] studied 112 insulin-dependent diabetics, 69 without retinopathy and 43 with retinopathy ranging from background to proliferative disease. Glare recovery was delayed for both groups compared to age-matched normals, and the retinopathy patients had significantly longer glare recovery times than the patients without retinopathy. However, there was considerable overlap between groups and the authors were only able to discriminate with 66% accuracy between retinopathy and no retinopathy, using glare alone. Nevertheless, the results are encouraging and prospective studies are now needed to determine whether glare recovery can help identify diabetic patients who are at increased risk for developing sight-threatening complications of the disease.


## Summary

Clinical glare tests are a useful adjunct to a complete ophthalmological examination. As a means of documenting visual disability caused by anterior segment disease, tests of disability glare are both more sensitive and more specific than other common clinical tests of visual function. More research is needed to relate disability glare findings to everyday visual problems associated with glare. Glare recovery shows promise as a simple, noninvasive method of assessing retinal function. If further work can establish that glare recovery is affected only by retinal disease, then the test could become a powerful tool for differentiating retinal disease from optic nerve disease in patients with unexplained vision loss. For both disability glare and glare recovery, additional research is needed to define the optimal vision test, the configuration of the glare source, its intensity and mode of presentation.



## References

1. Gawande AA, Donovan WJ, Ginsburg AP, Marmor MF. Photoaversion in retinitis pigmentosa. Br J Ophthalmol 1989; 73:115-120.
2. Wolf E, Gardiner JS. Studies on the scatter of light in the dioptric media of the eye as a basis of visual glare. Arch Ophthalmol 1965; 74:338-345.
3. Hirsch RP, Nadler MP, Miller D. Clinical performance of a disability glare tester. Arch Ophthalmol 1984; 102:1633-1636.
4. Elliott DB, Gilchrist J, Whitaker D. Contrast sensitivity and glare sensitivity changes with three types of cataract morphology: Are these techniques necessary in a clinical evaluation of cataract? Ophthal Physiol Opt 1989; 9:25-39.
5. Masket S. Reversal of glare disability after cataract surgery. J Cataract Regract Surg 1989; 15:165-168.
6. Miller D, Lazenby GW. Glare sensitivity in corrected aphakes. Ophthalmol Surg 1977; 8:54-57.
7. LeClaire J, Nadler MP, Weiss S, Miller D. A new glare tester for clinical testing—results comparing normal subjects and variously corrected aphakic patients. Arch Ophthalmol 1982; 100:153-158.
8. Nadler DJ, Jaffe NS, Clayman HM, Jaffe MS, Luscombe SM. Glare disability in eyes with intraocular lenses. Am J Ophthalmol 1984; 97:43-47.
9. Van der Hijde GL, Weber J, Boukes R. Effects of straylight on visual acuity in pseudophakia. Doc Ophthalmol 1985; 59:81-84.
10. Knighton RW, Slomovic AR, Parrish RK. Glare measurements before and after neodymium-YAG laser posterior capsulotomy. Am J Ophthalmol 1985; 100:708-713.
11. Hess RF, Carney LG. Vision through an abnormal cornea: a pilot study of the relationship between visual loss from corneal distortion, corneal edema, keratoconus and some allied corneal pathology. Invest Ophthalmol Vis Sci 1979; 18:476-483.
12. Carney LG, Jacobs RJ. Mechanisms of visual loss in corneal edema. Arch Ophthalmol 1984; 102:1068-1071.
13. Bourque LB, Cosand BB, Drews C, Waring GO III, Lynn M, Cartwright C. Reported satisfaction, fluctuation of vision, and glare among patients one year after surgery in the Prospective Evaluation of Radial Keratotomy (PERK) Study. Arch Ophthalmol 1986; 104:356-363.
14. Applegate RA, Trick LR, Meade DL, Hartstein J. Radial keratotomy increases the effects of disability glare: initial results. Ann Ophthalmol 1987; 19:293-297.
15. Verriest G, Uvijls A. Disability glare in normal and diseased eyes. Clin Vision Sci 1989; 4:253-256.
16. Deiter P, Wolf D, Geer S. Glare and the scatter of light in the vitreous. Arch Ophthalmol 1972; 87:12-15.
17. Rubin GS, Sunness JS. Assessing visual function in patients with macular edema. In Noninvasive assessment of the visual system, 1988 Technical Digest Series Vol 3. Washington, DC: Optical Society of America 1988:140-143.

18. Legge GE, Rubin GS, Luebker A. Psychophysics of reading. V. The role of contrast in normal vision. Vision Res 1987; 27:1165-1177.

19. Miller D, Jernigan ME, Molnar S, Wolf E, Newman J. Laboratory evaluation of a clinical glare tester. Arch Ophthalmol 1972; 87:324-332.

20. Abrahamsson M, Sjostrand J. Impairment of contrast sensitivity function (csf) as a measure of disability glare. Invest Ophthalmol Vis Sci 1986; 27:1131-1136.

21. Higgins KE, Jaffe MJ, Coletta NJ, Caruso RC, de Monasterio FM. Spatial contrast sensitivity. Importance of controlling the patient's visibility criterion. Arch Ophthalmol 1984; 102:1035-1041.

22. Rubin GS. Reliability and sensitivity of clinical contrast sensitivity tests. Clin Vis Sci 1988; 2:169-177.

23. Ferris FL III, Kassoff A, Bresnick GH, Bailey IA. New visual acuity charts for clinical research. Am J Ophthalmol 1982; 94:91-96.

24. Pelli DG, Robson JG, Wilkins AJ. The design of a new letter chart for measuring contrast sensitivity. Clin Vision Sci 1988; 2:187-199.

25. Odom JV, Weinstein GM, Chao GW. Preoperative prediction of postoperative visual acuity in patients with cataracts: a quantitative review. Doc Ophthalmol 1988; 70:5-17.

26. Rubin GS, Stark WS; Evaluation of visual function prior to cataract surgery. In Weinstock F, ed, Management and care of the cataract patient, Oxford and Boston, 1990, Blackwell.

27. Howes SC, Caelli T, Mitchell P. Contrast sensitivity in diabetics with retinopathy and cataract. Aust J Ophthalmol 1982; 10:173-178.

28. Hirsch RP, Nadler MP, Miller D. Glare measurement as a predictor of outdoor vision among cataract patients. Ann Ophthalmol 1984; 16:965-968.

29. Holladay JT, Trujillo J, Prager TC, Ruiz RS. Brightness acuity test and outdoor visual acuity in cataract patients. J Cataract Refract Surg 1987; 13:67-69.

30. Prager TC, Urso RG, Holladay JT, Stewart RH. Glare testing in cataract patients: instrument evaluation and identification of sources of methodological error. J Cataract Refract Surg 1989; 15:149-157.

31. Neumann AC, McCarty GR, Locke J, Cobb B. Glare disability devices for cataractous eyes: a consumer's guide. J Cataract Refract Surg 1988; 14:212-216.

32. Pulling NH, Wolf E, Sturgis SP, Vaillancourt DR, Dolliver JJ. Headlight glare resistance and driver age. Human Factors 1980; 22:103-112.

33. Wesemann W. Incoherent image formation in the presence of scattering eye media. J Opt Soc Am 1987; 4:1439-1447.

34. Legge GE, Rubin GS. Psychophysics of reading. IV. Wavelength effects in normal and low vision. J Opt Soc Am 1986; 3:40-51.

35. Legge GE, Rubin GS, Pelli DG, Schleske MM. Psychophysics of reading. II. Low vision. Vision Res 1985; 25:253-266.

36. Severin SL, Tour RL, Kershaw RH. Macular function and the photostress test 2. Arch Ophthalmol 1967; 77:163-167.

37. Glaser JS, Savino PJ, Sumers KD, McDonald SA, Knighton RW. The photostress recovery test in the clinical assessment of visual function. Am J Ophthalmol 1977; 83:255-260.

38. Sherman MD, Henkind P. Photostress recovery in chronic open angle glaucoma. Brit J Ophthalmol 1988; 72:641-645.

39. Smiddy WE, Fine SL. Prognosis of patients with bilateral macular drusen. Ophthalmology 1984; 91:271-277.

40. Zingirian M, Polizzi A, Grillo N. The macular recovery test after photostress in normal and diabetic subjects. Acta Diabetol Lat 1985; 169:169-172.

# 12 Treatment of Asymptomatic Retinal Breaks and Their Precursors

C. P. Wilkinson, MD
Ronald G. Michels, MD†

Gonin proved that retinal detachments were caused by retinal breaks by demonstrating that surgical closure of retinal breaks was followed by resolution of the subretinal fluid. However, the relationship of many retinal breaks, and their precursors, to subsequent clinical retinal detachment remains uncertain and controversial. Retinal breaks not associated with retinal detachment were thought to be unusual until autopsy reports, and clinical studies using the indirect ophthalmoscope, demonstrated retinal breaks in approximately 6% of the general population. The incidence of clinical retinal detachment is only about 0.01% per year in the same population.[1] Therefore, most retinal breaks do not cause retinal detachment and prophylactic therapy is not necessary for all retinal breaks.

Although rhegmatogenous retinal detachments are relatively uncommon, they are a significant cause of reduced vision and blindness. Between 5% and 10% of attempts at treatment are first surgical failures, and visual acuity returns to 20/50 or better in only about 50% of anatomically successful cases. Thus, attempts to prevent retinal detachment have been investigated since the time of Gonin, and numerous reports have attempted to identify the types of retinal breaks, and their precursors, which are most likely to benefit from prophylactic therapy.[2,3]

The risk of retinal detachment is substantially different among subgroups of eyes. For example, myopic aphakic or pseudophakic eyes with lattice degeneration, in patients with a history of retinal detachment in the fellow eye, have a far greater risk of subsequent retinal detachment than do otherwise normal eyes with lattice degeneration. To date, no studies have employed optimal prospective randomized trials to compare the natural course of retinal breaks and their precursors to the outcome of similar lesions treated with laser photocoagulation or cryotherapy. However, data are available to confirm the impression that the two most important factors associated with the likelihood of a retinal tear progressing to clinical retinal detachment are: 1) symptoms associated with an acute posterior vitreous detachment and 2) persistent vitreous traction on the edge of the retinal tear. Retinal detachment due to such symptomatic breaks occurs in 33% to 55%

---

†Deceased.

of cases, and retrospective studies have demonstrated the value of prophylactic therapy of symptomatic horseshoe tears.[4]

This report discusses prophylactic therapy of retinal breaks and their precursors in patients without symptoms of an acute posterior vitreous detachment. The lesions are usually discovered during routine examination of the peripheral retina, although retinal breaks and precursors not caused by posterior vitreous separation may be discovered at the time when a symptomatic vitreous detachment prompts ophthalmological examination. Treatment techniques, results, and complications of prophylactic therapy will not be discussed.

## ASYMPTOMATIC PATIENTS WITHOUT HIGH-RISK CHARACTERISTICS

Asymptomatic retinal breaks and their precursors can be subdivided as a function of additional factors that predispose to development of rhegmatogenous retinal detachment. Non-myopic phakic eyes in patients without a history of retinal detachment in the fellow eye are unlikely to develop retinal detachment, regardless of the presence or type of vitreoretinal pathology. Still, prophylactic therapy has sometimes been recommended to treat visible precursors of retinal breaks and asymptomatic retinal tears and holes, with or without subclinical retinal detachment.

## VITREORETINAL PRECURSORS OF RETINAL BREAKS

Visible precursors of retinal breaks include: 1) lattice degeneration, 2) cystic retinal tufts, and 3) degenerative retinoschisis. Lattice degeneration is the most common lesion predisposing to retinal breaks and detachment. Both lattice degeneration lesions and cystic retinal tufts can be sites of retinal tears caused by vitreoretinal traction. Atrophic retinal holes commonly occur within areas of lattice degeneration and also in the outer layer of degenerative retinoschisis.

### Lattice Degeneration

Lattice degeneration is present in about 8% of eyes in the general population, but it is present in 20% to 30% of retinal detachment cases.[5] Thus, the mere presence of lattice degeneration has sometimes been considered an indication for prophylactic therapy. However, lattice degeneration is a rare cause of retinal detachment in eyes without other predisposing factors. Byer[6] observed 176 untreated patients with lattice degeneration for 1 to 25 years (average, 10.8 years). Flap tears subsequently developed in 5 eyes (1.2%). All of these were successfully treated following the onset of symptoms. Clinical retinal detachment developed in 3 (0.7%) of the eyes in this series. One detachment was caused by a symptomatic flap tear, and atrophic holes within areas of lattice caused the other detachments. In another report, Byer[5] estimated the risk of progressive clinical detachment in patients with lattice degeneration and holes within the lattice lesions to be 1 in 365. Hyams et al[7] followed 278 eyes with lattice degeneration for one to six years, and retinal detachment occurred in four cases (1.4%).

Retinal detachments due to breaks in eyes with lattice degeneration are usually caused by: 1) a flap tear along the posterior or lateral edge of a lattice lesion, 2) similar tears at sites other than from visible lattice lesions, and 3) atrophic retinal holes within areas of lattice degeneration. The latter cases occur predominantly in young adult myopic patients without a clinically evident posterior vitreous detachment. The two former types of tears causing detachment usually occur after symptomatic posterior vitreous detachment in patients over age 50.

The value of prophylactic therapy for lattice degeneration, with or without round atrophic holes, is most difficult to document in phakic non-myopic eyes of patients without a history of retinal detachment in the fellow eye. Most authors studying prophylactic therapy have evaluated second eyes of patients with prior retinal detachment and have not separated symptomatic and asymptomatic cases. The reported rate of retinal detachment after prophylactic therapy appears to be little different than the natural history of lattice degeneration, with or without holes, in similar cases. Thus, prophylactic treatment is not recommended in asymptomatic patients without other high-risk factors.[3]

## Cystic Retinal Tuft

Retinal tears occurring in association with cystic retinal tufts may be responsible for up to 10% of clinical retinal detachments.[8] Cystic retinal tufts are associated with a firm vitreoretinal adhesion, and retinal breaks responsible for detachment usually occur at the time of symptomatic posterior vitreous separation. Byer[9] discovered retinal tears in 32% of phakic eyes with cystic tufts, but in only 11% of similar eyes without these vitreoretinal lesions, at the time of a symptomatic posterior vitreous detachment. In another report, Byer[8] calculated the chance of retinal detachment in eyes with a cystic retinal tuft to be approximately 1 in 357.

The natural course and effects of treatment for cystic retinal tufts have not been well studied. Routine prophylactic treatment of cystic retinal tufts in otherwise-normal eyes is not recommended.

## Degenerative Retinoschisis

Clinical retinal detachments are associated with degenerative retinoschisis in up to 6% of consecutive detachment cases.[3] Thus, retinoschisis with breaks in either layer has sometimes been considered an indication for prophylactic therapy. However, a recent long-term study of the natural history of retinoschisis demonstrated that clinical retinal detachments are unusual.[10] Byer[10] estimated asymptomatic subclinical detachments to be more frequent than symptomatic clinical detachments by a ratio of 178:1. Prophylactic therapy is not recommended in asymptomatic eyes with retinoschisis, with or without outer layer breaks or localized areas of retinal detachment, unless significant progression is documented or the fellow eye has had a retinal detachment.

## ASYMPTOMATIC RETINAL BREAKS

Autopsy and clinical studies have demonstrated that asymptomatic retinal tears and holes are not unusual, but they are an uncommon cause of clinical retinal detachment.[2,3] Retinal breaks are classically divided, on the basis of their cause, into retinal tears and retinal holes. Retinal tears are caused by vitreoretinal traction, whereas holes are believed to be caused by atrophic changes within the retina.

## Retinal Tears

Foos[11] observed flap tears in 89 (1.8%) of 4812 autopsy eyes, and these tears were associated with posterior vitreous detachment in 97% of these cases. Retinal tears appeared first in the third decade of life, and the incidence increased with advancing age thereafter. This was believed to be caused by the increased prevalence of posterior vitreous separation with increasing age. In a large clinical study, Byer[12] observed asymptomatic retinal breaks in 111 (3.3%) of 3400 eyes. Horseshoe tears accounted for only 10% of these breaks, and over 80% of patients with retinal breaks were over 40 years of age. Retinal detachments did not occur in a subsequent followup study of 50 horseshoe tears, 86% of which were followed for more than five years.[13] The prognosis in eyes with operculated holes is similar.[13]

The clinical course of retinal tears in asymptomatic eyes, regardless of their location, is benign; and retinal detachment is quite unusual. Thus, treatment of such lesions is not recommended in eyes without additional risk factors.

## Retinal Holes

Most retinal holes occur within areas of lattice degeneration. In autopsy eyes evaluated by Foos,[14] approximately three-fourths of retinal holes were associated with lattice degeneration, and the other retinal holes were associated with zonular traction tufts, prior chorioretinitis, meridional folds, or cobblestone degeneration. Only 6% of holes in this study were not associated with another retinal abnormality. In a clinical study, over 80% of 276 asymptomatic retinal holes were associated with lattice degeneration, and none progressed to clinical retinal detachment.[13]

Retinal holes with or without lattice degeneration are not considered dangerous in eyes without additional risk factors, and prophylactic therapy of these lesions is not recommended.

## SUBCLINICAL RETINAL DETACHMENT

*Subclinical retinal detachment* is a term employed by various authors to describe differing amounts of subretinal fluid associated with retinal breaks. We use the term to define localized detachments extending more than one disc diameter beyond the edge of the break, but not extending posteriorly to the equator.

Subclinical retinal detachments in otherwise asymptomatic eyes rarely progress to cause symptomatic retinal detachments, particularly in eyes without additional risk factors. The most common subclinical detachments that progress to clinical detachment are caused by round holes within lattice degeneration in young adult myopic patients.[3] Subclinical detachments in which retinal breaks are associated with persistent vitreoretinal traction are more likely to progress than are those caused by round holes not associated with traction forces.

Prophylactic therapy for subclinical retinal detachments in eyes without additional risk factors is usually not recommended unless progression of the detachment is observed. A single exception to this rule is a subclinical detachment associated with a retinal dialysis. These cases are usually slowly progressive and often remain symptomatic until macular involvement occurs.[3]

## ASYMPTOMATIC PATIENTS WITH HIGH-RISK CHARACTERISTICS

Factors associated with an increased risk of retinal detachment include myopia, prior cataract surgery, and a history of retinal detachment in the fellow eye. The latter is by far the most important variable, and some patients in this category also have a family history of retinal detachment. Asymptomatic retinal breaks and their precursors are considered more dangerous in eyes with these high-risk characteristics than in cases without them. However, the value of prophylactic therapy in many of these situations remains uncertain and controversial.

## MODERATE AND HIGH MYOPIA

Between 35% and 79% of eyes with retinal detachments are myopic, and this is significantly greater than the rate of myopia in the general population.[3] Myopia is associated with an increased risk of retinal breaks and retinal detachment, and this is probably caused by increased rates of vitreous liquification and posterior vitreous separation in myopic eyes. Because of the association between myopia and subsequent rhegmatogenous retinal detachment, some surgeons recommend that lesions associated with retinal detachment be treated prophylactically. Precursors of retinal breaks, retinal tears and holes, and subclinical retinal detachments have all been considered for therapy.

### Lattice Degeneration

Lattice degeneration is more common in myopic eyes than in emmetropic eyes. The incidence of posterior vitreous detachment is also significantly higher in myopic eyes and also in eyes with lattice degeneration. Byer[9] found that 69% of 39 eyes with lattice degeneration and a symptomatic posterior vitreous detachment were myopic, whereas 43% of 217 eyes with vitreous detachment but without lattice degeneration were myopic. These differences were statistically significant (P = 0.018). The incidence of retinal tears in phakic eyes with symptomatic posterior vitreous detachment was 11% in eyes without lattice degeneration and 22% in eyes with lattice degeneration (P = 0.023). Although retinal tears were significantly more common in eyes with myopia and lattice degeneration, 36% of tears in eyes with lattice degeneration occurred in locations other than at the sites of lattice. There are no data demonstrating the value of prophylactic therapy of lattice degeneration in myopic eyes without a history of retinal detachment in the fellow eye. Still, clinical retinal detachments have been reported as being caused by atrophic holes within lattice in up to 21% of phakic nontraumatic cases.[15]

Although prophylactic therapy is usually not recommended, patients with myopia and lattice degeneration should be informed about the relative risk of both visual field loss and symptomatic vitreous detachment.

## Cystic Retinal Tufts and Degenerative Retinoschisis

Neither cystic retinal tufts nor degenerative retinoschisis are statistically related to myopia. Although retinal tears are common following posterior vitreous detachment in eyes with cystic retinal tufts,[9] there are no data demonstrating the value of prophylactic therapy for these lesions in emmetropic or myopic eyes. Nevertheless, patients with cystic retinal tufts are instructed to return promptly, should symptoms of vitreous detachment occur. Similarly, retinoschisis in myopic eyes is managed in the same fashion as that described for emmetropic cases.

## Asymptomatic Retinal Breaks

Retinal breaks are more common in myopic eyes than in emmetropic or hyperopic cases, and there is a direct relationship between increasing axial length and the prevalence of retinal breaks.[3] Neumann et al[16] demonstrated that retinal breaks are more likely to cause retinal detachment in myopic eyes than are breaks in non-myopic eyes. However, Neumann and Hyams[17] demonstrated that clinical detachments due to asymptomatic breaks in myopic eyes are rare. Similarly, Byer[13] observed no clinical detachments in 29 such cases, most of which were followed for over five years. There are no data demonstrating that asymptomatic retinal breaks in myopic eyes should have prophylactic therapy.

## Subclinical Retinal Detachment

Subclinical retinal detachments associated with asymptomatic retinal breaks are not likely to progress to clinical detachment, unless there is persistent vitreoretinal traction on the retinal break or on the retina near the break. The most common type of subclinical retinal detachment associated with myopia is caused by atrophic holes within areas of lattice degeneration. In such cases, prophylactic treatment is recommended if significant progression of the detachment is documented by serial examinations.

## APHAKIC AND PSEUDOPHAKIC EYES

Removal of the crystalline lens is associated with a profound increase in the rate of subsequent retinal tears and retinal detachment, regardless of the method of cataract surgery. Approximately 2.9% of individuals in the United States have undergone cataract extraction, but up to 40% of retinal detachments occur in aphakic or pseudophakic eyes.[18] The relationships between cataract extraction and retinal detachment are complex, but the effects of lens extraction on the vitreous are probably the most important. The incidence of retinal detachment in aphakic and pseudophakic eyes is particularly high in myopic patients, and in those with a history of prior detachment in the fellow eye. Patients with prior retinal detachment in the fellow eye are discussed later in a separate section.

## Precursors of Retinal Breaks

Lattice degeneration occurs in aphakic and pseudophakic eyes with the same frequency as in phakic eyes, but retinal breaks causing clinical retinal detachment following cataract surgery are less likely to be associated with lattice lesions than in comparable cases of detachment in phakic eyes.[3] The prevalence of lattice degeneration associated with retinal tears in detachments after cataract extraction also decreases with advancing age. There are no studies demonstrating the value of prophylactic therapy of lattice degeneration in aphakic and pseudophakic eyes of patients without a history of retinal detachment in the fellow eye.

Similarly, there are no data dealing specifically with cystic retinal tufts or degenerative retinoschisis following cataract extraction. Although the increased rate of posterior vitreous separation might be expected to be associated with a higher rate of subsequent retinal detachment in eyes with cystic retinal tufts, cystic retinal tufts or retinoschisis are managed as noted above.

## Asymptomatic Retinal Breaks

Asymptomatic retinal breaks are more common in aphakic and pseudophakic eyes, but they are no more likely to cause retinal detachment than in comparable asymptomatic phakic cases.[3] The value of prophylactic therapy for asymptomatic retinal breaks in patients after cataract extraction but without prior detachment in the fellow eye, or in those about to undergo cataract extraction is unclear. This is because prior studies have not categorized cases as a function of: 1) symptoms, 2) refractive error, 3) presence of vitreous detachment, 4) history of retinal detachment in the fellow eye, and, 5) family history of retinal detachment. The limited studies available indicate that detachment occurs in many of these cases in spite of prophylactic therapy. Prophylactic therapy is not currently recommended for asymptomatic retinal breaks observed in aphakic and pseudophakic eyes. Horseshoe-shaped tears found prior to cataract extraction are often treated, but the relative benefit of treatment is unknown.

## Subclinical Retinal Detachments

There are few data describing the effects of prophylactic therapy for subclinical retinal detachments noted after cataract extraction in patients without prior detachment in the fellow eye. The decision to treat these localized detachments is based on the amount of subretinal fluid present and the type of retinal break. Subclinical detachments associated with horseshoe-shaped tears are usually treated, whereas those associated with operculated retinal breaks or atrophic holes within lattice degeneration are not treated unless there is significant progression of the detachment.

# ASYMPTOMATIC PHAKIC EYES IN PATIENTS WITH PRIOR RETINAL DETACHMENT IN THE FELLOW EYE

Abnormal vitreoretinal lesions often occur bilaterally, and patients with a history of retinal detachment in one eye have a substantially increased risk of retinal detachment occurring in the other eye. The incidence of retinal detachment in the second eye probably ranges from 25% to 40%.[3] Thus, attempts to prevent retinal detachment in the second eye have received considerable attention and most surgeons have attempted to prevent retinal detachment by creating a chorioretinal adhesion around retinal breaks or precursors of retinal breaks.

## Precursors of Retinal Breaks

Precursors of retinal tears considered for prophylactic therapy include lattice degeneration, cystic retinal tufts, and degenerative retinoschisis. Most data describe experience managing lattice degeneration.

Lattice degeneration is present in 9% to 34% of the fellow eyes of patients with retinal detachment, and the average prevalence is about 24%.[5] The incidence of subsequent retinal detachment in such eyes is far greater than in asymptomatic phakic eyes of patients with no history of prior retinal detachment. Available data indicate that 6% to 15% of phakic second eyes with lattice degeneration develop a retinal detachment during followup periods of three to ten years.[3]

Results of treating lattice degeneration in these cases are difficult to analyze because most studies have not categorized cases on the basis of refractive error, vitreous detachment, or the presence of atrophic holes. In a study comparing no treatment, partial treatment, and full treatment of areas of lattice degeneration, eyes with full treatment of lattice degeneration had fewer retinal tears and detachments than the partially treated and untreated groups (Table 12-1).[19] The beneficial effect was apparent at follow periods of three, five, and seven years. In this study the beneficial effect of treatment was statistically significant for all patient subgroups, except in eyes with myopia of six diopters or more and in eyes with both high myopia and more than six clock hours of lattice degeneration. In the latter subgroups, which have the highest risk of subsequent retinal detachment, prophylactic therapy did not reduce the occurrence of retinal detachment. Conversely, no detachments occurred after full treatment in eyes with less than six clock hours of lattice degeneration and less than 1.25 diopters of myopia.

In the study of Folk et al,[19] full treatment reduced the risk of detachment from 5.1% to 1.8% (see Table 12-1) during a seven-year period. This modest-treatment benefit is recommended for selected patients, including those with an anatomic failure or poor visual result after retinal reattachment surgery in the first eye, those who are incapable of recognizing symptoms of a posterior vitreous detachment, and in patients living in areas with limited access to ophthalmologic care.

Cystic retinal tufts are bilateral in only 6% of cases, and therefore they are not a common cause of bilateral retinal detachment. Still, eyes with cystic retinal tufts are more likely to develop a retinal tear at the time of posterior vitreous detachment.[15] Eyes with cystic retinal tufts are not routinely treated prophylactically, unless the retinal detachment in the first eye was associated with a retinal tuft. Similarly, bilateral retinal detachments are no more frequent in eyes with retinoschisis than in those without retinoschisis. However, if symptomatic retinal detachment due to retinoschisis occurs in one eye, prophylactic therapy of outer layer breaks, or treatment of subclinical retinal detachment associated with retinoschisis is recommended in the second eye.

**Table 12-1**  Outcome: Phakic Fellow Eyes with Lattice Degeneration

| Group | No. eyes | % new breaks excluding those with retinal detachment | New tears excluding those with retinal detachment | Retinal detachment |
|---|---|---|---|---|
| **All cases** | | | | |
| Untreated | 151 | 15.0 | 10 (6.6%) | 9 (5.9%) |
| Partial treatment | 73 | 20.0 | 7 (9.6%) | 5 (6.8%) |
| Full treatment | 164 | 5.5 | 5 (3.0%) | 3 (1.8%) |
| **7-year followup** | | | | |
| Untreated | | | | (5.1%) |
| Full treatment | | | | (1.8%) |

Adapted from Folk JC, Arrindell EL, Klugman MR: Ophthalmol, 1989; 96:72.

An uncommon situation in which prophylactic therapy is used to treat precursors of retinal tears in phakic fellow eyes is in cases in which an idiopathic giant retinal tear previously occurred in the first eye. In such eyes, particularly those with myopia, significant vitreous syneresis, and "white-without-pressure," prophylactic therapy is usually recommended for the entire circumference of the peripheral retina.[20]

## Asymptomatic Retinal Breaks

Asymptomatic retinal breaks in phakic second eyes of patients with prior retinal detachment are more likely to cause clinical retinal detachments than are similar lesions in phakic non-fellow eyes.[3] Asymptomatic horseshoe tears are more likely to cause retinal detachment than are other types of breaks; and round holes, with or without a free operculum, are unlikely to cause retinal detachment unless there is persistent vitreoretinal traction near the hole.

There are no satisfactory data proving the value of prophylactic therapy of asymptomatic retinal breaks in phakic fellow eyes. Thus, prophylactic therapy is usually recommended for horseshoe-shaped tears and round tears with nearby vitreoretinal traction. Prophylactic therapy for holes within lattice degeneration is recommended as mentioned earlier.

## Subclinical Retinal Detachments

Subclinical retinal detachments in asymptomatic phakic fellow eyes are more likely to progress to clinical detachments than are comparable retinal tears without subclinical detachment.[3] In such cases, prophylactic therapy is usually recommended for eyes with more than two disc diameters of subretinal fluid surrounding the break, particularly if there is residual vitreoretinal traction on the break.

## ASYMPTOMATIC APHAKIC OR PSEUDOPHAKIC EYES IN PATIENTS WITH PRIOR RETINAL DETACHMENT IN THE FELLOW EYE

All eyes have an increased risk of retinal detachment following cataract extraction and retinal tears, and detachments are significantly more common in aphakic and pseudophakic fellow eyes than in phakic eyes. Thus, prophylactic therapy of precursors of breaks, retinal breaks, and subclinical retinal detachments has been performed most extensively in this subgroup.

## Precursors of Retinal Breaks

Lattice degeneration is the only precursor of retinal tears that has been studied in aphakic and pseudophakic fellow eyes. Lattice degeneration in these cases occurs with a frequency equal to that in phakic eyes, but lattice degeneration is responsible for a smaller percentage of retinal detachments in aphakic and pseudophakic eyes. Nevertheless, lattice degeneration may be particularly dangerous in these eyes. In one study, retinal tears or detachment occurred in 11% of 265 phakic fellow eyes with "peripheral degeneration" and in 27% of 45 such aphakic cases.[21] In a subgroup of eyes in which the peripheral degeneration was associated with definite vitreoretinal adhesions or retinal tears, detachment occurred in 11% of 161 phakic eyes and in 45% of 11 aphakic cases. Later retinal detachments were more common in eyes without a posterior vitreous detachment at the time of the initial examination. However, all studies of this subject are limited because the presence or absence of vitreous detachment was not thoroughly evaluated and recorded.

Several studies have demonstrated that prophylactic therapy of lattice degeneration in aphakic fellow eyes is of value.[3] Nevertheless, none of these were prospective randomized trials with appropriate controls, and the cases were not stratified as to refractive error or the presence of vitreous detachment. Still, treatment appears to be effective in reducing the chance of retinal tears developing at sites of visible lattice lesions, and most treatment failures are caused by retinal tears occurring at previously "normal" sites. Prophylactic therapy of lattice lesions in aphakic and pseudophakic fellow eyes, and in phakic cases in which cataract surgery is planned, is reasonable if posterior vitreous separation is not already present. Nevertheless, subsequent retinal detachment occurs in up to 25% of cases.[3]

Cystic retinal tufts are only bilateral in about 6% of cases, and they are an unusual cause of bilateral retinal detachment. Since eyes with cystic retinal tufts have an increased risk of retinal tears following vitreous detachment, and since vitreous detachment is significantly increased after removal of the crystalline lens, prophylactic therapy of cystic retinal tufts in aphakic and pseudophakic eyes and in eyes prior to cataract extraction is recommended in patients in whom retinal detachment, due to a cystic retinal tuft, occurred in the first eye.

## Asymptomatic Retinal Breaks

Asymptomatic retinal breaks in non-phakic eyes of patients with a history of retinal detachment in the other eye have a relatively high rate of causing subsequent clinical detachment. Nevertheless, there are few studies demonstrating the efficacy of prophylactic therapy of these lesions.[3] Treatment usually prevents detachments from occurring, due to the visible break, but new tears are particularly likely in these cases. Treatment is recommended for all asymptomatic retinal breaks associated with persistent vitreoretinal traction. Other breaks are usually followed without treatment.

## Subclinical Retinal Detachment

The natural course of subclinical retinal detachments in aphakic or pseudophakic fellow eyes has not been studied extensively, perhaps because most such cases are treated. All such lesions associated with persistent vitreoretinal traction are usually treated. Detachments of two disc diameters or less, due to operculated tears or round atrophic holes unassociated with lattice degeneration, are usually not treated.

## SUMMARY

Prevention of retinal detachment is a worthy goal. However, prospective randomized controlled trials have not been performed to determine the results of prophylactic therapy compared to the natural history of the lesion being treated. Although available data demonstrate that symptomatic horseshoe tears should be promptly surrounded with a chorioretinal adhesion, the value of similar treatment for operculated retinal tears and asymptomatic retinal breaks and their precursors is questionable.

Prophylactic therapy of precursors of retinal breaks is of little value in emmetropic and myopic phakic non-fellow eyes. Therapy of lattice degeneration in phakic fellow eyes reduces the incidence of retinal detachment over the following seven years by about 3%. Treatment of lattice degeneration in aphakic and pseudophakic eyes is probably of little value in non-fellow eyes, but it may be worthwhile in fellow eyes. Nevertheless, subsequent detachments can be expected to occur from tears in otherwise normal areas in up to 25% of such cases.

Asymptomatic retinal breaks rarely cause retinal detachment in non-fellow eyes, even if the lesions are horseshoe tears. Still, such tears are treated prophylactically in eyes about to undergo cataract extraction. Treatment is recommended for retinal breaks associated with persistent vitreoretinal traction in phakic, aphakic, and pseudophakic fellow eyes.

Subclinical retinal detachments are treated in all cases in which significant progression is observed. Also, subclinical detachments, due to tears associated with persistent vitreoretinal traction, are treated at the time they are detected in fellow eyes. Most patients with asymptomatic lesions associated with retinal detachment can be successfully managed by providing an explanation of the problem, so the patient will come promptly for evaluation if symptoms of acute retinal tears or detachment occur.

## References

1. Wilkes SR, Beard CM, Kurland LT, et al. The incidence of retinal detachment in Rochester, Minnesota, 1970–1978. Am J Ophthalmol 1982; 94:670.

2. Benson WE. Prophylactic therapy of retinal breaks. Surv Ophthalmol 1977; 22:41.

3. Michels RG, Wilkinson CP, Rice T. Retinal Detachment. St Louis: Mosby–Year Book, 1990: 1059.

4. Shea M, Davis MD, Kamel I. Retinal breaks without detachment, treated and untreated. Mod Probl Ophthalmol 1974; 12:97.
5. Byer NE. Lattice degeneration of the retina. Surv Ophthalmol 1979; 23:213.
6. Byer NE. Long-term natural history of lattice degeneration of the retina. Ophthalmol 1989; 96:1396.
7. Hyams SW, Meir E, Ivry M, et al. Chorioretinal lesions predisposing to retinal detachment. Am J Ophthalmol 1974; 78:429.
8. Byer NE. Relationship of cystic retinal tufts to retinal detachment. Dev Ophthalmol 1981; 2:36.
9. Byer N. Fate of lattice degeneration of the retina following acute posterior vitreous detachment. Ophthalmol (in press).
10. Byer NE. Long-term natural history study of senile retinoschisis with implications for management. Ophthalmol 1986; 93:1127.
11. Foos RY. Postoral peripheral retinal tears. Ann Ophthalmol 1974; 6:679.
12. Byer NE. Clinical study of retinal breaks. Trans Am Acad Ophthalmol Otolaryngol 1967; 71:461.
13. Byer NE. The natural history of asymptomatic retinal breaks. Ophthalmol 1982; 89:1033.
14. Foos RY. Retinal holes. Am J Ophthalmol 1978; 86:354.
15. Murakami-Nagasako F, Ohba N. Phakic retinal detachment associated with atrophic hole of lattice degeneration of the retina. Graefes Arch Clin Exp Ophthalmol 1983; 220:175.
16. Neumann E, Hyams S, Barkai S, et al. The natural history of retinal holes with special reference to the development of retinal detachment and the time factor involved. Isr J Med Sci 1972; 8:1424.
17. Neumann E, Hyams S. Conservative management of retinal breaks: a follow-up study of subsequent retinal detachment. Br J Ophthalmol 1972; 56:482.
18. Goldberg MF. Clear lens extraction for axial myopia. An appraisal. Ophthalmol 1987; 94:571.
19. Folk JC, Arrindell EL, Klugman MR. The fellow eye of patients with phakic lattice retinal degeneration. Ophthalmol 1989; 96:72.
20. Freeman HM. Fellow eyes of giant retinal breaks. Trans Am Ophthalmol Soc 1978; 76:343.
21. Davis MD, Segal PP, McCormick A. The natural course followed by the fellow eye in patients with rhegmatogenous retinal detachment. In Pruett RC, Regan CDJ, eds, Retina Congress. New York: Appleton-Century-Crofts 1974:643.

# 13 Evaluation of the Swollen Disc

**Alfredo A. Sadun, MD, PhD**
**Vivian Rismondo, MD**

Swelling of the optic nerve head can be due to a variety of causes. Papilledema refers specifically to swelling of the optic disc secondary to increased intracranial pressure, so it is best to describe such swelling generically, as disc edema, until the intracranial pressure can be assessed. The term *papilledema* carries a powerful connotation to neurologists and neurosurgeons. Optic disc edema can be consequent to elevated intracranial pressure transmitted to the optic disc in the subarachnoid space; however, it can be caused by other pathologies of the posterior or anterior optic nerve. Disc edema can also be caused by abnormalities of the optic nerve head or the peripapillary fundus. Ocular anomalies, such as hypotony, can produce optic disc edema as well.

The principal pathophysiology of optic disc swelling is blockage of axoplasmic transport. Axoplasmic transport is a transport of materials responsible for maintaining the axon, consisting primarily of proteins and organelles formed in the cell body and transported along the axon. Axonal transport may depend on the microtubules that act as "railroad tracks." Orthograde axoplasmic transport occurs at various rates, with the slow component at between 0.5 mm and 3 mm per day, and rapid flow at between 200 mm to 1000 mm per day. In addition, there is also retrograde axoplasmic transport.[1] Mechanical and vascular etiologies can conjoin to produce a blockage of optic nerve axoplasmic flow. Such blockage at the level of the lamina choroidalis and lamina scleralis occurs when optic disc edema is produced experimentally through increased intracranial pressure, ocular hypotony, or increased intraocular pressure. In the experimental model, as well as in the clinical state, it is felt that local factors produce a stasis of axoplasmic flow. Optic disc edema can also be produced by an event that increases venous pressure at or near the lamina cribosa;[2-8] intrinsic tumors, extrinsic orbital masses, or abnormalities in blood flow all can cause an increase in venous pressure.

There are several mechanisms by which different diseases can produce disc edema: 1) *Compression* of tissues in the orbit such as that caused by tumors, infiltrations, or enlarged ocular muscles (e.g., Graves') can lead to increased venous pressure and generalized vascular congestion. Blockage of venous outflow leads to venous stasis of the disc. This contributes to axonal constipation that, in turn, further swells the crowded disc. If the compression is posterior (e.g., optic canal) it will cause optic nerve atrophy without disc edema. 2) *Ischemia,* at the disc, leads to infarction of axons, blockage of axonal transport, and the development of axonal constipation. 3) *Inflammation* can lead to both vascular congestion and ischemia, resulting in the same mechanisms described above. 4) *Toxic* agents can produce mild disc edema through inflammatory changes and also through interruption of axoplasmic transport by interfering with microtubule function (Ethambutol).

## ANATOMY

The optic nerve has four segments: intraocular (1 mm), intraorbital (25 mm), intracanalicular (9 mm), and intracranial (16 mm). The optic nerve head consists of retinal ganglion cell axons that penetrate an opening in the retina, retinal pigment epithelium, choroid, and sclera. The horizontal disc diameter is 1.76 +/− 0.3 mm; the vertical diameter is 1.92 +/− 0.3 mm; and the mean cup to disc ratio is 0.39 and 0.34 in horizontal and vertical diameters, respectively. The retinal ganglion cell axons pass through the perforations of the lamina cribrosa. Since the optic nerve consists primarily of myelinated axons and astrocytes, it can be considered analogous to the white matter tracts of the brain.[9] The subarachnoid space is continuous from optic nerve head to intracranial cisterns and ventricles.

The surface of the optic disc is supplied by branches of the central retinal artery. The laminar and prelaminar portions of the optic nerve head are supplied by an anastomotic arterial complex (circle of Zinn-Haller) that derives blood from the posterior ciliary arteries, the peripapillary choroid, and the pial arterial network. The retrobulbar nerve receives its blood supply from branches of the ophthalmic artery and from the pial arterioles.

## SIGNS OF DISC EDEMA

In general, there are ten clinical signs of optic disc edema:
- hyperemia of nerve head
- blurring of optic disc margins
- filling of optic disc cups
- anterior extension of nerve head (3 diopters = 1 mm of elevation)
- edema of the nerve fiber layer
- venous congestion
- hemorrhages
- nerve fiber layer infarcts
- retinal or choroidal folds
- hard exudates of the optic disc

Some authors have distinguished between mechanical and vascular signs in optic disc edema. The five mechanical signs consist of the following:
- blurring of disc margins
- filling in of physiological cup
- anterior extension of nerve head
- edema of the nerve fiber layer
- retinal/choroidal folds

The five vascular signs consist of the following:
- hyperemia of the disc
- venous congestion
- hemorrhages

- nerve fiber layer infarcts
- exudates

In addition, the signs of optic disc swelling are useful in characterizing the disc edema as being early, fully developed, chronic, or late. In early disc edema, one sees disc hyperemia, disc swelling, blurring of the disc margins, and blurring of the nerve fiber layer. In fully developed disc edema there is gross elevation of the optic nerve head; the veins are engorged and dusky; there are peripapillary splinter hemorrhages and choroidal folds, and retina striae can be seen (Figure 13-1). In chronic papilledema there are fewer hemorrhages; the optic disc cup is completely obliterated; there is less disc hyperemia; and there are hard exudates within the nerve head (Figure 13-2). In late disc edema there is secondary optic atrophy; disc swelling subsides; retinal hemorrhages have narrowed or become sheathed; and the disc appears dirty, gray, and blurred, secondary to gliosis (Figure 13-3).

## CAUSES OF DISC EDEMA

- Compressive optic neuropathies that can produce disc edema can be caused by a variety of mass lesions. The space-occupying lesion tends to be in the anterior orbit, or so large as to displace all orbital contents forward. Neoplasms of the optic nerve itself (gliomas) or its sheaths (meningiomas) and masses from the orbital tissues or paranasal sinuses may impinge on the anterior optic nerve leading to disc edema. Inflammatory and infiltrative lesions can also present as masses. Distal malignancies can also involve the optic nerve and it sheaths by metastasizing. The history is usually one of slow progressive visual loss; the visual field defect is often a centrocecal scotoma, and the triad of optic nerve functions is impaired (afferent pupillary defect, poor color vision, decreased brightness sense).
- Papillitis often has a component of disc edema. Inflammatory papillitis is thought to sometimes be associated with a prodromal viral illness. The inflammation may extend beyond the confines of the optic disc and can develop into a neuroretinitis. Cells are frequently seen in the vitreous; deep retinal exudates may form a star or a half-star figure between the disc and the macula. Inflammatory papillitis and neuroretinitis are often seen in young, healthy adults. Although the disease is usually self-limiting, it resolves faster with steroids. In some cases progressive optic atrophy may ensue regardless of therapy.
- Ischemic optic neuropathy often manifests as sectoral disc edema with peripapillary hemorrhages. The visual loss is usually abrupt and the visual field loss may take on an altitudinal shape. Anterior ischemic optic neuropathy occurs most often in patients 50 to 75 years of age who have hypertension or diabetes.[10]
- Central retinal vein occlusion (CRVO) or impending central retinal occlusion can lead to congested optic nerve heads. Central retinal vein occlusions generally occur in middle-aged or older individuals who sometimes have hypertension or, less often, hyperviscosity syndrome. Venous stasis retinopathy is sometimes a manifestation of retinal ischemia, that may be secondary to poor anterior cerebral circulation.[9] Diabetes, chronic glaucoma, and underlying inflammation may be associated with CRVO.
- Juvenile diabetic papillopathy may manifest as disc edema, occurring unilaterally

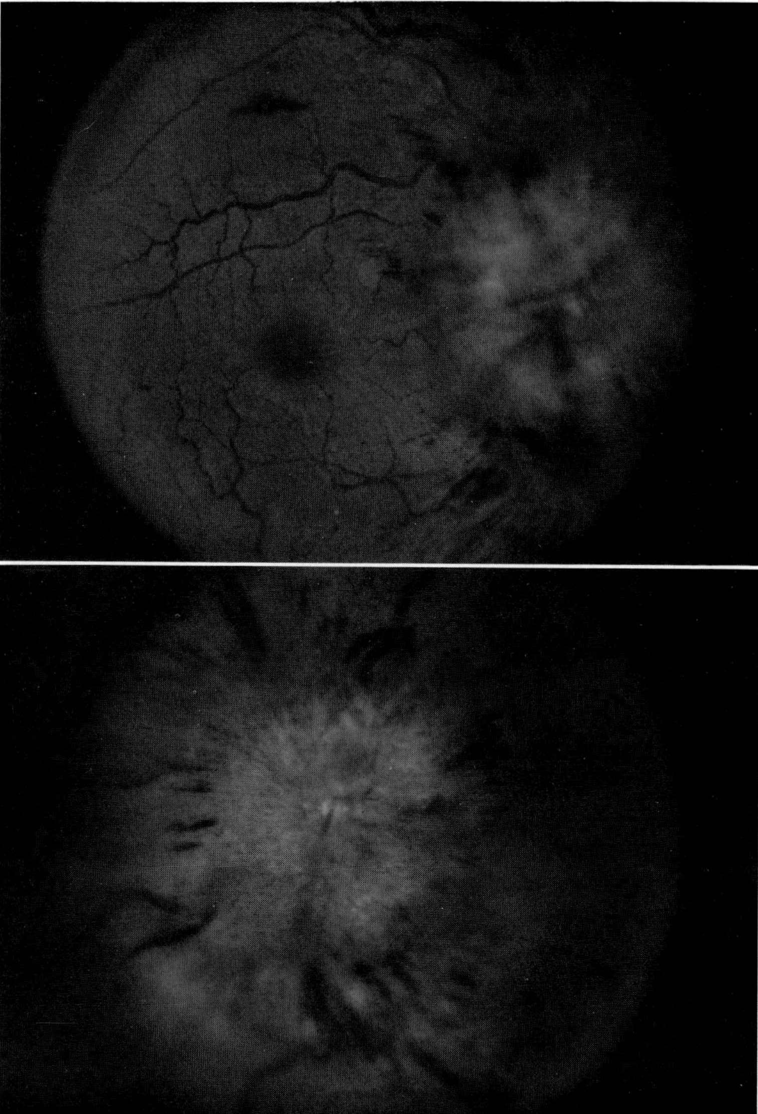

**FIGURE 13-1**    A 16-year-old boy 2 weeks after first noting blurred vision. Fully developed disc edema present. Note engorged veins, peripapillary hemorrhages, choroidal folds, and retinal striae.

or bilaterally. The visual symptoms are usually minimal, although there may be a modest loss of visual acuity. Progressive painless loss of vision is characteristic. Visual fields may show peripheral constriction or central scotomas. Fundus examination reveals dilated telangiectatic vessels over the discs that appear very much like optic disc neovascularization, but that disappear when the disc edema resolves spontaneously four to eight weeks later.[9] Corticosteroids are usually not indicated.

- Optic disc vasculitis or, more globally, uveitis, may produce optic disc edema. Papillophlebitis, optic disc vasculitis, benign retinal vasculitis, and "the big blind-spot syndrome" are all variations on this theme. This condition is usually uni-lateral in young, healthy adults with only minimal visual impairment. The optic

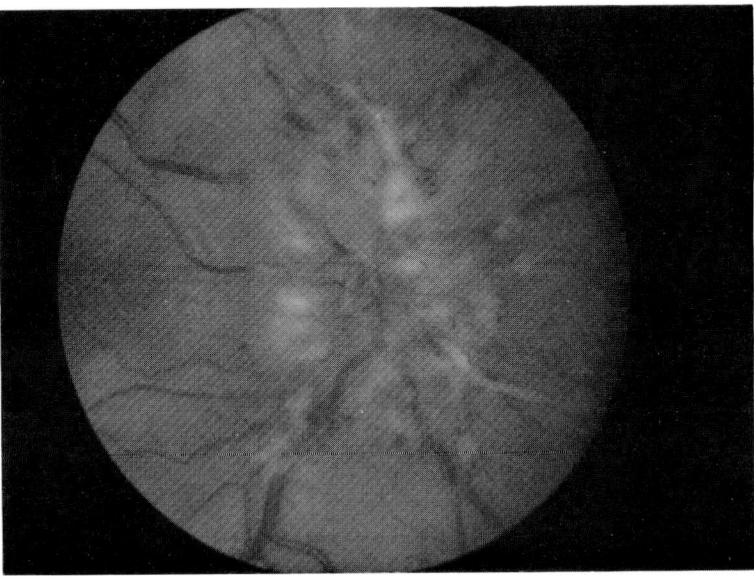

**FIGURE 13-2**    Same patient as Figures 13-1 and 13-2 seen 5 weeks after ICP reduced. There remains a picture of chronic papilledema with less disc hyperemia. The disc cup is obliterated and there are hard exudates present.

disc edema is seen in association with engorged retinal veins and occasionally with retinal hemorrhages. There is spontaneous resolution of the signs and symptoms over several months; however, resolution can be accelerated through the use of systemic steroids.

- Other causes of disc edema include Graves' disease, hypertension, and hypotony. Graves' disease causes orbital congestion and proptosis, and the optic disc is encroached upon by swollen extraocular muscles. Malignant processes, such as carcinoma, lymphoma,[11] or leukemia,[12] as well as uremia[13] and sarcoid granuloma, can cause swelling of the optic disc. Toxic and nutritional optic neuropathies can be caused by drugs such as ethambutol, isoniazid, streptomycin, chloramphenicol, digitalis, Amiodarone,[14] or Antabuse. A variety of disc anomalies can mimic disc edema (pseudopapilledema). Orbitocranial trauma, radiation, and burns can also cause swelling of the disc. Usually optic nerve involvement after radiation or burns is delayed. In several cases, visual loss can be an early complication of burns secondary to hypoxia and diffuse cerebral edema.

## COMMON OPTIC NEUROPATHIES

Two types of optic neuropathies are particularly likely to present as disc edema. In young patients, optic neuritis is common; in older patients, ischemic optic neuropathy should always be considered.

Optic neuritis may be retrobulbar, in which case optic disc changes are not seen. Bulbar optic neuritis may present as simple papillitis or, in some cases, other features of disc edema may be seen. Causes of optic neuritis are multiple. In addition to an idiopathic etiology, inflammations associated with the orbit, adjacent paranasal sinuses,[15] cranial base, brain, meninges, granulomatous dis-

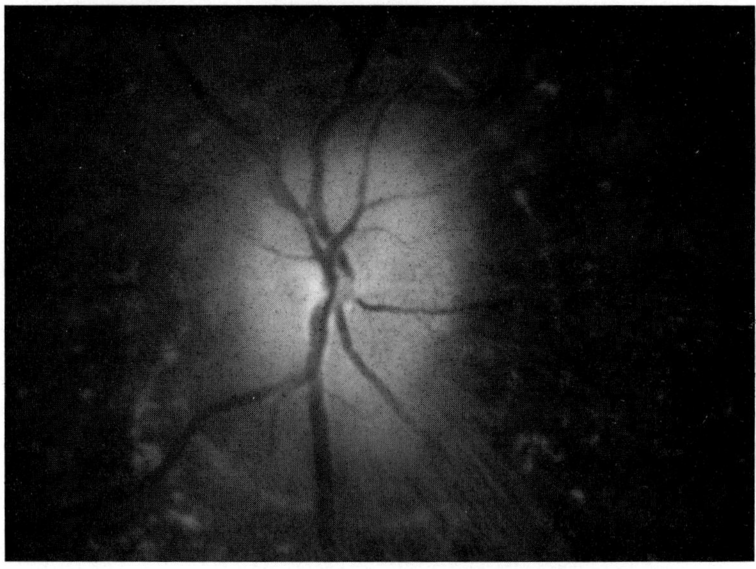

**FIGURE 13-3**  Three months later. Secondary optic atrophy has fully developed. The disc margins appear hazy or "dirty."

eases, or other systemic diseases (syphilis, AIDS, Lyme disease, sarcoidosis, tuberculosis) need to be considered. Optic neuritis can be immune-mediated (systemic lupus erythematosus), or a sign of a demyelinating illness,[16-18] or can occur following cataract surgery.[19]

Patients with optic neuritis usually present with acute, progressive loss of vision over several days often associated with phosphenes, pain and tenderness of the globe, and orbit on eye movement. Optic neuritis may be bilateral, especially in children, in Devic's syndrome. Devic's syndrome or neuromyelitis optica is a clinical syndrome characterized by acute bilateral optic neuritis and transverse myelitis. The two syndromes may occur simultaneously, or they may be separated in time (days or weeks). It may be a manifestation of post-infectious encephalomyelistis or a variant of multiple sclerosis. Patients with optic neuritis will usually complain of monocular dimness of vision and color deterioration.[20] There is no anisocoria, but an afferent pupillary defect is present on the side of the neuritis. Patients with papillitis present with some degree of disc swelling, flame hemorrhages, and cells in the vitreous. Visual field defects vary from small central and centrocecal scotomas, to arcuate and altitudinal defects and, less often, severe constriction. Vision usually improves dramatically over two to three months.

Anterior ischemic optic neuropathy (AION) is most commonly associated with hypertension, diabetes, or cataract extraction in patients over 50 years of age,[10,21] and with giant cell arteritis in older patients. The vision loss may be sudden, or it can progress in a stepwise fashion over days or weeks. An afferent pupillary defect is present. Patients with AION usually demonstrate an altitudinal field defect. The optic disc is swollen; however, swelling is usually segmental, involving only a part of the disc. Sectoral involvement of the optic disc is further evidenced by small flame hemorrhages along a portion of the optic nerve head.

Patients with cranial (temporal) arteritis have other systemic symptoms, such as weakness, weight loss, headache, myalgia, jaw claudication, and pain and tenderness of the temples and scalp. An erythrocyte sedimentation (ESR) rate should be checked promptly and, if found to be elevated, a temporal artery biopsy is probably indicated. The patient suspected of having cranial arteritis must be started on high doses of corticosteroids (prednisone, 80–100 mg daily) and maintained on this regimen until the diagnosis is ruled out. High doses of steroids should be continued for several weeks and the sedimentation rate closely monitored and kept below about 40 mm per hour. Steroids can be adjusted accordingly.[22,23]

## PAPILLEDEMA

Elevation of intracranial pressure due to an intracranial mass lesion, meningitis, or pseudotumor cerebri[24] causes an elevation of pressure in the subarachnoid space that is transmitted along the optic nerve. This pressure at the optic nerve head impinges on axons at the lamina cribrosa resulting in axoplasmic flow blockage (optic axon "constipation"). This also causes stagnation of venous return from the retina and nerve head. The abnormalities of intraaxonal fluid mechanics result in swelling of axons and subsequent leakage of water, protein, and other substances. Papilledema is principally a mechanical phenomenon followed by venous obstructions, vascular telangiectases and nerve fiber hypoxia.[3-8]

Optic disc edema from increased intracranial pressure may take several hours to develop and often takes days to weeks to resolve. Normal cerebral spinal fluid pressures vary between 100 and 200 mm of water. However, the intracranial pressure may vary a great deal and a single low reading may be misleading in a patient with papilledema. In the event that disc edema is noted in a patient in whom the physician can not be sure whether this represents papilledema or not, neuro-radiological studies (CT or MRI) should be obtained initially, followed by a lumbar puncture with manometry, if appropriate. The ophthalmoscopic appearance of papilledema depends upon the stage and the duration of the process. Initially there may be minimal hyperemia of the optic disc. In early papilledema one can also see blurring of the peripapillary nerve fiber layer, optic disc swelling manifested later by obliteration of the physiological optic cup, extension of the optic disc anteriorly, and a blurring of the optic disc margins. Although venous pulsations are usually absent in early disc edema, sometimes they are not seen in normal optic nerves as well. In longer standing papilledema, the more fully developed disc edema manifests as an optic disc that is grossly elevated above the retina. The veins of the retina become engorged, tortuous, and dusky. Peripapillary splinter hemorrhages are also seen. Choroidal folds can be noted in patients with severe papilledema. (See Figures 13-1 and 13-2.) In chronic papilledema, fewer hemorrhages are seen but capillary telangiectases and optocilliary shunt vessels develop. Exudations within the disc substance coalesce into hard, shiny crystaloids resembling optic disc drusen, hence the description of pseudodrusen in "old" or chronic disc edema (see Figure 13-3). The final stage of papilledema is atrophy with disc pallor.[25] Once atrophy develops, the disc edema diminishes. Dead axons do not swell. Ultimately, postpapilledema atrophy develops as the disc swelling subsides. The disc becomes atrophic in a characteristic fashion. Funduscopy reveals a dirty gray blurred appearance on the surface of the optic disc caused by glial proliferation and disorganized axonal degeneration. The retinal veins are narrowed and may be sheathed. This is termed *secondary optic atrophy* and is important in revealing the history of an optic nerve head that was once swollen. (See Figure 13-3.)

Papilledema is almost always bilateral. Rarely, a congenital nerve sheath anomaly may not enable transmission of pressure so that the ipsilateral disc appears normal, despite increased intracranial pressure.[26] In cases of chronic compression of the optic nerve by a subfrontal tumor, the optic disc will appear atrophic and the opposite disc will appear swollen, due to a generalized increase in intracranial pressure.[27] This is known as the Foster-Kennedy syndrome.

Symptoms of transient visual obscurations (TOVs) are characteristic of increased intracranial pressure, but they may occur in other causes of disc edema and even in pseudo disc edema.[8,28] Bilateral VI nerve involvement, headache, nausea, and vomiting often accompany increased intracranial pressure that causes papilledema. Visual field defects begin with enlargement of the blind spot, and often progress to constriction of the visual fields. However, almost any pattern of visual field loss can be seen in advanced papilledema.[29,30] Patients with chronic disc edema must be followed closely for visual impairments, since central acuity loss may not herald the problem. In addition to regular visual field testing, assessments of color vision, and Amsler grid and contrast sensitivity testing can be very helpful. The treatment of disc edema associated with visual loss depends on the etiology, symptoms, signs, and progression. Attempts should be made to redress the pathophysiology. In general, medical treatment consists of repeated lumbar punctures, corticosteroids, carbonic anhydrase inhibitors, and weight reduction.[31] If medical treatment is not sufficient, optic nerve sheath decompression[32,33] or a lumboperitoneal shunt[34] should be done.

## PSEUDOPAPILLEDEMA (PSEUDO DISC EDEMA)

The optic nerve head can appear elevated and irregular due to a variety of causes that can mimic disc edema. Hyaline bodies (optic disc drusen) are often embedded deeply in the optic nerve head at the level of the lamina or just anterior to it. Optic disc drusen are sometimes inherited as an autosomal dominant trait with variable penetrance. They are often calcified and are thought to represent axoplasmic derivatives from retinal ganglion cell axons. Congenital anomalies of the optic nerve head, such as tilted disc or Fuch's coloboma, may be difficult to assess and can lead to misdiagnosis of disc edema. The optic nerve head in hyperopic eyes often appears full and may even extend a small distance anterior to the plane of the retina. Patients with pseudo disc edema may have transient obscurations of vision that are indistinguishable from those seen in patients with true disc edema, since the normal architecture of the lamina cribrosa is disturbed.[35]

## SUMMARY

In short, swelling of the optic disc can be characterized by about ten signs. Disc edema may reflect increased intracranial pressure (papilledema) and requires neurological consultation. Disc edema is caused, primarily, by stasis of axoplasmic flow. Hence, atrophic nerves do not swell. Usually, early disc edema minimally impacts visual function. However, chronic disc edema can lead to severe and permanent visual impairments. It behooves the clinician to detect, characterize, monitor, and, when necessary, treat swelling of the optic disc.

## References


1. Brady ST, Lasek RJ, Allen RD. Video microscopy for fast axonal transport of extruded axoplasm: a new model for study of molecular mechanisms. Cell Motil 1985; 5:81-101.
2. Minckler DS, Bunt AH. Axoplasmic transport in ocular hypotony and papilledema in the monkey. Arch Ophthalmol 1977; 95:1430-1436.
3. Hayreh MS, Hayreh SS. Optic disc edema in raised intracranial pressure. I. Evolution and resolution. Arch Ophthalmol 1977; 95:1237-1244.
4. Hayreh SS, Hayreh MS. Optic disc edema in raised intracranial pressure. II. Early detection with fluorescein fundus angiography and stereoscopic color photography. Arch Ophthalmol 1977; 95:1245-1254.
5. Tso MOM, Hayreh SS. Optic disc edema in raised intracranial pressure. III. A pathologic study of experimental papilledema. Arch Ophthalmol 1977; 95:1448-1457.
6. Tso MOM, Hayreh SS. Optic disc edema in raised intracranial pressure. IV. Axoplasmic transport in experimental papilledema. Arch Ophthalmol 1977; 95:1458-1462.
7. Hayreh SS. Optic disc edema in raised intracranial pressure. V. Pathogenesis. Arch Ophthalmol 1977; 95:1553-1565.
8. Hayreh SS. Optic disc edema in raised intracranial pressure. VI. Associated visual disturbances and their pathogenesis. Arch Ophthalmol 1977; 95:1566-1579.
9. Glaser J. Neuro-ophthalmology. ed 2 Philadelphia: JB Lippincott, 1990:64-68; 95-97; 107-108; 135-140.
10. Green GJ, Lessell S, Loewenstein JI. Ischemic optic neuropathy in chronic papilledema. Arch Ophthalmol 1980; 98:502-504.
11. Kline LB, Garcia JH, Harsh GR III. Lymphomatous optic neuropathy. Arch Ophthalmol 1984; 102:1655-1657.
12. Currie JN, Lessell S, Lessell IM, et al. Optic neuropathy in chronic lymphocytic leukemia. Arch Ophthalmol 1988; 106:654-660.
13. Knox DL, Hanneken AM, Hollows FC, et al. Uremic optic neuropathy. Arch Ophthalmol 1988; 106: 50-54.
14. Feiner LA, Younge BR, Kozmier FJ, et al. Optic neuropathy and amiodarone therapy. Mayo Clin Proc 1987; 62:702-717.
15. Goldberg RA, Weisman JS, McFarland JE, et al. Orbital inflammation and optic neuropathies associated with chronic sinusitis of intranasal cocaine abuse: possible role of continguous inflammation. Arch Ophthalmol 1989; 107:831-835.
16. Johns K, Lavin P, Elliot JH, et al. Magnetic resonance imaging of the brain in isolated optic neuritis. Arch Ophthalmol 1986; 104:1486-1488.
17. Sandberg-Wollheim M, Bynke H, Cronqvist S, et al. A long-term prospective study of optic neuritis: evaluation of risk factors. Ann Neurol 1990; 27: 386-393.
18. Eidelberg D, Newton MR, Johnson G, et al. Chronic unilateral optic neuropathy: a magnetic resonance study. Ann Neurol 1988; 24:3-11.
19. Michaels DD, Zugsmith GS. Optic neuropathy following cataract extraction. Ann Ophthalmol Mar 1973; 5:303-306.
20. Sadun AA, Lessell S. Brightness-sense and optic nerve disease. Arch Ophthalmol 1985; 103:39-43.
21. Guyer DR, Miller NR, Auer CL, et al. The risk of cerebrovascular and cardiovascular disease in patients with anterior ischemic optic neuropathy. Arch Ophthalmol 1985; 103:1136-1142.
22. Cox TA, Woolson RF. Steroid treatment of optic neuritis. Arch Ophthalmol 1981; 99:338.
23. Burde RM, Savino PJ, Trobe JD. Clinical decisions in neuro-ophthalmology. St. Louis: CV Mosby Company, 1985:41-46.
24. Grant DN. Benign intracranial hypertension: a review of 79 cases in infancy and childhood. Arch Disease of Childhood 1971; 46:651-655.
25. Frisen L. Swelling of the optic nerve head: a staging scheme. J of Neurology Neurosurgery and Psychiatry 1982; 45:13-18.
26. To KW, Warren FA. Unilateral papilledema in pseudotumor cerebri. Arch Ophthalmol 1990; 108:644-645.
27. Sanders MD, Sennhenn RH. Differential diagnosis of unilateral optic disc oedema. Trans Ophthalmol Soc UK 1980; 100:123-131.
28. Orcutt JC, Page NGR, Sanders MD. Factors affecting visual loss in benign intracranial hypertension. Ophthalmol 1984; 91:1303-1312.
29. Baker RS, Carter D, Hendrick EB, et al. Visual loss in pseudotumor cerebri of childhood: a follow-up study. Arch Ophthalmol 1985; 103:1681-1686.

30. Smith TJ, Baker RS. Perimetric findings in pseudotumor cerebri using automated techniques. Ophthalmol 1986; 93:887-894.
31. Corbett JJ, Thompson HS. The rational management of idiopathic intracranial hypertension. Arch Neurol 1989; 46:1049-1051.
32. Brourman ND, Spoor TC, Ramocki JM. Optic nerve decompression for pseudotumor cerebri. Arch Ophthalmol 1988; 106:1378-1383.
33. Corbett JJ, Nerad JA, Tse DT, et al. Results of optic nerve sheath fenestration for pseudotumor cerebri: the lateral orbitotomy approach. Arch Ophthalmol 1988; 106:1391-1397.
34. Tytla ME, Buncic JR. Recovery of spatial vision following shunting for hydrocephalus. Arch Ophthalmol 1990; 108:701-704.
35. Apple DJ, Rabb MF, Walsh PM. Congenital anomalies of the optic disc. Surv Ophthalmol 1982; 27:3-41.

# 14 Sedation for Ophthalmic Surgery

**G. Edward Morgan, Jr., MD**

One of the most dramatic transformations in health care delivery during the past decade has been a shift from inpatient surgery to outpatient and office surgery. As would be expected, the trend toward same-day surgery has affected the practice of ophthalmology. One result has been an increased utilization of local anesthesia with intravenous sedation in eye surgery. This article provides a review of the goals of sedation, patient and case selection, pharmacologic and nonpharmacologic techniques of sedation, monitoring standards, and the treatment of complications.

## GOALS OF SEDATION

The goals of sedation depend upon many factors including patient personality, surgical procedure, and physician preference. Decreasing anxiety is usually the major goal of sedation for ophthalmic surgery in adults. While anxiety is a normal emotional response to impending surgery, its degree varies greatly from patient to patient. In general, younger patients are more anxious and more resistant to anxiolytic drugs. In fact, unconsciousness is often necessary for the examination of infants or children. Immobilization is a more important objective in some surgical procedures than in others. For example, minimizing patient movement is critical during cataract surgery, but less significant during a blepharoplasty. Finally, physicians vary in their own definition of an "ideal" level of sedation. Some like to keep their patients responsive and cooperative, while others prefer them asleep and unaware of their surroundings. Other goals of sedation include perioperative pain relief and amnesia.

Two conclusions can be made from this discussion of goals. First, a perfect level of sedation is difficult to define, let alone achieve. Second, the goals of sedation often contradict one another. For example, it would be ideal to achieve complete analgesia yet maintain adequate patient cooperation during a retrobulbar block. This specificity of effect is difficult, if not impossible, with currently available drugs. Thus, providing sedation must always be individualized to each patient and often represents a compromise of conflicting goals. Nonetheless, one important objective holds true for all sedated patients: maintaining an effective airway. Cyanosis, vomiting, or coughing must be avoided.

## PATIENT AND CASE SELECTION

Not every patient is a candidate for local anesthesia with sedation. Unless rendered unconscious, some patients are obviously going to be uncooperative. These include children, the mentally retarded, and patients suffering from involuntary movements (e.g., tic douloureux) or chronic cough. Except for very brief procedures (e.g., suture removal or tonometry), general anesthesia is probably a better choice for these patients. Other patients adamantly reject even the thought of being awake during surgery. Unless general anesthesia is specifically contraindicated, it is usually a mistake to try to change the minds of these individuals. There is a final group of patients that do not tolerate local anesthesia with sedation, but are very difficult to identify in advance. This group includes patients that become claustrophobic under drapes, that talk incessantly, or that seem to wiggle continuously once surgery has begun. Controlling these patients intraoperatively poses a great challenge.

Similarly, not every surgical procedure lends itself to local anesthesia. Clearly, the patient should not be allowed to experience more than minor discomfort. This would preclude surgeries such as orbital reconstruction or decompression. Because of psychological considerations, enucleation is rarely performed under local anesthesia in the United States. Procedures lasting longer than three hours will test the duration of currently available local anesthetic agents, not to mention the patient's endurance for lying on an operating-room table. Nonetheless, most ophthalmic surgery is suitable for local anesthesia with supplemental sedation.

## NONPHARMACOLOGIC SEDATION TECHNIQUES

Successful intraoperative sedation is part of the art of medicine. As such, it requires more than merely administering medications according to a "cookbook formula." No tranquilizer can replace the confidence and trust that constitutes the patient-physician relationship.

Patients fear surgery. Every facet of their intraoperative experience is out of their control: from the duration of the surgery, to the clothes they are allowed to wear. The operating room is an alien environment: It is cold, sterile, and uncomfortable. During the typical outpatient experience, patients will meet an average of five to ten strangers in whom they are expected to place their trust. How could anyone relax in this situation?

Many techniques are helpful in allaying patient fears. Foremost is properly explaining what can be expected during the perioperative period.[1] There is no value in surprise injections of local anesthetic or unrealistically short time estimates. However, more important than what is said to patients, is how it is said.[2] An example of inappropriate word choice is; "I'm going to give you an injection behind your eye, and it's going to hurt like a killer bee sting. But don't squint!" Words such as needle stick, pain, hurt, and injection all trigger an immediate stress response, which is often significant enough to cause a rise in heart rate. This sounds better: "Relax your eye lids and eye muscles as much as you can. I'm just rubbing a little cold alcohol here. Now I'm going to give you that numbing medication we talked about before so that you will be completely comfortable during the operation. The more you relax, the better you will feel." Relaxation techniques such as hypnosis and behavior modification have been successfully used during ophthalmologic surgery.[2,3]

During surgery, many patients enjoy the relaxation that music can provide. Miniaturized stereo cassette or compact disc players with small headphones are becoming increasingly popular in the operating room. I have even recorded a relaxation tape that some patients have wanted to take home after surgery. Most patients appreciate having someone hold their hand, if only intermittently during the procedure.[4] The power of these simple maneuvers can not be overstated.

## PHARMACOLOGIC SEDATION TECHNIQUES

There is a plethora of pharmacologic agents suitable for sedation. Many of these have become available during the past five years and are still finding their place in clinical usage. The properties of an ideal sedative would include: 1) a rapid onset of action; 2) a short duration of action or the availability of a specific reversal agent; 3) no effect on cardiovascular, pulmonary, or upper airway function; 4) no effect on ocular function; 5) an antiemetic effect; and 6) sedative effects consistent with the goals outlined above. It is not surprising that no drug has proven to be the ideal agent in all situations. Factors that influence the choice of a specific drug include its effects on vital organs, effects on the eye, and other clinical considerations.

## Barbiturates

Barbiturates are barbituric acid derivatives that depress the reticular activating system, a complex polysynaptic network of neurons and regulatory centers located in the brain stem that controls several vital functions including consciousness. Alterations in structure determine hypnotic potency and pharmacokinetics. For example, thiopental and thiamylal have greater potency, a more rapid onset of action, and a shorter duration of action compared to pentobarbital and secobarbital. There is no specific barbiturate antagonist available.

### Effects on vital organs

Large doses of intravenously administered barbiturates can cause a fall in blood pressure and an elevation in heart rate. In the presence of some medical conditions such as hypovolemia, congestive heart failure, or beta-adrenergic blockade, cardiac output and arterial blood pressure may fall dramatically due to uncompensated peripheral pooling and unmasked direct myocardial depression. Patients with poorly controlled hypertension are particularly prone to wide swings in blood pressure during intravenous administration. Thus, the cardiovascular effects of barbiturates vary depending on volume status, baseline sympathetic tone, and preexisting cardiovascular disease.

Barbiturate depression of the medullary ventilatory center decreases the ventilatory response to hypercarbia and hypoxia. Apnea usually follows intravenous administration of anything but a small dose of barbiturate. Bronchospasm in asthmatic patients or laryngospasm in lightly anesthetized patients is not uncommon. Laryngospasm and hiccuping may be more common after methohexital than thiopental.

The degree of central nervous system depression induced by barbiturates ranges from mild sedation to unconsciousness, depending on the dose administered. Unlike narcotics, barbiturates do not selectively impair the perception of pain. In fact, they sometimes appear to have an antianalgesic effect by lowering the pain threshold. Small doses occasionally cause a state of excitement and disorientation that can be disconcerting when sedation is the objective. Barbiturates do not produce muscle relaxation, and some agents, such as methohexital, induce involuntary skeletal-muscle contractions. Ethanol, narcotics, antihistamines, and other central nervous system depressants potentiate the sedative effects of barbiturates.

## Ocular effects

Ocular effects of barbiturates include nystagmus, impairment of convergence, and changes in electroretinography and visually evoked response testing.[5,6] Barbiturates lower intraocular pressure.

## Clinical considerations

In ophthalmology, short-acting barbiturates (e.g., methohexital and thiopental) are frequently administered intravenously, immediately before performing retrobulbar and facial nerve blocks (Table 14-1).[7,8] Patients become unconscious within one to two minutes and awaken within five to ten minutes. An anesthesiologist should be present during intravenous administration of barbiturates in case of apnea.

Another use of barbiturates in ophthalmology is for heavy sedation of children during brief examinations. Rectally administered methohexital typically produces unconsciousness within 10 minutes. The child will usually be completely awake within 30 to 60 minutes. Intramuscular injection is appropriate for moderate sedation of children. The onset of action of intramuscular pentobarbital or secobarbital is usually within 30 to 60 minutes, but their effects can linger for several hours.

---

# Benzodiazepines

Benzodiazepines interact with specific receptors in the central nervous system, particularly in the cerebral cortex. Benzodiazepine-receptor binding enhances the inhibitory effects of neurotransmitters such as gamma-aminobutyric acid. The chemical structure of benzodiazepines includes a benzene ring and a seven-member diazepine ring. The insolubility of diazepam and lorazepam in water requires commercial preparations containing propylene glycol, which has been associated with venous irritation.

## Vital organ effects

The benzodiazepines display minimal cardiovascular depressant effects, even at high doses. Arterial blood pressure, cardiac output, and peripheral vascular resistance usually decline slightly, while heart rate sometimes rises. Midazolam tends to lower blood pressure and peripheral-vascular resistance more than diazepam.

Although apnea may be less common than following barbiturate induction, *even small intravenous doses of diazepam and midazolam have resulted in*

**Table 14-1**   Uses and Dosages of Barbiturates in Ophthalmology

| Clinical use | Drug | Dosage |
| --- | --- | --- |
| During retrobulbar and facial nerve block | 1.0% Methohexital | 0.2-0.5 mg/kg IV |
| | 2.5% Thiopental | 0.5-1.5 mg/kg IV |
| Heavy sedation in children | 10.0% Methohexital | 20-30 mg/kg rectally |
| | 5.0% Secobarbital | 2-4 mg/kg IM* |
| | 5.0% Pentobarbital | 2-4 mg/kg IM* |

*up to a maximum dose of 150 mg

*respiratory arrest.* The steep dose-response curve and high potency of midazolam necessitates careful titration. Ventilation must be monitored in all patients receiving intravenous benzodiazepines and resuscitation equipment must be immediately available.

Oral sedative doses often produce antegrade amnesia, an extremely useful property. The antianxiety, amnesic, and sedative effects seen at low doses progress to stupor and unconsciousness at higher doses. Like many sedative drugs, benzodiazepines can cause paradoxical excitatory behavior.[9] Benzodiazepines do not have direct analgesic properties.

Ethanol, barbiturates, and other central nervous system depressants potentiate the sedative effects of the benzodiazepines. A specific benzodiazepine-receptor antagonist (flumazenil) effectively reverses most of the central nervous system effects.

## Ocular effects

Ocular effects of benzodiazepines include nystagmus and diplopia.[6] Attacks of narrow-angle glaucoma have been reported, although benzodiazepines usually decrease intraocular pressure.[5]

## Clinical considerations

Benzodiazepines are commonly administered orally, intramuscularly, and intravenously (Table 14-2). Diazepam and lorazepam are well absorbed from the gastrointestinal tract with peak plasma levels usually achieved in one and two hours, respectively. Midazolam is not available for oral administration. Intramuscular injection of diazepam is painful and absorption is unreliable. In contrast, midazolam and lorazepam are well absorbed after intramuscular injection with peak levels achieved in 30 and 90 minutes, respectively.

Diazepam is quite lipid-soluble and rapidly penetrates the blood-brain barrier. Although midazolam is water soluble at a low pH, its imidazole ring closes at physiologic pH, causing an increase in its lipid solubility. The moderate lipid solubility of lorazepam accounts for its slower brain uptake and the onset of action. None of the benzodiazepines can match the rapid onset and short duration of action of thiopental.

Small doses of benzodiazepines provide relatively safe sedation in situations where an anesthesiologist is not available. Because of its shorter duration of action and less tendency to cause pain on injection, parenterally administered midazolam has largely replaced diazepam as a sedative in ophthalmic procedures.[10] However, the risk of respiratory depression following intravenous midazolam must be ap-

**Table 14-2**   Dosages of Benzodiazepines Commonly Used for Sedation in Ophthalmology

| Agent | Route | Sedative dose |
|---|---|---|
| Diazepam | Oral | 0.20-0.5  mg/kg* |
|  | Intravenous | 0.02-0.2  mg/kg |
| Midazolam | Intramuscular | 0.07-0.1  mg/kg |
|  | Intravenous | 0.01-0.1  mg/kg |
| Lorazepam** | Oral | 0.05 mg/kg*** |
|  | Intramuscular | 0.03-0.05 mg/kg |
|  | Intravenous | 0.02-0.04 mg/kg |

*maximum dose 15 mg
**not recommended for children
***maximum dose 3 mg

preciated, especially since the dose required for individual patients is somewhat unpredictable.[11]

## Chloral Hydrate

Chloral hydrate is a relatively safe and effective hypnotic drug. Its therapeutic action is caused by an active metabolite (trichloroethanol). This metabolite has a long half-life that can exceed nine hours.

### Vital organ effects

Chloral hydrate has little effect on respiration or blood pressure in the recommended dosage range. However, overdosage can result in severe respiratory depression. Undesirable central nervous system effects may include paradoxical excitement, disorientation, and paranoid behavior.

### Ocular effects

The effects of chloral hydrate on intraocular pressure appear to be minimal.[12]

### Clinical considerations

Chloral hydrate has become a popular sedative for children undergoing brief ophthalmic examinations or procedures.[5,12] Because of its relatively high margin of safety and minimal ocular effects, chloral hydrate is probably the best choice for congenital glaucoma examinations in the absence of an anesthesiologist. The recommended oral dosage depends upon age and physical health, as shown below. If there is no response after 30 minutes, one-half of the initial dose may be repeated. Maximum effect is usually within one hour, but sedation may last anywhere from two to several hours. Oral ingestion is characterized by an unpleasant taste and gastric irritation. Possible side effects include vomiting (15% of patients), delirium, bradypnea, and airway obstruction. Vomiting may result in insufficient sedation. Rectal suppositories are also available.

## Propofol

Propofol (2,6-diisopropylphenol) consists of a phenol ring with two isopropyl groups attached. Propofol's mechanism of action has not been described. Propofol

**Recommended Dosages of Chloral Hydrate**

---

Healthy children and > 4 weeks old      50-100 mg/kg PO*
Unhealthy child or < 4 weeks old        25-50   mg/kg PO

*maximum recommended dose varies from 1 to 3 grams.

is not water soluble, but a 1% aqueous solution (10 mg propofol/ml) is available as an oil-in-water emulsion containing soybean oil, glycerin, and egg lecithin. This formulation can cause pain during injection. Propofol is only available for intravenous administration.

## Vital organ effects

The major cardiovascular effect of propofol is a decrease in arterial blood pressure caused by a drop in systemic vascular resistance. Factors exacerbating the hypotension include large doses, rapid injection, and old age. Changes in heart rate and cardiac output are usually transient and insignificant in healthy patients.

Like the barbiturates, propofol is a profound respiratory depressant that usually causes apnea following a large dose. Induction is occasionally accompanied by excitatory phenomena, such as muscle twitching, spontaneous movement, or hiccuping.

## Ocular effects

Propofol decreases intraocular pressure.

## Clinical considerations

The high lipid solubility of propofol results in an onset of action that is almost as rapid as thiopental (one arm-brain circulation time). Awakening from a single bolus dose is also rapid because of a very short initial distribution half-life (two to eight minutes). Some investigators feel that the recovery from propofol is more rapid and accompanied by less "hangover" than methohexital or thiopental. This would make it a good agent for outpatient use.

Because of its rapid onset and extremely short duration of action, a small bolus of propofol can be administered immediately before retrobulbar and facial nerve block to produce a brief state of unconsciousness. The risk of potential complications such as airway obstruction or apnea is similar to the risk with thiopental or methohexital. Thus, equipment and personnel for resuscitation should be immediately available. Propofol can also be given as a continuous infusion (1 to 3 mg/kg/hr) for prolonged intraoperative sedation.[11,13] When used in this fashion, the patient must be continuously monitored by an anesthesiologist for signs of excessive sedation.

---

## Opioid Agonists and Agonist-Antagonists

Opioids bind to specific receptors located throughout the central nervous system and other tissues. The pharmacodynamic properties of specific opioids depend upon which opioid receptor type is bound, the binding affinity, and whether the receptor is activated. Although both opioid agonists and antagonists bind to opioid receptors, only agonists are capable of receptor activation. Agonist-antagonists, such as nalbuphine, nalorphine, butorphanol, and pentazocine, are drugs that have opposite actions at different receptor types.

## Vital organ effects

In general, sedative doses of opioids do not seriously impair cardiovascular function. Opioids depress ventilation, particularly respiratory rate. Resting arterial carbon dioxide partial pressure ($P_aCO_2$) increases and the response to a carbon dioxide challenge is blunted, resulting in a shift of the carbon dioxide response curve downward and to the right. These effects are mediated through the respiratory centers in the brain stem. The apneic threshold, the highest $P_aCO_2$ at which a patient remains apneic, is elevated and hypoxic drive is decreased. Opioids (particularly fentanyl, sufentanil, and alfentanil) can induce chest wall rigidity that is severe enough to prevent adequate ventilation. This centrally mediated muscle contraction is most frequent after large drug boluses. Stimulation of the medullary chemoreceptor trigger zone is responsible for a high incidence of nausea and vomiting.

## Ocular effects

Ocular side effects of opioid administration include nystagmus and miosis. Intraocular pressure is decreased.

## Clinical considerations

Opioids are excellent analgesics, but relatively large doses are required to render patients unconscious. Regardless of dose, opioids do not reliably produce amnesia. Many drugs with opioid receptor activity have been used for sedation during ophthalmologic surgery. Morphine, meperidine, and the other longer-acting agonists have fallen from popularity since the introduction of fentanyl. A small intravenous dose of fentanyl (25 to 100 mcg) provides analgesia and will supplement the sedation of a benzodiazepine.[7] A new ultrashort acting opioid agonist, alfentanil, may prove useful as a bolus injection during retrobulbar blockade or as an infusion for prolonged sedation.

Opioid agonists are sometimes combined with sedative drugs that possess antiemetic properties in a fixed ratio mixture. For example, meperidine (25 mg/ml), promethazine (6.25 mg/ml), and chlorpromazine (6.25 mg/ml) have been administered intramuscularly at a dose of 0.07 ml/kg. The prolonged effect of this "cocktail" detracts from its use with outpatients.[5] Innovar is a commercially available combination of fentanyl (50 mcg/ml) and droperidol (2.5 mg/ml), a butyrophenone that is structurally related to phenothiazines. Droperidol is a tranquilizer, and it does not produce analgesia, amnesia, or unconsciousness at usual doses. However, the combination of fentanyl with droperidol produces a state characterized by analgesia, immobility, and variable amnesia known as *neuroleptanalgesia*. Because of the longer-lasting effects of droperidol, many clinicians feel that a fixed combination is not as valuable as administering the components separately as needed. Droperidol should not be administered without an opioid drug because of its tendency to cause dysphoric reactions. Several agonist-antagonists (e.g., butorphanol, nalbuphine) have been examined for conscious sedation, since they may cause less respiratory depression than opioid agonists following unintentional overdosage.[7,14]

The combination of opioids, particularly meperidine, and monoamine oxidase inhibitors may result in respiratory arrest, hypertension or hypotension, coma, and hyperpyrexia. The cause of this dramatic interaction is not understood. Barbiturates, benzodiazepines, and other central nervous system depressants can have synergist cardiovascular, respiratory, and sedative effects with opioids. A distinct advantage of opioids is the availability of a specific opioid antagonist (naloxone).

## Ketamine

Ketamine has multiple effects throughout the central nervous system, including blocking polysynaptic reflexes in the spinal cord and inhibiting excitatory neurotransmitter effects in selected areas of the brain. In contrast to the depression of the reticular activating system induced by the barbiturates, ketamine functionally "dissociates" the thalamus from the limbic cortex. Clinically, this state of dissociative anesthesia causes the patient to appear conscious (e.g., eye opening, swallowing, muscle contracture) but unable to process or respond to sensory input.

Ketamine is a structural analogue of phencyclidine (PCP). It is one-tenth as potent, yet retains many of phencyclidine's "psychotomimetic" effects. Ketamine is administered intravenously or intramuscularly. Peak plasma levels are usually achieved within 10 to 15 minutes of intramuscular injection.

### Vital organ effects

In sharp contrast to other sedative agents, ketamine increases arterial blood pressure, heart rate, and cardiac output. These indirect cardiovascular effects are caused by central stimulation of the sympathetic nervous system. For these reasons, ketamine should be avoided in patients with coronary artery disease, uncontrolled hypertension, congestive heart failure, and arterial aneurysms.

Ventilatory drive is minimally affected by sedative doses of ketamine, although rapid intravenous bolus or pretreatment with opioids may occasionally produce apnea. Undesirable psychotomimetic side effects such as illusions, disturbing dreams, and delirium during emergence and recovery are less common in children and patients premedicated with benzodiazepines.

### Ocular effects

Ketamine has multiple effects on the eye, including nystagmus, blepharospasm, diplopia, and a variable effect on intraocular pressure.[15,16]

### Clinical considerations

Because of the high incidence of hallucinations and other emergence phenomena in adults, ketamine is usually reserved for use in children (1 to 2 mg/kg intravenously or 5 to 10 mg/kg intramuscularly) or uncooperative, combative adults. As an added precaution against emergence reactions, a benzodiazepine is usually administerd prior to ketamine administration. This combination produces a true anesthetic state and should only be administered by an anesthesiologist. A small dose of intravenous ketamine (0.25 mg/kg) may be useful during brief, painful stimulation in adults, such as local anesthetic infiltration during plastic surgical procedures.

## MONITORING STANDARDS

It is obvious from the above discussion that sedation is associated with potential side effects. Detection of these complications depends upon effective monitoring techniques. The extent of monitoring indicated depends upon three factors: 1) the invasiveness of the surgical procedure; 2) the health of the patient; and 3) the degree of sedation. For example, a healthy 30-year-old undergoing a minor plastic procedure with minimal sedation probably requires no special monitoring beyond observation by the surgeon. On the other hand, an elderly patient with heart disease having cataract surgery under local anesthesia with considerable intravenous sedation may require a level of monitoring approaching that for general anesthesia. Recently, a fourth factor has emerged that influences monitoring standards: regulations published by states and professional organizations.

Note that location is irrelevant: Monitoring standards do not depend upon whether the patient is being treated in a hospital, an outpatient clinic, or a physician's office. Any of the agents discussed in this review can be administered outside the hospital environment, *if* appropriate personnel and monitoring equipment are available. Surgeons often request the presence of an anesthesiologist to continuously monitor patients and to be prepared to convert to general anesthesia if necessary. The term *standby anesthesia* is a misnomer that has been replaced with *monitored anesthesia care* (MAC). Whether or not an anesthesiologist needs to be involved in patient sedation usually depends upon the health of the patient, the extent of the proposed surgery, and the degree of sedation desired. Most ophthalmologists are uncomfortable administering anything more than minimal amounts of intravenous sedation to patients in the absence of an anesthesiologist. This is probably particularly true for thiopental, methohexital, propofol, and ketamine. Conversely, all agents, including the benzodiazepines, can be lethal if given in inappropriate doses or without adequate monitoring.

Adequacy of oxygenation can be grossly assessed by observation of skin and nail color. Continuous auscultation of breath sounds with a precordial stethoscope will identify airway obstruction caused by excessive sedation. Electrocardiography, intermittent noninvasive blood pressure, and palpation of a peripheral pulse will help to ensure adequate circulation. These cardiovascular monitors are particularly important during procedures that may elicit the oculocardiac reflex. Conversation with the patient assesses level of consciousness.

Noninvasive monitoring of arterial oxygen saturation with pulse oximetry should be considered in most, if not all, procedures. However, while pulse oximetry will warn of hypoxia, it will not detect hypoventilation until it interferes with oxygenation. Aspiration end-tidal carbon dioxide analyzers can be adapted to local cases by connecting the collection tubing to a location near the patient's mouth. Although entrainment of room air precludes exact measurements, this technique provides a qualitative indicator of ventilation. In addition to providing information regarding the circulation, keeping a finger on the radial pulse will help to reassure an anxious patient.

If the case needs to be converted to general anesthesia, additional monitors

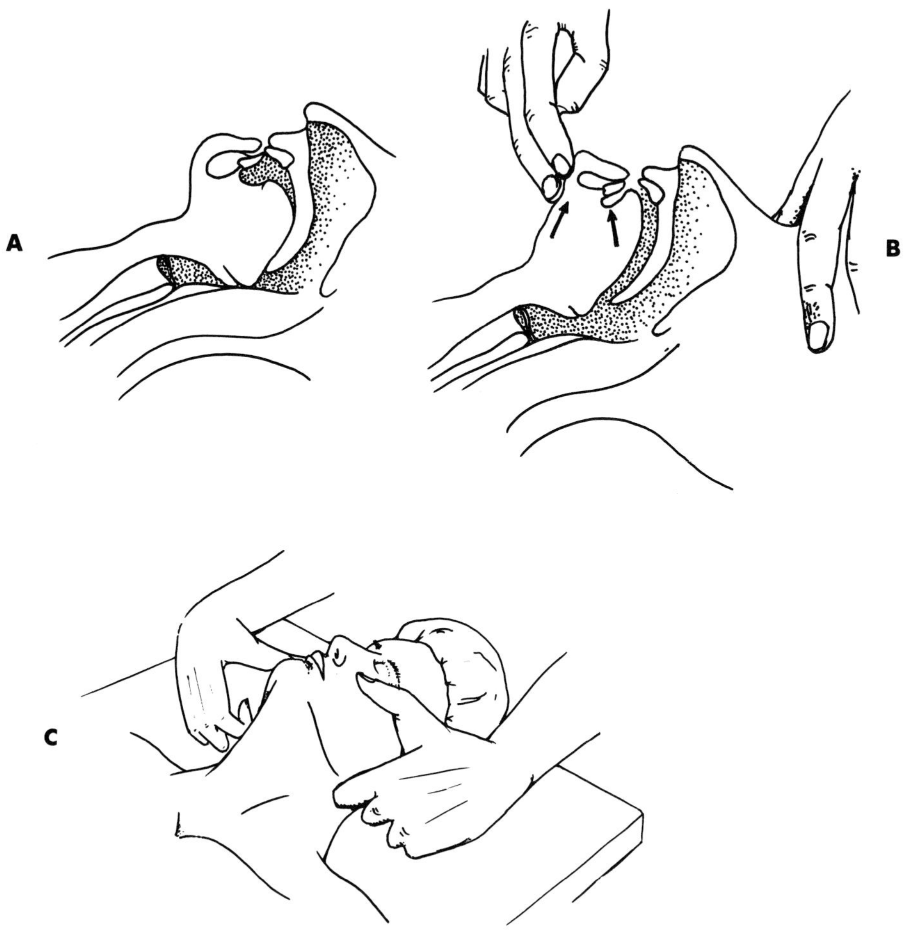

**FIGURE 14-1**  The airway, which is most commonly obstructed by posterior displacement of the tongue **(A)**, is easily opened by retroflexion of the neck **(B)** or a jaw thrust **(C)**. *(Reproduced with permission from Morgan GE, Mikhail MS: Clinical anesthesiology, Norwalk, Conn., 1992, Appleton and Lange.)*

will be required. The oxygen concentration of the patient's inspired or expired gas should be measured. Some method to continuously monitor temperature must be available. If a ventilator is used, it must be equipped with a disconnect alarm. These monitors can be added when the decision is made to convert to general anesthesia.

## TREATMENT OF COMPLICATIONS

Hypoxemia, due to apnea, is the most serious complication of sedation. Recognition by conscientious monitoring is a crucial, but only initial, step toward treatment. Relieving upper-airway obstruction by retroflexion of the neck and jaw thrust is often the only therapy required (Figure 14-1). Respiratory arrest, due to overdose of sedative or retrobulbar apnea syndrome,[17] must be aggressively treated by positive pressure ventilation with 100% oxygen (Figure 14-2). If respiratory depression is caused by an opioid agonist, it can be readily reversed with

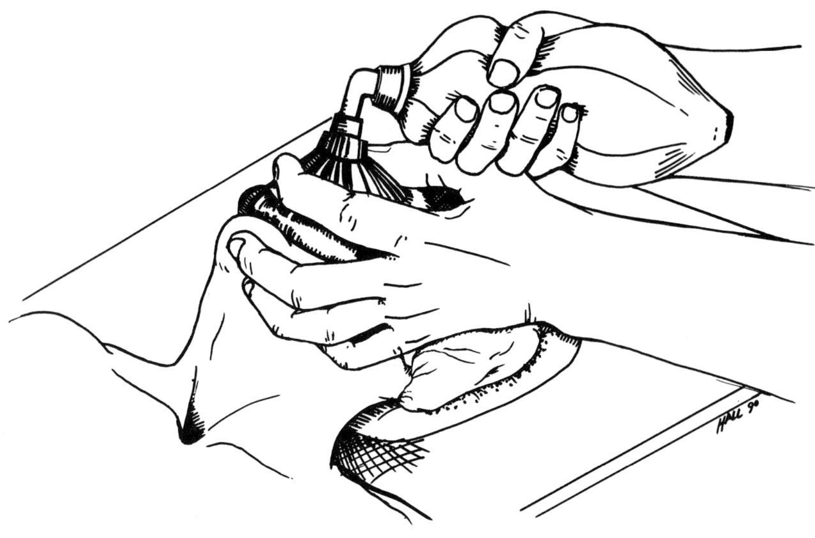

**FIGURE 14-2**   While a mask is held with the left hand, the right hand generates positive pressure ventilation by squeezing the breathing bag. The mask is held against the face by downward pressure exerted on the mask body with the left thumb and index finger. The middle and ring fingers grasp the mandible to extend the atlanto-occipital joint. The little finger slides under the angle of the jaw and thrusts it anteriorly. *(Reproduced with permission from Morgan GE, Mikhail MS: Clinical anesthesiology, Norwalk, Conn., 1992, Appleton and Lange.)*

naloxone (0.1 to 0.4 mg). The longer-acting opioids have a longer duration than naloxone and require repeated intravenous administration of the antagonist. All equipment necessary for airway management, such as resuscitation breathing system, oral and nasal airways, oxygen source, and the like, must be immediately available anywhere sedation is being administered. Likewise, personnel trained in airway management must be in close proximity.

Nausea and vomiting are side effects of many sedative agents. Suction equipment should be available to prevent aspiration of gastric contents in the sedated patient. Antiemetic drugs such as metoclopramide (10 to 20 mg parenterally) or droperidol (1.25 to 2.5 mg parenterally) may be of benefit.

A serious complication of sedation is uncontrollable patient movement during intraocular surgery. This is more commonly caused by excessive sedation rather than insufficient sedation. If this is recognized prior to opening the globe, serious consideration should be given to converting to general anesthesia. Obviously, this alternative requires the attendance of an anesthesiologist.

## SUMMARY

Local anesthesia with sedation provides an excellent alternative to general anesthesia for many types of ophthalmologic surgery. Success depends upon understanding the goals of sedation, good case and patient selection, utilization of relaxation techniques, familiarization with the sedative drugs, adequate monitoring, and the capability to treat potential complications.

## References


1. Egbert LD, Battit GE, Turndorf H, Beecher HK. The value of the preoperative visit by the anesthetist: a study of the patient-doctor rapport. JAMA 1963; 185:553-555.
2. Morgan GE. Hypnosis in ophthalmology. ed 1. Birmingham, Ala.: Aesculapius Publishing Company, 1980.
3. Shane MS. Conscious sedation and behavior modification with local standby anesthesia for ophthalmologic surgery. Ophthal Surg 1982; 13:50-52.
4. Frandsen JL. Nursing approaches in local anesthesia for ophthalmic surgery. J Ophthal Nurs Technol 1989; 8:135-138.
5. Whitacre MM, Ellis PP. Outpatient sedation for ocular examination. Surv Ophthalmol 1984; 28: 643-652.
6. Schalen L, Pyykko I, Korttila K, Magnusson M, Enbom H. Effects of intravenously given barbiturate and diazepam on eye motor performance in man. Adv Otorhinolaryngol 1988; 42:260-264.
7. Gilbert J, Holt JE, Johnston J, Sabo BA, Weaver JS. Intravenous sedation for cataract surgery. Anaesthesia 1987; 42:1063-1069.
8. Vindhya PKC, Sheets JH, Tolia NH, Tomlinson LJ. Retrobulbar block using pentothal as a sedative for ambulatory cataract surgery. J Cataract Refract Surg 1987; 13:321-322.
9. Greenblat KJ, Kock-Weser J. Adverse reactions to intravenous diazepam. Am J Med Sci 1973; 266:261-266.
10. Mayhew JF. Midazolam as a sedative for cataract surgery (letter). J Cataract Refract Surg 1987; 13:689.
11. Fanard L, Van Steenberge A, Demeire X, van der Puyl F. Comparison between propofol and midazolam as sedative agents for surgery under general anesthesia. Anaesthesia 1988; 43:87-89.
12. Judisch GF, Anderson S, Bell WE. Chloral hydrate sedation as a substitute for examination under anesthesia in pediatric ophthalmology. Am J Ophthalmol 1980; 89:560-563.
13. Valtonen M, Salonen M, Forssell H, Scheinin M, Viinamaki O. Propofol infusion for sedation in outpatient oral surgery: a comparison with diazepam. Anaesthesia 1989; 44:730-734.
14. Day OL, Nespeca JA, Ringgold C, Behr DA, Evens RP. Outpatient sedation for oral surgery: a comparison of butorphanol and fentanyl. Acute Care 1988; 12:63-69.
15. Yoshikawa K, Murai Y. The effect of ketamine on intraocular pressure in children. Anesth Analg 1971; 50:199-200.
16. Ausinch B, Rayborn RL, Munsen ES, Levy NS. Ketamine and intraocular pressure in children. Anesth Analg 1976; 55:773-775.
17. Morgan GE, Hales K. Retrobulbar apnea syndrome. West J Med 1988; 149:78.

# 15   Enucleation Surgical Techniques and the Management of Complications

**David B. Soll, MD**

The incidence of enucleation procedures has decreased since the advent of sophisticated surgical techniques for salvaging the globe following trauma or complications occurring during intraocular surgery. There is, however, still a significant number of eyes that require enucleation because of intraocular tumors, chronic pain, and also the possibility of sympathetic ophthalmia. It is important for the ophthalmic surgeon to realize that although the patient may initially be grateful for relief of the pain or removal of the tumor, the long-term adjustment process invariably involves an awareness of the functional and cosmetic defect that occurs following an enucleation operation. As time progresses, most patients adjust to the monocular status but become more aware of the cosmetic blemish if, in fact, it is obvious. The middle one-third of the face is the facial region that attracts the attention of most people when they look at another person. Even a patient with an excellent initial cosmetic enucleation result will eventually develop some cosmetic asymmetry. Many of these problems are inevitable, but many can be prevented.

This section deals with the surgical technique that I use when performing an enucleation, which is somewhat different from the ones usually described in basic ophthalmic textbooks; however, recently more and more eye plastic surgeons have adopted it.

It is important for the ophthalmologist to be aware of the pathophysiology of the anophthalmic orbit, when corrective surgery is necessary, and of the various procedures available for correction of anophthalmic orbital deformities.

The normal eye is a living structure with metabolic requirements. Metabolic activity takes place in diseased eyes and also in eyes with tumors, so that when any eye is enucleated, there are some immediate, uncontrollable orbital effects.

The orbital metabolic requirements are immediately decreased and the orbital blood flow is, therefore, also decreased. This is documented and demonstrated by thermographic patterns when normal and anophthalmic sides are compared. The anophthalmic orbit is always cooler than the normal orbit, indicating decreased blood flow and decreased metabolic activity.

There is also an immediate change in the anatomic relationship of the levator muscle to the roof of the orbit. A space develops between the periosteum and the roof of the orbit and the levator muscle complex. This space has been experimentally demonstrated in animal studies and occurs at the time of enucleation and/or evisceration, and cannot be prevented.

The normal globe has a volume of approximately 7 cc, and a combination of an 18-mm implant and a prosthesis has a combined volume of approximately 5 cc, so even at best, when this size of implant and prosthesis are used, some enophthalmos occurs.

In the average adult, Tenon's capsule will accept an 18-mm implant—occasionally a 20-mm implant. Most often if anything larger is used, it eventually extrudes.

The decreased orbital circulation accounts for eventual orbital fat atrophy that is most pronounced in the superior eyelid sulcus area, due to atrophy of the preaponeurotic fat pad.

A prosthesis, no matter how light it is, rests and is supported by the lower eyelid and eventually some stretching of the medial and lateral canthal tendons occurs. In some instances, this is so great that a dropped socket appearance occurs and an upper eyelid ptosis is accentuated.

If too heavy an intraorbital implant is used, the gravitational forces associated with this implant eventually cause compression of the orbital tissue below the implant, and this also contributes to a dropped socket appearance along with additional dropping of the levator complex and the development of more ptosis.

Displacement of too large an implant inserted within Tenon's capsule affects the motility of the prosthesis and also contributes to atrophy of orbital fat, enophthalmos, and superior eyelid sulcus defects.

The motility of the prosthesis is primarily dependent upon the movement and depth of the fornices and only minimally dependent upon the movement of the posterior socket wall when a buried, nonintegrated, orbital implant is used. When the patient looks to the right, if the right orbit is anophthalmic, the right lateral fornix deepens, the right medial fornix becomes shallower, and the prosthesis is pushed towards the deeper lateral fornix; the edge of the prosthesis drops into this deeper lateral fornix, and the edge of the prosthesis is pushed laterally by the shallower medial fornix. This same mechanism of prosthesis movement takes place in all directions.

Recently, a new type of orbital implant made out of hydroxyapatite has been developed. The surgical technique and postoperative management are different from those used with the usual or more common standard enucleation techniques.

Using a hydroxyapatite implant significantly enhances prosthesis motility. The implant is manufactured from a form of calcium phosphate, a naturally occurring substance in the body. This mineral forms the hard portion of human bone and eventually becomes fully vascularized so that the implant actually becomes a living part of the orbit. After the implant is fully vascularized, a hole which accepts a peg is drilled in its anterior surface, through overlying conjunctiva, Tenon's fascia, and donor sclera, if the implant was encased in sclera. The initial peg inserted has a flat surface; however, this is eventually replaced with a peg which has a rounded, ball-like, anterior tip which coordinates with a corresponding drilled out area in the artificial eye as a ball and socket joint. The movement of the implant is transmitted to the prosthesis, and motility is significantly improved. Even when using this type of implant it is very important to have deep fornices (Figure 15-1, *A-E*).

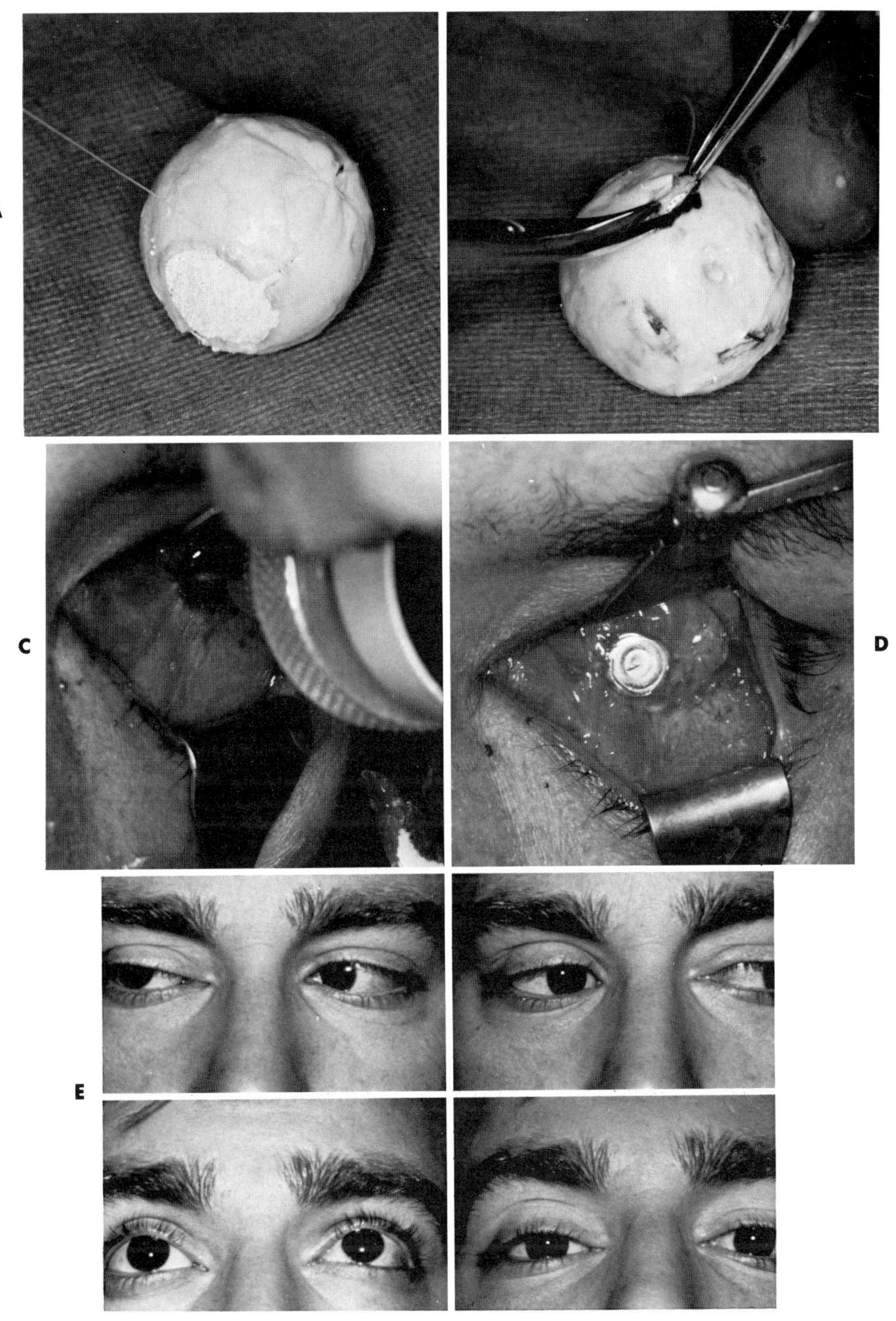

**FIGURE 15-1** **A,** Hydroxyapatite implant encased in sclera with posterior portion exposed. **B,** Four windows are cut in the scleral shell. The four recti muscles are sutured in these areas. **C,** Postoperative drilling of the vascularized hydroxyapatite implant. **D,** A flat peg is inserted immediately after the drilling. This is eventually replaced with a ball-type peg. **E,** Example of final motility. *(Slide courtesy of Arthur C. Perry, MD.)*

## SURGICAL TECHNIQUE

The technique I now use for primary enucleation when using spherical silicone or plastic implant is as follows:

1. A superior fornix, 4-0 black silk mattress suture is inserted and hung by a hemostat. This pulls up the levator muscle complex and, during the surgical procedure, aids in the prevention of injury to this complex.

2. The globe is enucleated and only the medial and lateral rectus muscles are tagged with double-armed 6-0 vicryl sutures. As much conjunctiva and Tenon's tissue as possible is preserved.

3. The opening in Tenon's fascia where the optic nerve passes through is identified (Figure 15-2, *A*). A 20-mm spherical implant, either encased in fascia lata or donor sclera, is inserted through this opening into the fatty tissue of the muscle cone (Figure 15-2, *B-D*). Three double-armed 4-0 vicryl mattress sutures are then passed through the anterior surface of the implant, each suture imbricates the edge of Tenon's over the implant, thus fully enclosing the implant within the muscle cone; the edges of posterior Tenon's fascia being imbricated one above the other. The Tenon's fascia between the exits of the four recti muscles and the opening where the optic nerve went through is called *posterior Tenon's* and this tissue is thinner than the anterior portion of Tenon's, which is between the four recti muscles and the conjunctival edge.

   When there is a deficiency of Tenon's or conjunctiva, or a congenitally small bony orbit, I prefer to use a deepithelialized dermal fat graft. In these instances, it is not necessary to insert the deepithelialized dermal fat graft posterior to the posterior layers of Tenon's fascia.

4. Anterior Tenon's is separated from conjunctiva by sharp dissection. The dissection is carried to the medial, inferior, and lateral orbital wall and superiorly as high as possible without damaging the levator muscle complex. Anterior Tenon's is now closed edge-to-edge with interrupted 5-0 vicryl sutures. During the separation of anterior Tenon's from overlying conjunctiva, it is often desirable to inject either saline or a local anesthetic subconjunctivally to separate these two tissues.

5. The vicryl sutures, which were previously placed in the tendons of the medial and lateral rectus muscles, are now passed through the medial and lateral conjunctival fornices and tied.

   The superior and inferior rectus muscles are allowed to retract. There are enough connections between Tenon's fascia and the superior and inferior rectus muscles to give superior and inferior movement to the prosthesis. If the superior rectus muscle were brought forward, it would create a ptosis because of the connections between the superior rectus muscle and the levator muscle complex.

   Conjunctiva is closed with 6-0 plain-gut interrupted sutures and a conformer inserted.

   Antibiotic solution is instilled and a mild pressure bandage is applied for two to three days after which the patient is instructed to use compresses and an antibiotic ointment once or twice daily for an additional

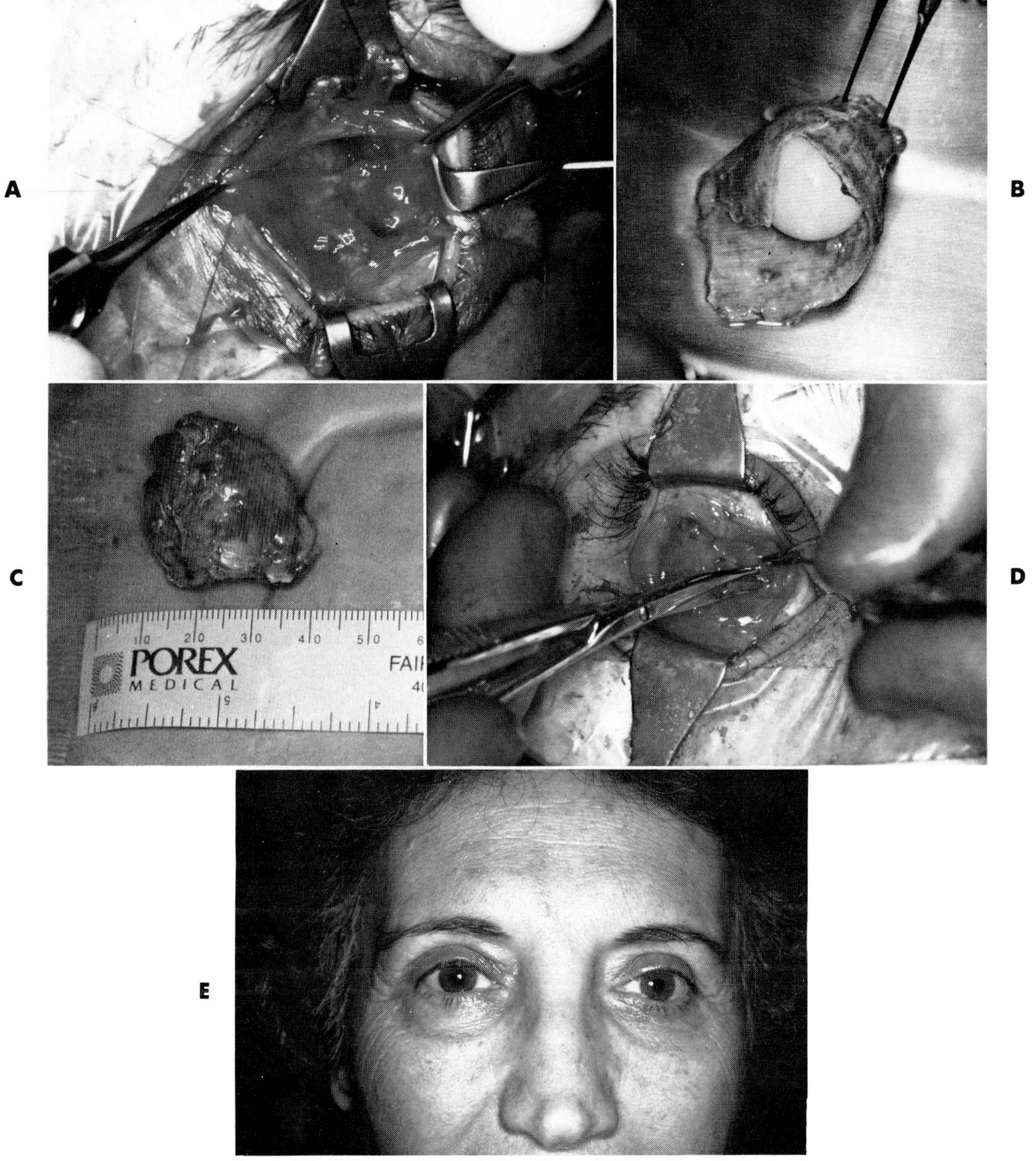

**FIGURE 15-2**   **A,** The posterior layer of Tenon's fascia being held by two forceps. The fatty tissue of the muscle cone is visible through the opening in the posterior layer of Tenon's fascia where the optic nerve originally passed through. **B, C,** Enucleation implant being encased in fascia lata. **D,** Fascia lata–covered enucleation implant being inserted behind the posterior layer of Tenon's capsule within the fatty tissue of the muscle cone. **E,** Appearance of the patient 2½ years after enucleation of the right eye with insertion of a fascia lata–encased implant.

three to four weeks. After that, the patient is fitted with a prosthetic eye (Figure 15-2, *E* ).

When a hydroxyapatite implant is used, the technique is somewhat different. The implant is encased in a scleral shell with the posterior portion of the hydroxyapatite implant exposed. Windows on the sides of the scleral shell are cut for the four rectus muscles, and these muscles are sutured to the sclera at these windows. The windows are in approximately the position of the four recti muscles in the normal eye.

Suturing of the superior and inferior oblique muscles to the scleral shell is optional. I have not found that this step makes much difference in the final motility. When a sclera-encased hydroxyapatite implant is used, it is placed within Tenon's fascia. Usually after four to six months, a bone scan or MRI with contrast is ordered. If the implant is fully vascularized, a hole for the peg is drilled through the anterior portion of the implant. Initially, a flat peg is inserted, which is then replaced with a peg with a rounded ball anterior portion to coordinate with the prosthesis.

Patients are instructed not to remove their artificial eyes, but rather always to leave them in position and twice daily to apply a soaking tepid compress of plain water to the open eyelids. A wash cloth is used for this. If necessary, the patient can also use an antibiotic drop, once or twice daily, should there be socket discharge. Occasionally, a patient will have to add a steroid drop several times weekly. Patients are told not to remove the prosthesis, and not to pull down on the lower eyelid—rather to elevate the upper eyelid when inserting a drop.

## TREATMENT OF POSTOPERATIVE COMPLICATIONS

The development of a superior sulcus eyelid deformity associated with some ptosis is one of the most common complications. It is best corrected by the subperiosteal injection of room-temperature vulcanizing silicone (Dow Corning RTV silicone 382). The vulcanization time of the silicone can be adjusted prior to injecting the material. The approach is through a lateral canthal incision or a blepharoplasty incision with elevation of the periosteum. The RTV silicone is injected subperiosteally, the potential space being held open by malleable retractors. Some overcorrection is desirable and the patient's prosthesis should be left in position during this procedure.

If the superior sulcus defect is not great, a deepithelialized dermal fat graft may be inserted on the posterior surface of the eyelid above the superior border of the tarsus. This also facilitates eyelid closure (Figure 15-3, *A-E*).

## PTOSIS

If the ptosis is severe, it should be managed with either a fascial sling or a silastic sling. If only 1 or 2 mm of ptosis is present and it is not helped by adjustment of the prosthesis, an aponeurotic advancement or a very conservative tarsoconjunctival resection can be performed. The repair camouflages the appearance of a deep sulcus as does a blepharoplasty on the opposite side.

## LAXITY OF THE LOWER EYELID

Laxity of the lower eyelid is corrected by resection or imbrication of the medial and lateral canthal tendons. It is usually not advisable to resect eyelid tissue. Nonabsorbable 4-0 suture material should be used to secure the resected or

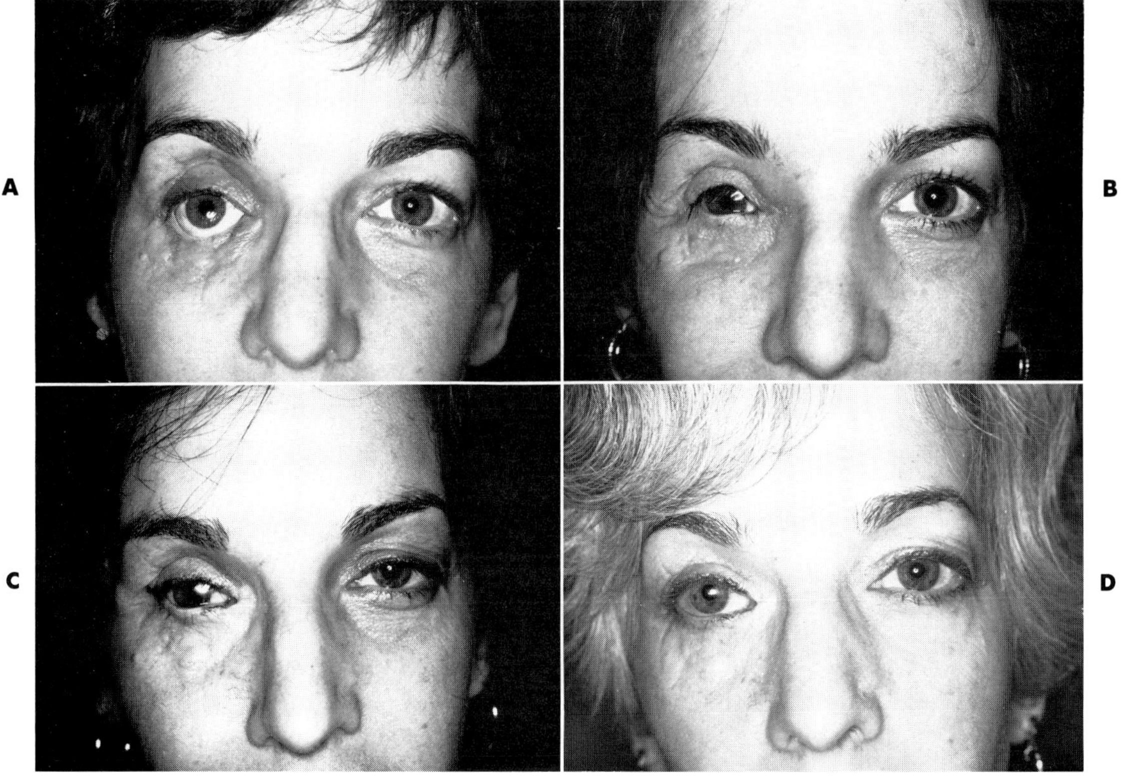

**FIGURE 15-3**　　**A,** Appearance of a patient following severe facial trauma with previous evisceration, right side. **B,** Appearance of the patient after the following procedures: elevation of lower eyelid, insertion of molded subperiosteal implant, fascia lata sling to lower eyelid. **C,** Appearance of the patient after deepithelialized dermal fat-graft insertion to the upper eyelid and scar revision. **D,** Final appearance of the patient, 7 years after completion of surgical procedures.

imbricating tendons in position. Correcting a lax lower eyelid frequently improves the cosmesis when there is a superior eyelid sulcus defect and dropped sulcus deformity.

## DISPLACED ORBITAL IMPLANT

This can only be corrected by removal and replacement of the implant. Extensive dissection is not necessary and the secondary implant should be inserted within the muscle cone. If there is deficiency of Tenon's or conjunctival tissue, it is advisable to use a deepithelialized dermal fat graft as a secondary implant.

## INABILITY OF THE SOCKET TO HOLD THE PROSTHESIS

A socket that cannot retain a prosthesis usually exhibits poor motility and shallow fornices. These problems can only be corrected with mucous-membrane grafting.

## SUMMARY

The above are some of the more common problems related to the anophthalmic orbit that the ophthalmologist encounters and has to deal with. These and less common problems can usually be prevented, to a large extent, by proper initial surgery.

The ophthalmic surgeon should approach every enucleation as both a functional and cosmetic challenge.

## Suggested Reading

Dutton, JJ. Coralline hydroxyapatite as an ocular implant. Ophthalmol 1991; 98(3):370-377.

Perry, AC. Integrated orbital implants. Ophthal Plast Recon Surg 1990; 8:75-81.

Soll DB. The anophthalmic socket. Ophthalmol 1982; 89:407-423.

Soll DB. Evolution and current concepts in the surgical treatment of the anophthalmic orbit. Ophthal Plast Recon Surg 1986; 2(3):163-171.

# 16 Using Computerized Perimetry

Anders Heijl, MD
Peter Åsman, MD

With automation, visual field testing can be performed in a much more predictable and reproducible way than was previously possible. The quality of standard clinical visual field determinations has been strikingly improved and good perimetry is available to all ophthalmologists. Still, however, the physician has to choose among test procedures and to interpret the printout given by the perimeter. The aim of this chapter is to describe some principles of automated field testing; special attention is given to modern aids in interpretation of its results.

## TEST PROCEDURES

Most automated perimeters offer a variety of test programs. The selection among these is influenced by the needs and equipment of the individual physician, but some general guidelines can be given.

## Tested Area

In glaucoma patients field loss can occur anywhere, including the temporal parts.[1] In early stages, there is a predominance of nasal defects,[2] and as a rule defects start in the central 30° field.[3] There is no doubt that tests aiming at detecting glaucomatous field loss should concentrate on the central 30° field. Only a small percentage (0% to 11%)[4,5] of field defects will be missed if a careful examination is performed, but limited to this area. It is valuable to examine the nasal field out to 30° from fixation, even if testing is otherwise restricted to 20° to 25° or less. Testing for neurologic diseases should also concentrate on the central field.[6]

Test-point patterns with points located on the horizontal or vertical meridians should be avoided, since such patterns are nonoptimal for detection of nasal steps and hemianopic defects.

## Principles of Testing

Two principally different test strategies are available in most perimeters: threshold measuring tests and screening algorithms.[7]

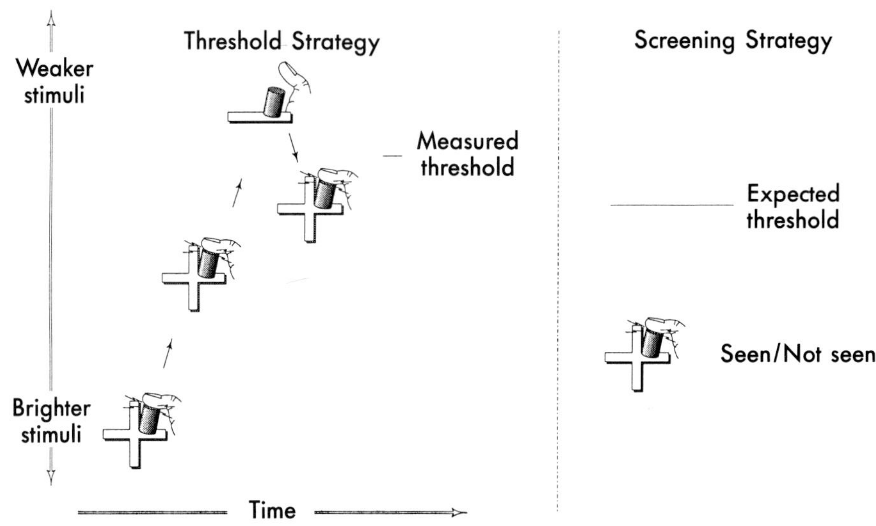


**FIGURE 16-1**    Threshold and screening strategies. Threshold determination (left) based upon last responses in up-down sequence of stimulus exposures. Other locations tested between exposures to provide randomness. Screening strategies (right) present stimuli approximately 6 dB brighter than expected threshold. Normally only one exposure needed at each test location.

## Threshold measuring

For the very earliest detection of field loss, it is always better to rely on threshold perimetry than on supraliminal screening. Almost all current visual field research is conducted with static threshold perimetry. Presenting several stimuli, above as well as below the threshold, allows a more precise estimation of the hill of vision than does supraliminal screening. Currently used methods employ up-and-down staircase procedures; that is, if the first stimulus at a test location is not seen, then the intensity of following stimuli is increased in a stepwise fashion until the stimulus is perceived and subsequently decreased until it is not seen, and vice versa. The threshold value is estimated from these responses (Figure 16-1).

## Screening

Visual field screening can be performed rapidly with a computer handling the test situation. Screening tests present stimuli that are intended to be bright enough to be readily perceived by normal subjects. Therefore, a single stimulus presentation is usually sufficient at each location (Figure 16-1). It is crucial that appropriate stimulus intensities are used, slightly higher than those of the actual threshold levels. Stimulus intensities approximately 6 dB higher than the expected threshold are common. At the individual test these brightnesses are usually derived from initial threshold determinations at a few preselected central locations, or they may be based on age-corrected normal values.

The results of the test are given in the form of a matrix of seen/not seen points. The shape of any "missed areas" can then help the examiner in the interpretation of the field.

With increasing knowledge of variability of the frequency-of-seeing curve among subjects and within the field, a better selection of intensity levels may be possible in the future. It is likely that stimulus intensities in the center of the field can be closer to the expected threshold than in the periphery, where variability is larger.

While supraliminal screening is very fast, it will occasionally miss shallow but important field defects; it is also not suited for follow-up of known visual field defects.

Both screening and threshold measuring strategies save technician time compared to manual perimetry, since several field examinations can be monitored simultaneously by one single technician, and also because the technician can perform some other tasks while intermittently supervising the perimetric test. Much more time is saved with screening strategies than by threshold measuring tests, but at the cost of obtaining less accurate information about the field.

In conclusion, a threshold measuring test covering the central 30° is almost always a good clinical choice. If demands on fast testing are very high or if poor cooperation is expected from the patient, a screening test in the same area may be preferable.

## INTERPRETING A SINGLE VISUAL FIELD

Two important aspects have to be considered when single fields are interpreted. First, one has to judge the reliability of the test results. Second, one must judge the presence and extent of field defects.

### Reliability of Patient Responses

Inadequate patient behavior may reduce the reliability of the test results. Most often this reliability is estimated from results of catch trials, which are presented more or less randomly during the test. False positive (FP) catch trials are performed in the same way as ordinary stimulus exposures, but the stimulus shutter is left closed and no stimulus is actually presented. The patient is, of course, expected not to respond to such questions. Certain field tests can immediately be seen to contain nonsense data caused by "trigger happiness," that is, when the patient continues to press the response button when not seeing stimuli (Figure 16-2). Characteristic for such tests are high percentages of answers in FP catch trials and/or areas with extremely high sensitivity values. Such field charts cannot be interpreted; instead, the patient should be reinstructed and tested again.

The degree of attentiveness is often estimated by means of false negative (FN) catch trials. These are presented at locations where the threshold has already been estimated. Such catch trials are performed with strong suprathreshold stimuli; the patient is expected to see the targets and respond by pressing the button. There are several different reasons for high rates of false negative answers, however, and a high rate of such answers in a seriously disturbed field does not necessarily indicate an inattentive patient; high rates of FN answers are common in seriously disturbed fields. Therefore, the technician's subjective evaluation of the alertness may be of great help. If the patient has been truly inattentive one should regard the individual measurements with skepticism and the patient should be reinstructed and motivated to do his or her best. If inattentiveness persists in subsequent tests it may be a good idea to resort to a shorter threshold test covering a smaller area or to screening tests, which are much easier for patients.

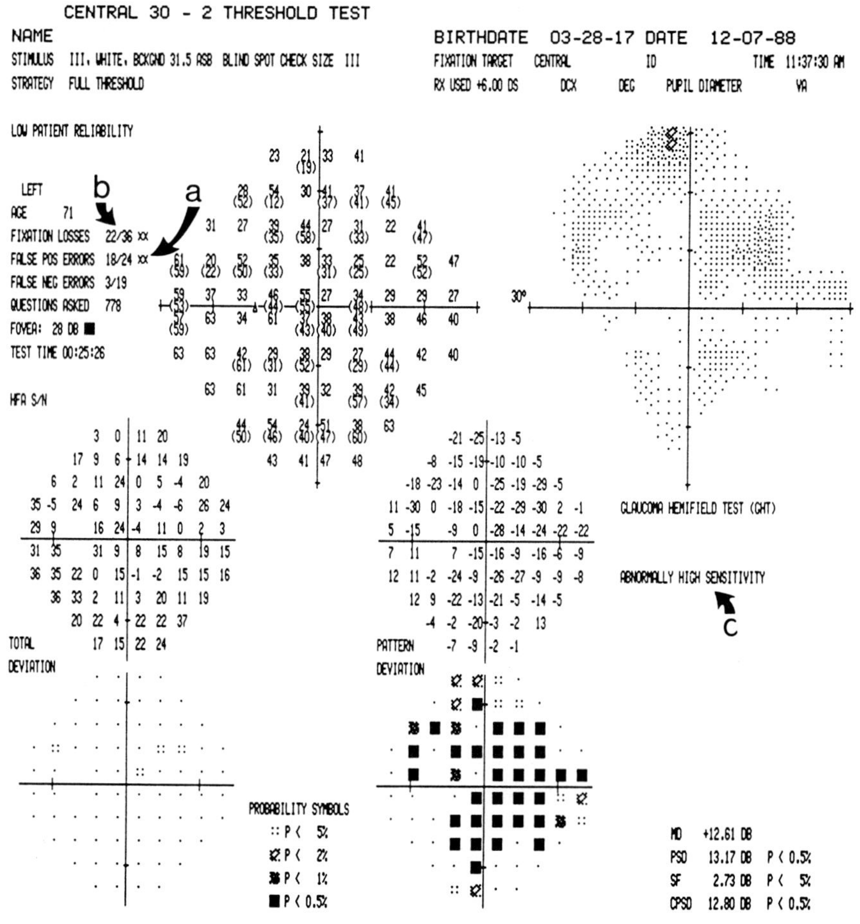


**FIGURE 16-2**    Visual field in "trigger happy" patient. Multiple responses also when stimuli have not been seen result in many abnormally high sensitivity values and/or high false-positive catch trial ratio **(a)**. Field cannot be interpreted. Numerous false positive answers lead to high fixation loss ratio **(b)**. Glaucoma Hemifield Test indicates abnormally high sensitivity **(c)**.

Fixation can be monitored in a variety of ways. The most common method is the blind spot technique.[8] Bright stimuli are presented at the assumed location of the blind spot. If the patient is not fixating properly he or she may see these targets. Misleading high rates of fixation losses may result if the blind spot has not been correctly located. In such cases the field chart usually has a well-delineated blind spot despite the indicated high rate of fixation losses. If fixation has really been poor, small defects may be easily missed, making comparisons with previous test results difficult.

## Judging Field Status

In manual perimetry the human examiner filters and averages the individual measurements, consciously or subconsciously. The technician's ideas of visual fields in general and the field tested will clearly influence the chart. Therefore the estimated field chart is often smoothened with beautifully outlined defects.

Computerized visual fields are obtained without such filtering. Small irregularities, due to physiologic and pathologic variability, are not eliminated and the measured hill of vision is slightly irregular. This often leads to difficulties in interpretation; one has to decide whether irregularities are caused by true pathology or if they are merely the result of random or physiologic variability. Several statistical approaches have addressed this problem.

## Visual field indexes

Results of computerized perimetry can be reduced into single numbers: visual field indexes. The simplest such index is the sum of all threshold values within the field.[9] Several indexes have been suggested but only a few have gained clinical acceptance. The most important are MD, which is the average deviation of measured threshold values from age-corrected normal threshold values, and PSD and LV, which are irregularity indexes intended to detect local defects.[10,11] Both of these index categories have been used for detection and for followup of field loss.[10,12] MD, PSD, and LV do not take any spatial factors into account and therefore do not reflect the relevance of any apparent defects. Thus, they are not optimal for diagnostic purposes and, in our opinion, diagnosis should not be based primarily upon currently available visual field indexes even though they permit a crude classification of test results. Indexes are of greater value for followup, however. Certainly, in the future other indexes will be developed that may indicate more specifically the existence of meaningful field defects.

## Visual field maps

At present, when interpreting a single visual field, the physician can gain more information from looking carefully at the field chart than from relying on global indexes.

Visual field results are influenced by factors such as random variability, method of testing, test duration, etc. The accuracy of measurements is not as high as the numerical threshold values may indicate. A good understanding of normal, automated, visual field results and the amount of expected variability is of great value for the ability to efficiently interpret visual fields. The physician's knowledge is based upon clinical experience. The computer may be equipped with data reflecting similar experience, and it has the unique ability to absorb, retain, and effectively use much more detailed numerical knowledge of this type than can the human mind.

Threshold measurements are subjected to variation not only among normal subjects and between test sessions but also within one test session. Localized increase in threshold variability, during and between tests, may be an early perimetric sign in glaucoma.[13]

Intuitive judgements of fields are probably most commonly based upon *grayscale maps* of the measured threshold values. Such maps resemble manual kinetic field charts. Interpretation may be facilitated if the measured field is compared to a normal, standard field. Pointwise differences between the measured field and age-corrected normal reference fields can be plotted in *deviation maps.* These have been used for a number of years and have proven quite helpful.[11,14] With such maps, however, one still has to judge the importance of the displayed pointwise differences. It has sometimes been assumed that deviations of equal depth are equally important regardless of location, and depressions of 5 dB or

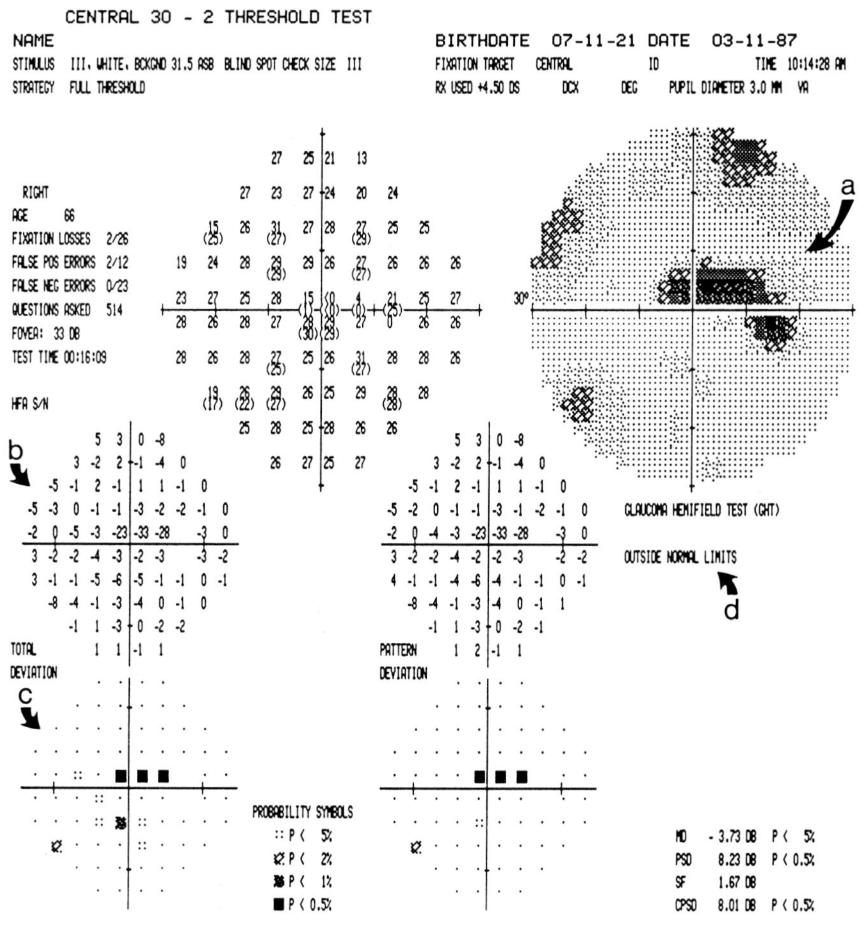



**FIGURE 16-3**  Glaucomatous visual field. Obvious paracentral defect seen in grayscale **(a)**. Deviations from age-corrected normal threshold values **(b)** found in scotoma are very uncommon among normal subjects. Hence, probability maps confirm defect **(c)**. Further support for significant finding is given by Glaucoma Hemifield Test **(d)**.

more have frequently been regarded as pathological. Studies have shown, however, that threshold variability is highly dependent on location[15-18] increasing with eccentricity. These results have been translated into a new and improved empiric model of the normal visual field. Using this model, perimetric *probability maps* have been devised.[19,20] Such maps show, graphically, the significance of the measured threshold values. They can deemphasize common test artifacts, and highlight shallow defects in areas where normal variability is small (Figure 16-3).

The use of such graphic printouts has made interpretation of automated visual fields less complicated, but the new maps require a fair amount of experience. Clusters of points with diminished sensitivity have often, and correctly, been considered a good sign of pathology.[21,22] However, shallow clusters may also occur in normal subjects.[23,24] Therefore, one should refrain from judging small or shallow clusters of significant points in probability maps as indications of glaucoma if there are no confirming clinical signs. The total area involved in a cluster is less important than the volume and shape of it.[25]

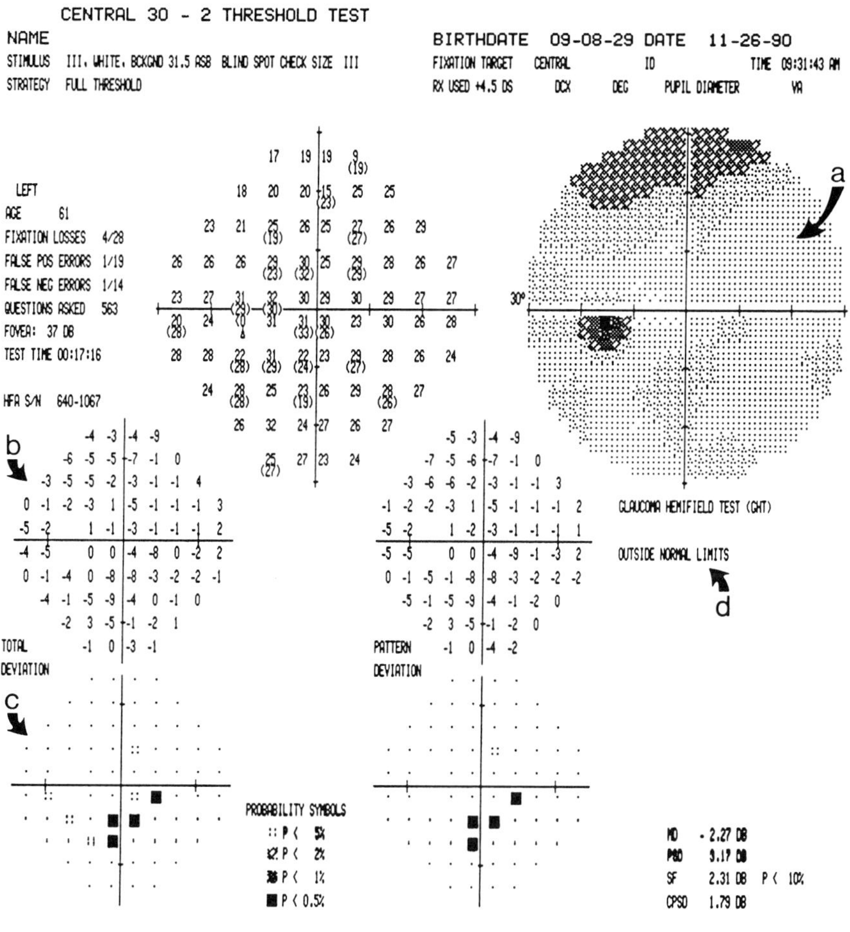



**FIGURE 16-4** Glaucomatous visual field. Grayscale looks quite normal **(a)**. Deviations from age-corrected normal threshold values **(b)** found in lower paracentral area are uncommon among normal subjects. Probability maps **(c)** therefore show defect in that region, and Glaucoma Hemifield Test indicates significant defect **(d)**.

## Computer-assisted plain text evaluation

An ultimate goal for computer-assisted interpretation may be a written statement that summarizes all relevant information about the field in a few words or sentences. It is unlikely that such a tool will ever be constructed, but efforts have been made at presenting visual field results in a more comprehensive way. These methods have often been constructed as expert systems.[26-28] The benefits from expert systems are greatly diminished, and written statements may be misleading if they are only based upon what is shown on the printout and do not take empiric knowledge of normal visual field behavior into account. The Glaucoma Hemifield Test (GHT) of the Humphrey perimeter is an expert system that incorporates such knowledge. The GHT compares the results from the probability map in the upper hemifield with results in the lower hemifield and identifies differences large enough to be uncommon in normal populations. A short written statement about visual field status indicates the presence of localized or generalized abnormalities in the measured field[29] (Figures 16-2 through 16-4). Further improvements in

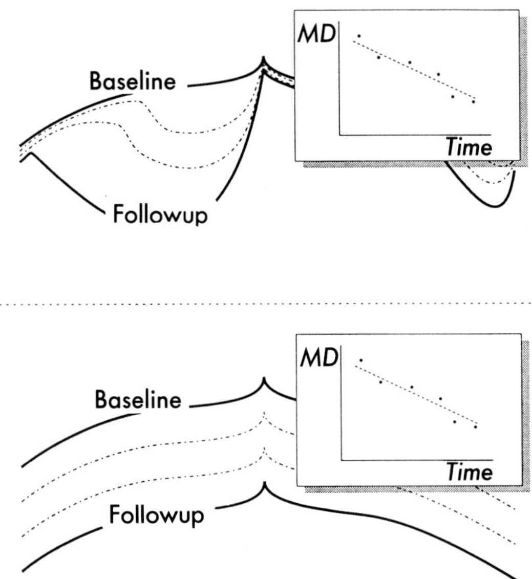



**FIGURE 16-5**    Linear regression analysis of mean deviation (MD) over time. Significant negative slope indicates deterioration. Analysis helpful when several tests are available but provides no help in differentiating between localized (top) and generalized (bottom) decay.

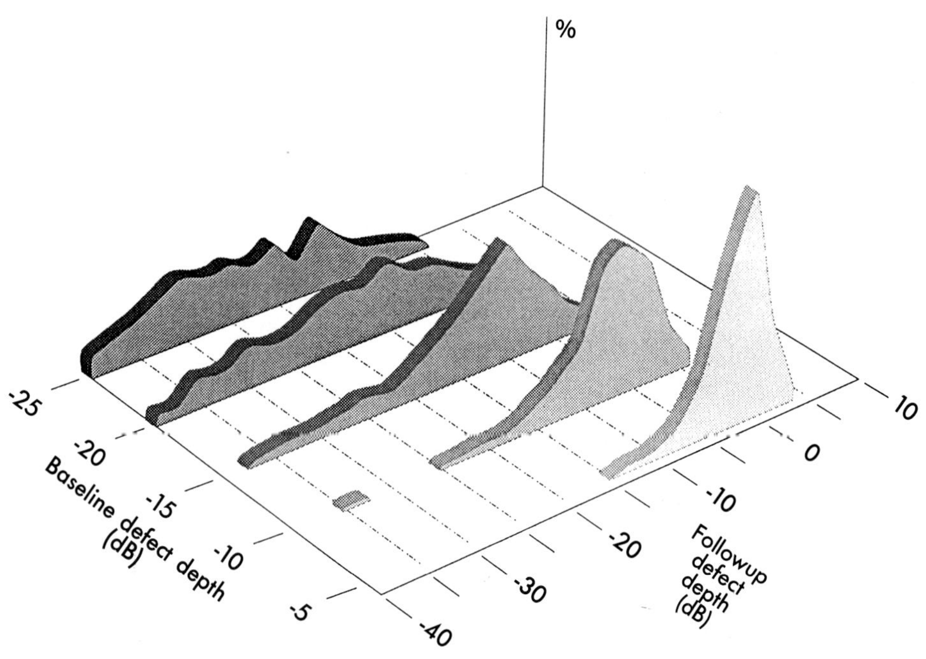



**FIGURE 16-6**    Distribution of defect depth in single-tested points at followup for different baseline defect depths. Intertest variability increases with increasing initial defect depth.

plain text analysis are expected and may considerably facilitate the interpretation of single and multiple visual fields in glaucoma and other disease entities.

## JUDGING FIELD CHANGE OVER TIME
### Basic Techniques

In glaucoma management, much interest centers around the question of whether or not the visual field is stable over time. Obviously, this has direct implications for the patient's treatment. Looking through the printouts of all measured fields in sequence is a simple method for judging field change. This approach can be severely hampered by small mistakes; field charts that are not stored in perfect order in the patient records, or if different test procedures have been used at different visits, etc. Some logical arrangement of the fields offered by the computer may be helpful, for instance, results printed in a condensed format permitting easy overview.

More practical and precise methods of judging change have been developed and several statistical tools have been used. Linear regression techniques are suitable when several field tests are available,[30] but they cannot, at present, differentiate between focal glaucomatous decay and generalized deterioration (Figure 16-5). The latter is often caused by increasing media opacities. Regression analysis is also not useful when fewer than five tests have been obtained, and actually requires a larger number of examinations to be really helpful. When only few tests are available, it is often very difficult to tell intuitively whether true progression has occurred, and one has to rely on other methods (c.f. below).

### Variability in Glaucoma

Threshold variability causes problems of interpretation in normal visual fields. The difficulties are even larger in glaucoma followup.

Threshold variability is higher in glaucomatous fields than in normal fields.[31-33] Inter-test changes increase with increasing defect depth[33] (Figure 16-6). In fact, an initially, moderately disturbed point may show almost any measured threshold value at the next visit because of random variability alone. Further, test-retest variability is higher in the midperiphery than more centrally, and it increases with greater abnormality of the field at large.[34] Prospective studies have provided knowledge about the factors influencing threshold variability in manifest glaucoma and have made possible the construction of probability maps for point-by-point changes over time[29] (Figure 16-7). Such maps are similar to probability maps for single fields in that they help deemphasize seemingly large changes that are small enough to fall within the limits of random variation. These printouts give geographic information about significant field decay, or improvement, and can be used as early as at the second test session.

## OPTIMIZING THE TEST PROCEDURE

Test algorithms currently used in threshold perimetry are not optimal. Much of the information given by the patient as he or she presses the response button is

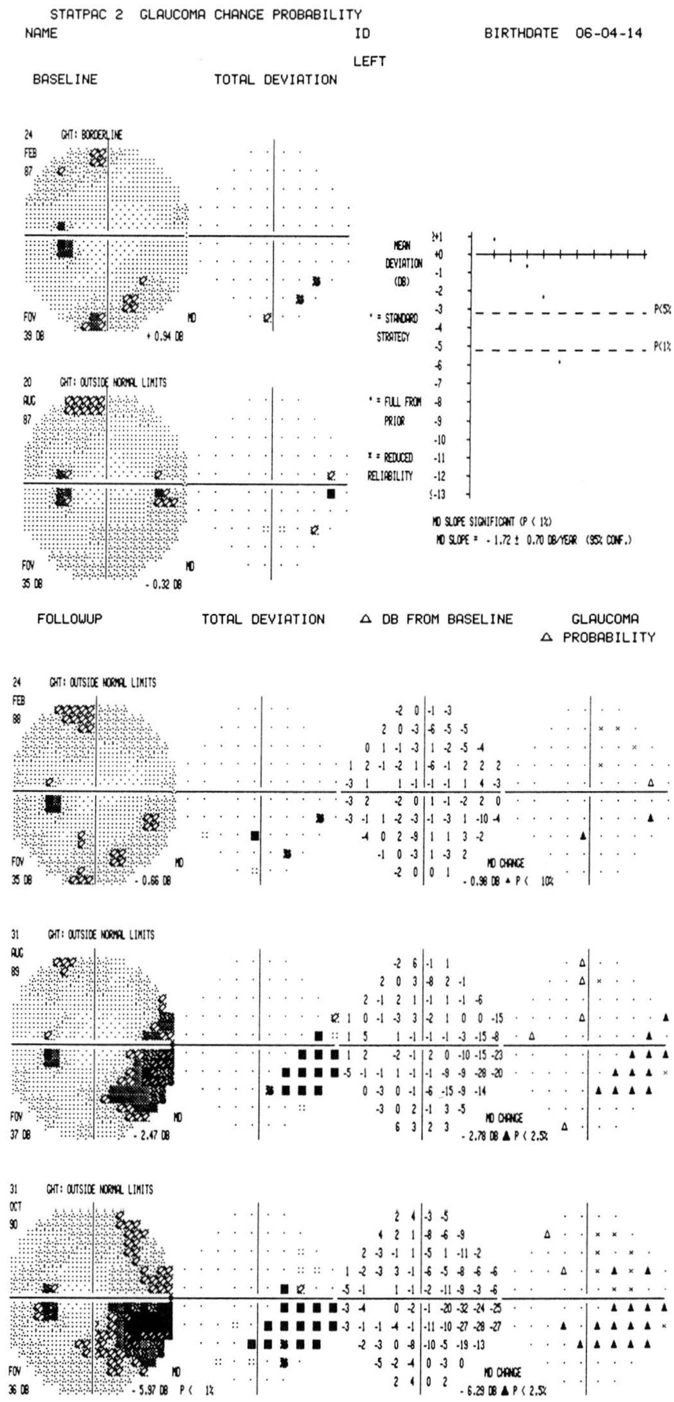

**FIGURE 16-7** Change probability map in glaucoma patient. Progression of field loss in inferior nasal area seen in grayscale printouts. Dark triangles in change probability map naturally support finding.

not utilized. Instead, usually only the very last patient responses at each location are used. If all responses can be efficiently used, it will be possible to develop new test algorithms that are as accurate as the algorithms of today but permit shorter tests. This would not only ease the task of the patient, but also make automated threshold perimetry more practical, more readily available, and more attractive as a choice in private practice.

## References

1. Brais P, Drance S. The temporal field in chronic simple glaucoma. Arch Ophthalmol 1972; 88:518-522.

2. Drance SM, Fairclough M, Thomas B, Douglas GR, Susanna R. The early visual field defect in glaucoma and the significance of nasal steps. Documenta Ophthalmol Proc Ser 1979; 19:119-126.

3. Aulhorn E, Harms M. Early visual field defects in glaucoma. In Glaucoma, Tutzing symposium. ed. Leydhecker W. Basel, Switzerland: Karger 1966:151-186.

4. LeBlanc RP, Lee A, Baxter M. Peripheral nasal field defects. Documenta Ophthalmol Proc Ser 1985; 42:377-381.

5. Caprioli J, Spaeth GL. Static threshold examination of the peripheral nasal visual field in glaucoma. Arch Ophthalmol 1985; 103:1150-1154.

6. Hård-Broberg AL, Wirtschafter JD. Evaluating the usefulness in neuro-ophthalmology of visual field examinations peripheral to 30 degrees. Documenta Ophthalomol Proc Ser 1985; 42:197-206.

7. Greve EL. Single and multiple stimulus static perimetry. In Glaucoma: the two phases of visual field examination. The Hague: Junk Publishers 1973.

8. Heijl A, Krakau CET. An automatic static perimeter, design and pilot study. Acta Ophthalmol 1975; 53:293-310.

9. Holmin C, Krakau CET. Visual field decay in normal subjects and in cases of chronic glaucoma. Graefe's Arch Klin Exp Ophthalmol 1980; 213:291-298.

10. Flammer J, Drance SM, Augustiny L, Funkhouser A. Quantification of glaucomatous visual field defects with automated perimetry. Invest Ophthalmol Vis Sci 1985; 26:176-181.

11. Heijl A, Lindgren G, Olsson J. A package for the statistical analysis of visual fields. Documenta Ophthalmol Proc Ser 1987; 49:153-168.

12. Enger C, Sommer A. Recognizing glaucomatous field loss with the Humphrey STATPAC. Arch Ophthalmol 1987; 105:1355-1357.

13. Werner EB, Drance SM, Schultzer M. Early visual field defects in glaucoma. Arch Ophthalmol 1977; 95:1173-1175.

14. Bebié H. Computerized techniques of visual field analysis. In Drance SM, Anderson DR, eds, Automatic Perimetry in Glaucoma: A practical guide. New York: Grune and Stratton. 1985:147-160.

15. Heijl A, Lindgren G, Olsson J. Normal variability of static perimetric threshold values across the central visual field. Arch Ophthalmol 1987; 105:1544-1549.

16. Katz J, Sommer A. Asymmetry and variation in the normal hill of vision. Arch Ophthalmol 1986; 104:65-68.

17. Brenton RS, Phelps CD. The normal visual field on the Humphrey Field Analyzer. Ophthalmologica 1986; 193:56-74.

18. Lewis RA, Johnson CA, Keltner JL, et al. Variability of quantitative automated perimetry in normal observers. Ophthalmol 1986; 93:878-881.

19. Statpac User's Guide. San Leandro, CA: Allergan Humphrey, 1986.

20. Heijl A, Lindgren G, Olsson J, Åsman P. Visual field interpretation with empirical probability maps. Arch Ophthalmol 1988; 107:204-208.

21. Anderson DR. Interpretation of automatically plotted visual fields. In Drance SM, Anderson DR, eds, Automatic perimetry in glaucoma. Orlando: Grune and Stratton 1985:141-145.

22. Lewis RA, Johnson CA, Keltner JL, et al. Variability of quantitative automated perimetry in normal observers. Ophthalmol 1986; 93:878-881.

23. Heijl A, Åsman P. Clustering of depressed points in the normal visual field. Perimetry Update 1988/89: Proc of the 8th Internat Perimetric Soc Meeting. Amstelveen, Kugler Ghedini 1988:185-189.

24. Åsman P, Britt J, Mills RP, Heijl A. Evaluation of adaptive spatial enhancement in suprathreshold visual field screening. Ophthalmol 1988; 95:1656-1662.

25. Åsman P, Heijl A. Spatial considerations in cluster analysis for detection of glaucomatous field loss. Perimetry Update 1990/91 (in press), 1991.

26. Bebié H. Computer-assisted evaluation of visual fields. Graefe's Arch Klin Exp Ophthalmol 1990; 228:242-245.

27. Nagata S, Kani K, Sugiyama A. A computer-assisted visual field diagnosis system using neural network.

Accepted for publication. Perimetry Update 1990/91 (in press), 1991.

28. Kelman S, Perell H, D'Autrechy L, Scott RJ. A neural network can differentiate glaucoma and optic neuropathy visual fields through pattern recognition. Perimetry Update 1990/91 (in press), 1991.

29. Heijl A, et al. Extended empirical statistical package for evaluation of single and multiple fields in glaucoma. Perimetry Update 1990/91 (in press), 1991.

30. Holmin C, Krakau CET. Regression analysis of the central visual field in chronic glaucoma cases. Acta Ophthalmol 1982; 60:267-274.

31. Flammer J. Fluctuations in the visual field. In Automatic Perimetry in Glaucoma. A Practical Guide. eds. Drance SM, Anderson DR. Orlando: Grune and Stratton, 1985:161-174.

32. Werner EB et al. Visual field variability in stable glaucoma patients. Documenta Ophthalmol Proc Ser 1987; 49:77-84.

33. Heijl A, Lindgren A, Lindgren G. Inter-test variability of computer-measured individual differential light threshold values in glaucomatous visual fields. In Heijl A ed, Perimetry Update 1988/89. Amsterdam, Kugler and Ghedini Pub 1989:165-172.

34. Heijl A, Lindgren A, Lindgren G, Patella M. Inter-test threshold variability in glaucoma: importance of censored observations and general field status. Perimetry Update 1990/91 (in press), 1991.

**Lanning B. Kline, MD**
**John J. Wasenko, MD**

$S$ince the 1970s the advances in neuroimaging have been spectacular. Computed tomography (CT) was the first modality to allow direct visualization of intracranial and intraorbital contents. In less than a decade, refinements in CT technology, with increased spatial and contrast resolution, thin section tomograms, and reformatted images, rendered early CT scanners obsolete. The impact of CT was so great that its inventors were awarded the Nobel Prize in Physiology or Medicine in 1979.

The 1980s witnessed the introduction of another exciting neuroimaging technique, magnetic resonance (MR) imaging. Not only can this technique provide images of the central nervous system, but MR is performed without exposing the patient to ionizing radiation. In less than five years there have been continued improvements in MR technology, including the use of intravenous contrast, faster scanning times, and fat suppression techniques. Appropriately, MR has been described as "one of the miracles of imaging of the 1980s."[1]

The tremendous impact of MR as a neurodiagnostic modality has been felt in ophthalmology. MR has proved helpful in evaluating virtually all aspects of the visual apparatus. It is the purpose of this report to illustrate the preeminent role that MR currently plays in evaluation of ophthalmologic disease. However, CT is still of great value and specific indications for its use will be discussed.

## TECHNIQUE OF MR IMAGING[2]

Protons, electrons, and neutrons are the basic particles which compose atoms. The proton is positively charged and the electron negatively charged. These particles rotate about their axes and, as a result, generate a magnetic field with north and south poles, acting like tiny magnets. As they revolve, they have a magnetic moment, a vector that describes the direction and strength of the magnetic field (Figure 17-1). The neutron, while electrically neutral, possesses a net magnetic moment and generates a magnetic field as a result of its subatomic composition. Atoms that contain an odd number of protons and neutrons possess larger magnetic moments than those that do not, because the individual magnetic moments do not cancel each other. Hydrogen possesses a large magnetic moment because of its single-proton nucleus. This property, plus its abundance in human tissue, makes hydrogen an ideal element to measure with magnetic resonance.

Individual nuclei are randomly arranged in a given substance, and as a result

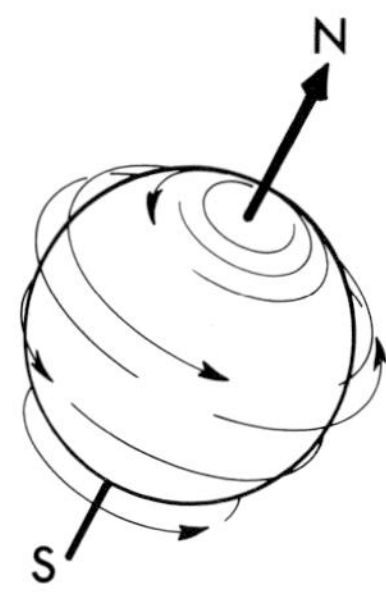

**FIGURE 17-1**    A moving charged particle generates a magnetic field with north and south poles. Arrow indicates direction of the magnetic field.

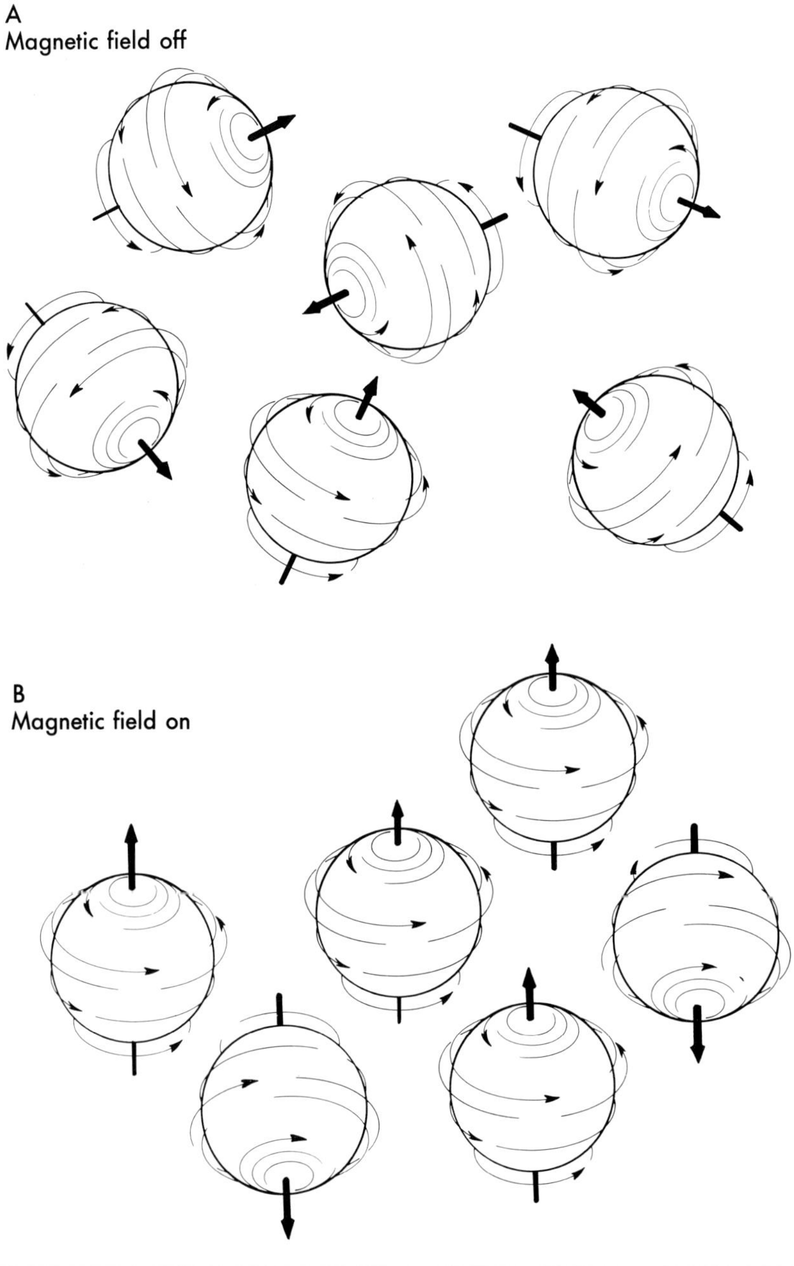

**FIGURE 17-2**    **A,** Nuclei are oriented at random with individual magnetic moments cancelling each other. **B,** When placed in a magnetic field, nuclei align parallel with or antiparallel with the magnetic field. A slightly larger number of nuclei align parallel with the magnetic field.

there is no net magnetic moment (Figure 17-2, *A* ). If a substance is placed in an external magnetic field, the nuclei will align with and rotate or precess around the external magnetic field (Figure 17-2, *B* ). The nuclei possess one of two energy states, either parallel (aligned with) or antiparallel (aligned against) the external magnetic field. Nuclei will at random exchange energy with each other and change from a higher to a lower energy state, and vice-versa. A slightly larger number of nuclei are in the lower energy state, and as a result there is a net magnetic vector. In addition to aligning with the magnetic field, the nuclei rotate or precess about it at a frequency dependent on the strength of the external magnetic field.

The nuclei precess in a random manner at an angle of zero, transcribing a cone (Figure 17-3). As previously stated, there is a net magnetic vector in the direction of the external magnetic field. This vector is made up of two components, one along the longitudinal axis $[M_z]$ and one in the transverse plane $[M_{xy}]$. Because of the random precession of individual nuclei, there is no net magnetization in the transverse plane, and the individual vector components cancel each other.

To generate a signal, energy in the form of a radiofrequency (RF) pulse is utilized to stimulate the substance to be imaged. The frequency of the RF pulse must equal the precessional frequency of the nuclei. When this condition exists, the nuclei begin to resonate. As the nuclei resonate, energy is radiated at a frequency equal to that of the incident RF pulse. The energy, often referred to as an "echo," induces a current in a nearby wire or receiver coil that can be measured. The measured current is then processed by a computer into an image.

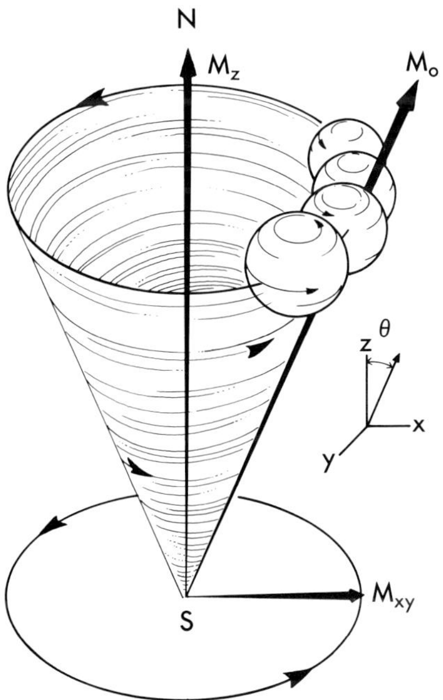


**FIGURE 17-3**  When placed in a magnetic field, nuclei precess about the magnetic field at an angle 0. The magnetization vector ($M_o$) of a nucleus is composed of longitudinal ($M_z$) and transverse ($M_{xy}$) components. A net longitudinal magnetization vector exists while there is no net transverse magnetization.

The RF pulse displaces or rotates the precessing nuclei 90° into the transverse (XY) plane (Figure 17-4). Two processes now occur simultaneously. The first is $T_1$ relaxation. The nuclei in the transverse plane begin to realign with the external magnetic field along the Z axis. The rate at which this process occurs is the $T_1$ relaxation rate. $T_1$ is defined as the time for a substance to recover 63.2% of its longitudinal magnetization (Figure 17-5). This process of $T_1$ relaxation is also called spin-lattice relaxation, and is caused by interactions of the nuclei with their surrounding environment.

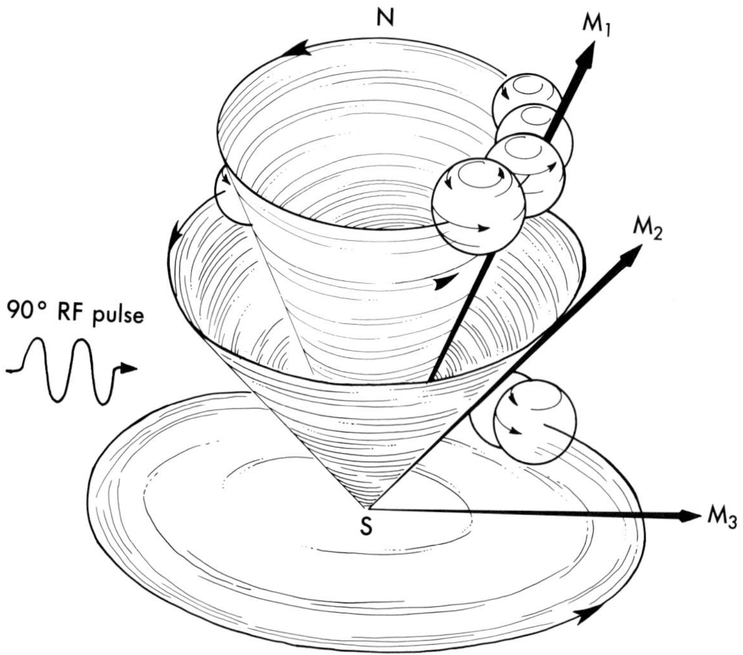


**FIGURE 17-4**   A 90-degree RF pulse rotates the magnetization vector, ($M_1$) into the transverse plane ($M_3$) where the longitudinal magnetization is zero. The nuclei will begin to recover longitudinal magnetization ($M_2$) and realign with the magnetic field. The vector eventually returns to the original position and recovers full longitudinal magnetization.

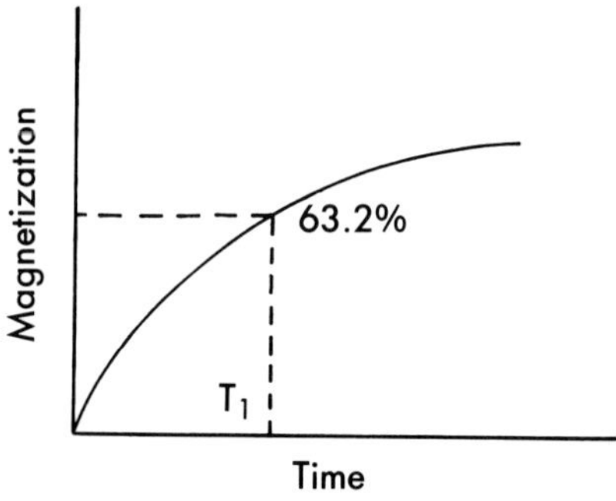


**FIGURE 17-5**   Following a 90-degree radiofrequency pulse, longitudinal magnetization recovers at an exponential rate. $T_1$ is the time for the vector to recover 63.2% of initial longitudinal magnetization. Longitudinal magnetization is fully recovered after four $T_1$ periods have elapsed.

The second process that occurs simultaneously is $T_2$ relaxation, or spin-spin relaxation. This process occurs as a result of interactions of nuclei with each other. Nuclei precess at random about the external magnetic field (Z axis). A 90° RF pulse is applied, which displaces the nuclei into the transverse plane. At this instant the nuclei are in phase; that is, they are aligned along the same direction in the transverse plane. The nuclei rapidly dephase, or lose coherence, and point in random directions in the transverse plane (Figure 17-6). The rate of dephasing in the transverse plane is the $T_2$ relaxation rate. $T_2$ is defined as the time for a tissue to possess only 36.8% of its original transverse magnetization (Figure 17-7). In general, $T_2$ values of tissues are much shorter than $T_1$ values.

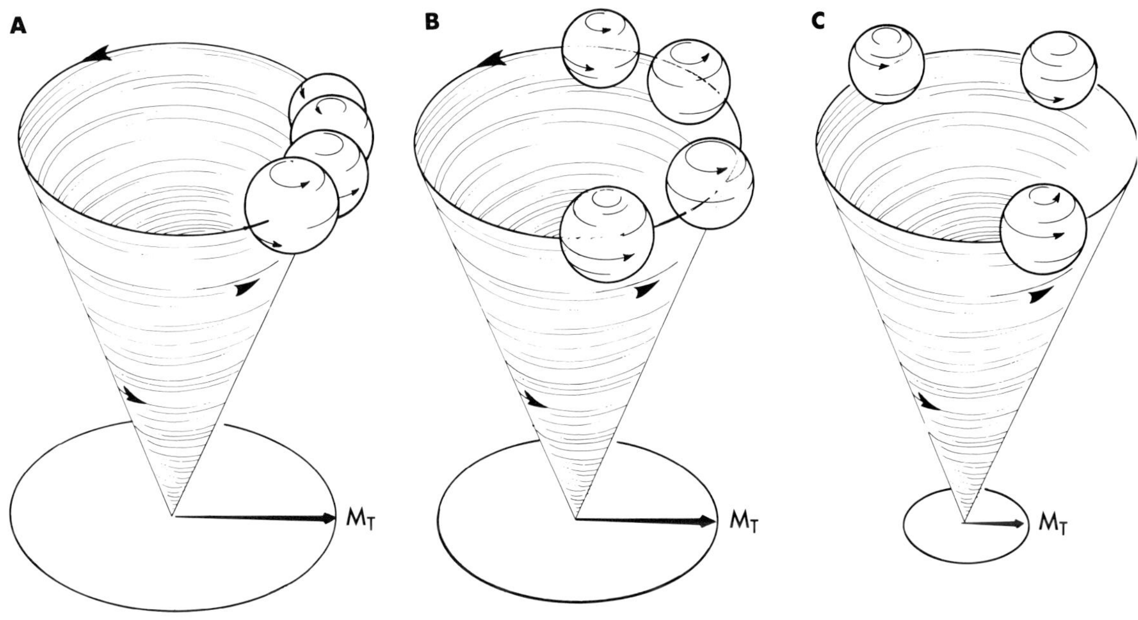

**FIGURE 17-6**     **(A)** The nuclei are in phase in the transverse plane at the echo time with maximum transverse magnetization ($M_T$). **(B,C)** Loss of transverse magnetization occurs rapidly as nuclei dephase and become oriented at random.

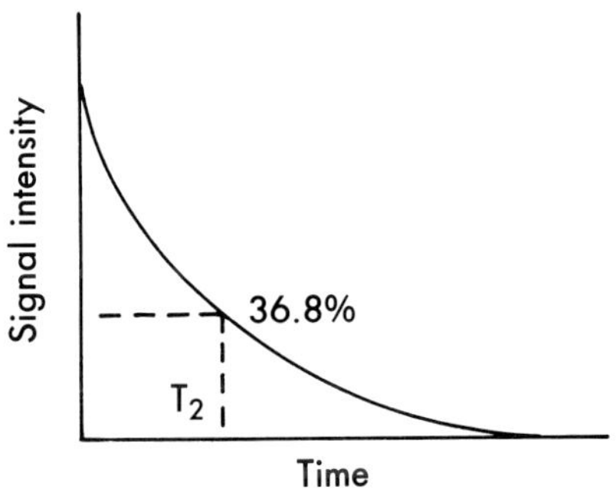

**FIGURE 17-7**     After application of 180-degree RF pulse, transverse magnetization decreases at an exponential rate. $T_2$ is the time at which 36.8% of the initial transverse magnetization remains.

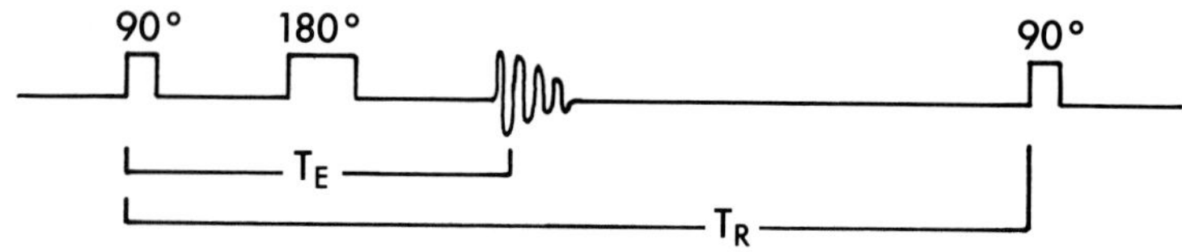



**FIGURE 17-8**    Spin-echo sequence: 90-degree and 180-degree pulses produce a spin-echo. Repetition time (TR) is the time between 90-degree pulses. The time between a 90-degree pulse and when the receiver coil is turned on to listen for a signal (echo) is the echo time (TE).

### Types of Spin-echo MR Scans

| Image | TR | TE |
|---|---|---|
| $T_1$-weighted | Short | Short |
| Proton density | Long | Short |
| $T_2$-weighted | Long | Long |

| TR (msec) | TE (msec) |
|---|---|
| Short: 200–1000 | Short: 20–30 |
| Long: 2000–2500 | Long: 50–1000 |

The most commonly used pulse sequence in MR is spin-echo. This consists of a 90° RF pulse, which displaces nuclei into the transverse plane, followed by a 180° pulse, which rephases nuclei in the transverse plane. The time between the 90° pulses is called the repetition time (TR). The time between a 90° pulse and when the receiver coil is turned on to listen for a signal ("echo") is the echo time (TE) (Figure 17-8). By altering TR and TE values, several MR images are obtained: $T_1$ weighted, $T_2$ weighted, and proton or spin density. (See box above.)

Various tissues have different signal intensities on each pulse sequence (Table 17-1). Gray matter is decreased in signal intensity compared with white matter on $T_1$-weighted images, while it is increased in signal intensity relative to white matter on $T_2$-weighted images. This is caused by the higher water content of gray matter, which prolongs relaxation times. Cortical bone is decreased in signal intensity on both $T_1$- and $T_2$-weighted images. The paucity of mobile protons results in the low signal intensity observed in cortical bone. Rapid blood flow is decreased in signal intensity on $T_1$- and $T_2$-weighted scans. A tissue must be exposed to both 90° and 180° pulses to emit a signal. If the velocity of blood is high enough that it passes through a tissue volume without being exposed to both pulses, no signal will be emitted. Thus, blood will appear as decreased signal intensity on both types of scans. This is referred to as "flow void" phenomenon.

Pulse sequences utilized in the evaluation of the orbit are fat saturation[3] and short-time inversion recovery (STIR).[4] In the fat saturation technique, a 90° pulse is applied at the frequency of fat prior to initiating the imaging sequence. This places the magnetization vector of fat in the transverse plane. An RF pulse of equal magnitude but opposite in direction, is applied, which eliminates the signal from fat. In the STIR sequence, a 180° pulse inverts the magnetization vector into the

**Table 17-1**   Relative signal intensity of different tissues in $T_1$- and $T_2$-weighted MR scans.[24]

|  | $T_1$-weighted | $T_2$-weighted |
|---|---|---|
| Brain |  |  |
|    White matter | Bright | Darker |
|    Gray matter | Darker | Brighter |
| CSF*/H$_2$O | Dark | Bright |
| Vitreous/aqueous | Dark | Bright |
| Fat | Bright | Dark |
| Rapidly flowing blood | Black** | Black** |
| Cortical bone | Black | Black |
| Air | Black | Black |

*CSF—cerebrospinal fluid
**Exquisitely dependent on pulse sequence and time parameters used

Z plane. An appropriate inversion time is chosen such that the magnetization vector of fat is approximately zero at the echo time, and as a result the signal from fat is eliminated.

Gadolinium-diethylene triamene pentacetic acid is a paramagnetic contrast material developed for use in MR. Gadolinium is similar to iodinated contrast utilized in CT, in that it crosses a defect in the blood-brain barrier. Gadolinium has seven unpaired electrons. The large magnetic moment of the electrons produces inhomogeneities in the local magnetic field that increases $T_1$ and $T_2$ relaxation rates. The increase in relaxation rates results in increased signal intensity on $T_1$-weighted images.

Direct multiplanar imaging is a great advantage of MR over other imaging techniques. Axial, coronal, and sagittal views are obtained with MR without repositioning the patient's head in the scanner. As is illustrated below, the direct sagittal view is helpful in the assessment of ocular, orbital, and intracranial disease.

## AREAS OF OPHTHALMOLOGIC INTEREST
### Globe

Ultrasonography and CT are excellent methods for visualizing a variety of ocular abnormalities, including tumors and foreign bodies. These techniques are of even greater value in eyes with opaque media. The advent of MR with standard cylindrical RF coils provided suboptimal images of these ocular conditions. However, if a surface coil is used, the MR signal received is stronger. The signal-to-noise ratio is improved, allowing thin sections with increased spatial resolution.[5] With MR, choroidal melanomas can be differentiated from effusions and nonpigmented tumors. Characteristic bright signal on $T_1$ and dark signal on $T_2$ scans should be seen (Figure 17-9). However, this is not pathognomonic for a melanoma.[6] MR is superior to CT in detection and differential diagnosis of the majority of ocular tumors.[7] However, retinoblastoma is imaged to greater advantage with CT because of CT's ability to demonstrate calcifications.

Evaluation of intraocular foreign bodies with neuroimaging studies should be done cautiously. The presence of ferromagnetic intraocular foreign bodies

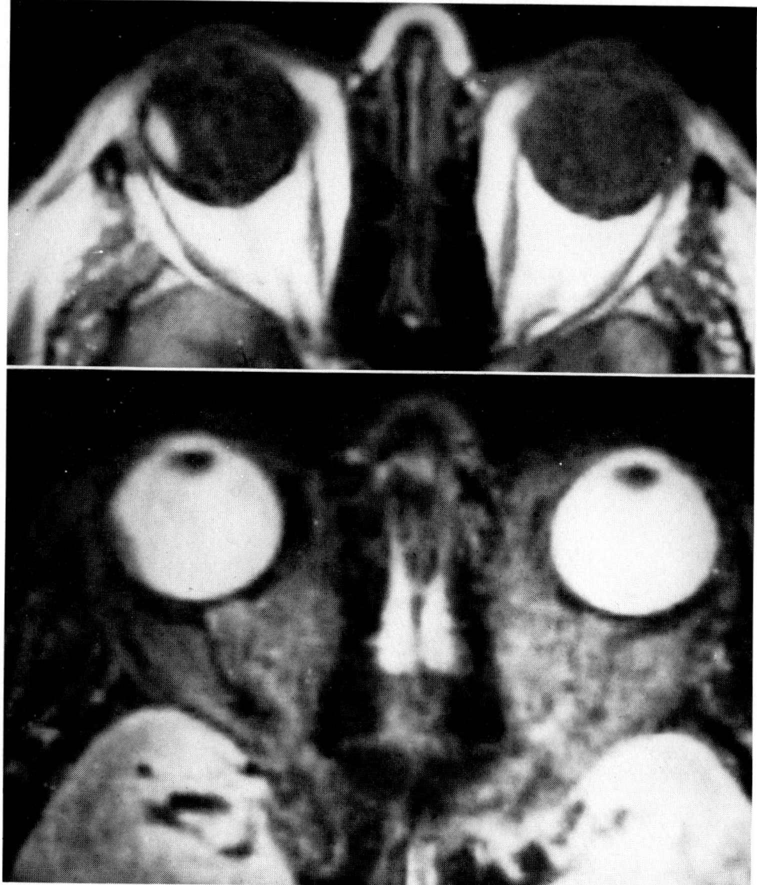

**FIGURE 17-9**    Choroidal melanoma. Top, Axial $T_1$ (500/30) image demonstrates a mass of increased signal intensity in right eye. Bottom, Melanoma is decreased in signal on $T_2$ (2000/80) image. Signal characteristics are those of subacute hemorrhage and/or melanin.

such as BBs or metallic intraocular foreign bodies of unknown composition are contraindications for MR imaging.[8] The presence of nonferromagnetic materials such as retinal tacks made of titanium or cobalt-nickel and intraocular lens loops of platinum or titanium are not contraindications.[9]

## Orbit

Currently, CT and MR are often complementary studies in the evaluation of orbital disease. While soft-tissue detail and vascular structures are better imaged with MR, bone changes and areas of calcification are seen more readily with CT. Thus, in cases of orbital trauma, bone fractures can be optimally seen with CT, and in tumors of the skull base, paranasal sinuses, and metastases, bone erosion is best imaged with CT. CT is superior to MR for detecting small amounts of calcification, as with optic nerve meningioma (Figure 17-10).

The resolution of orbital lesions with MR continues to improve with improvements in MR technology. High magnetic field strength (1.5 Tesla) and small-

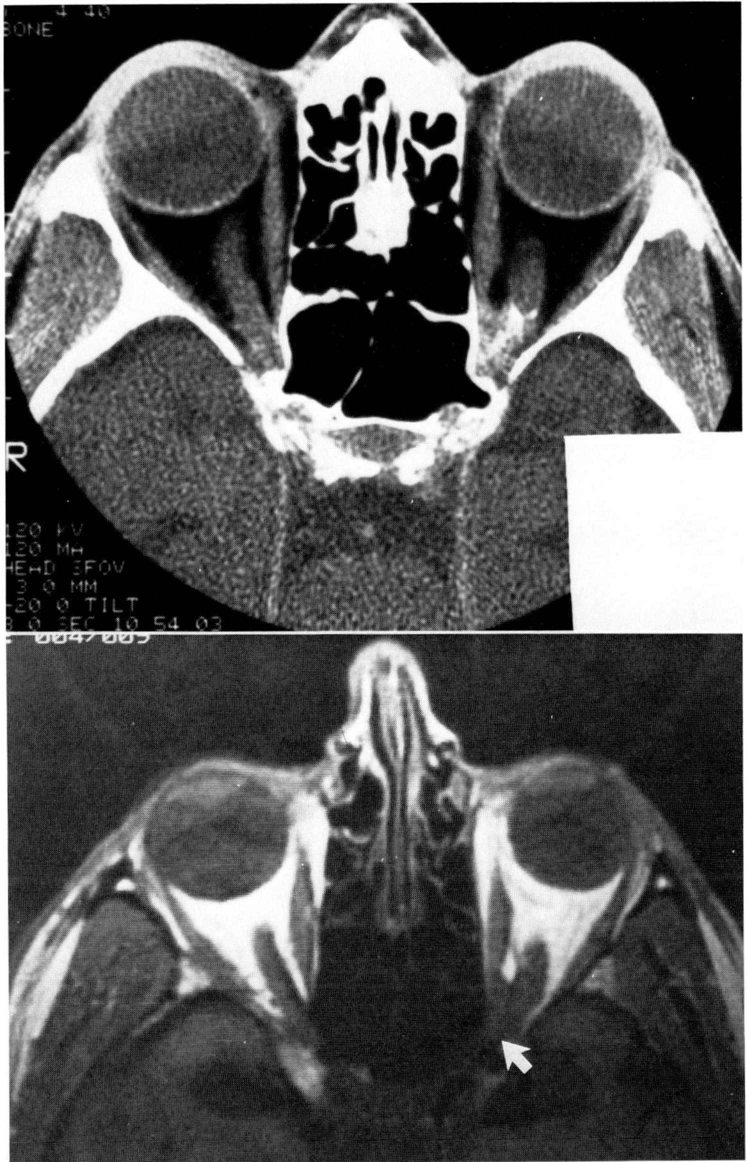

**FIGURE 17-10**  Optic nerve meningioma. Top, CT demonstrates calcification in the left optic nerve. Bottom, With MR, calcification is not visualized on axial $T_1$ (500/20) image, but enlargement of the left optic nerve is evident (arrow).

diameter surface coils are two of these advances. MR is superior to CT in identifying lesions in the orbital apex and in distinguishing nonspecific orbital inflammation (pseudotumor) from malignancy in clinically similar patients (Figure 17-11).[10] In addition, flow in the superior ophthalmic vein can be assessed with MR. In cases of dural-cavernous or carotid-cavernous fistulas, this flow is increased (Figure 17-12). When the fistula undergoes thrombosis, whether spontaneous or via embolization, reduced flow within the superior ophthalmic vein can be detected with MR.

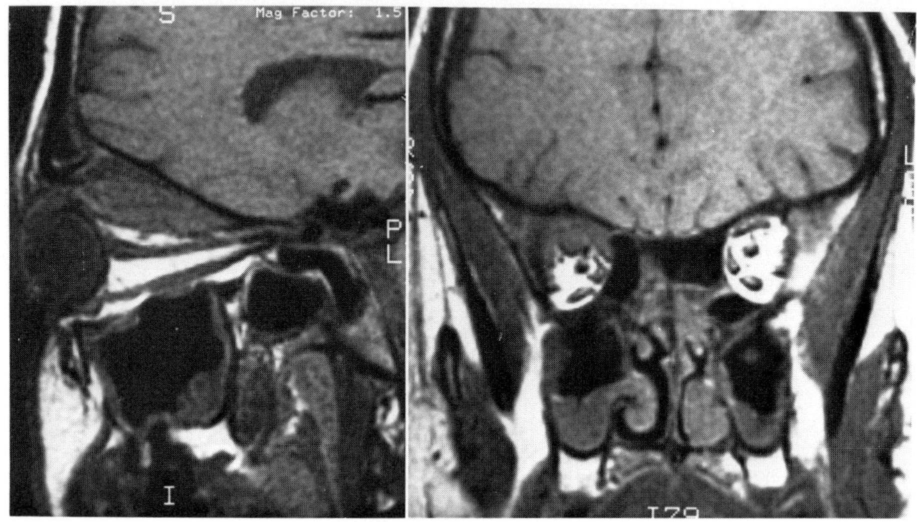



**FIGURE 17-11** Nonspecific orbital inflammation. Sagittal (left) and coronal (right) $T_1$ (700/30) images reveal mass in superior right orbit extending to the apex. Signal is isointense with brain. The mass was isointense with fat on $T_2$-weighted images consistent with orbital pseudotumor.

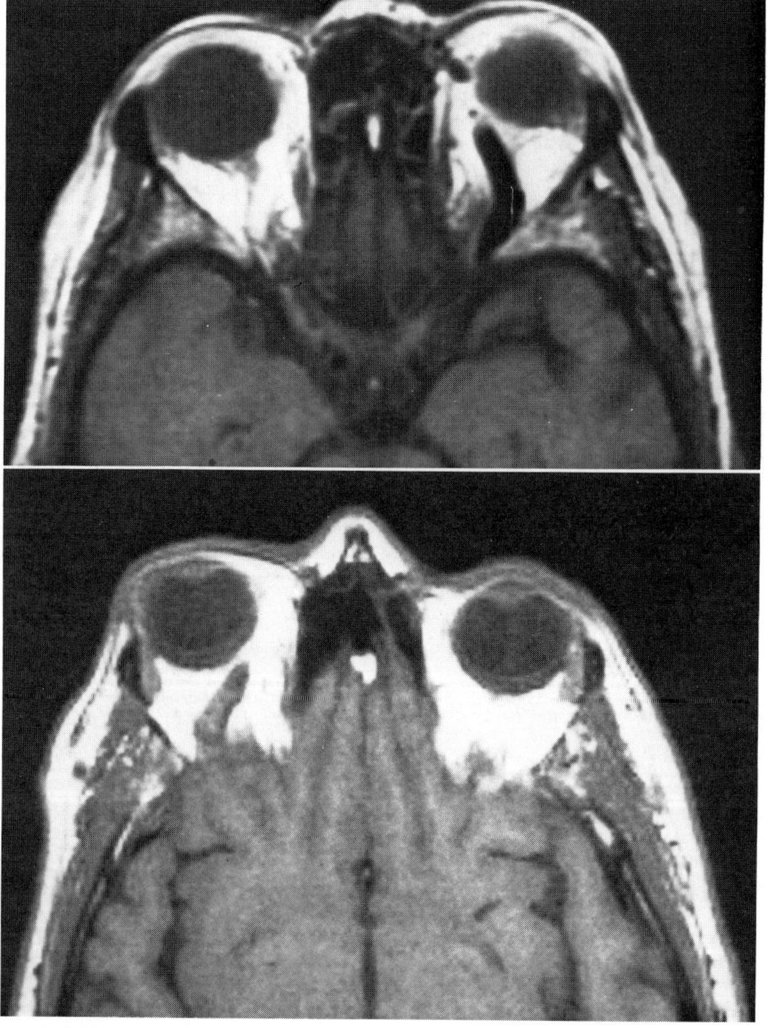

**FIGURE 17-12** Top, Angiographically proven carotid-cavernous fistula. Axial $T_1$ (500/20) image shows enlarged left superior ophthalmic vein of decreased signal intensity due to rapidly flowing blood. Bottom, Patient with spontaneous resolution of dural-cavernous fistula. Superior ophthalmic vein contains isointense signal on $T_1$ (500/15) image, indicating thrombosis.

Orbital MR is also improving because of the above mentioned techniques that suppress orbital fat. This is necessary because of the hyperintense signal of fat on $T_1$-weighted images (Figure 17-13). Limitations related to the presence of fat are loss of contrast of orbital structures and loss of anatomic detail as a result of chemical shift artifact.[3] This artifact may obscure small lesions in the orbit. It appears as adjacent bands of increased and decreased signal intensity (Figure 17-13). The artifact occurs because fat-bound water molecules are partially shielded from the external magnetic field, and therefore precess at a slower frequency than other water molecules. As a result, during image reconstruction, the computer places the fat-bound water molecules in a position corresponding to their slower frequency rather than their true position.

Figure 17-14 illustrates improved definition of orbital detail with fat suppression. Important retrobulbar structures, including extraocular muscles and the optic nerve/sheath complex, are seen more clearly with fat suppression imaging.

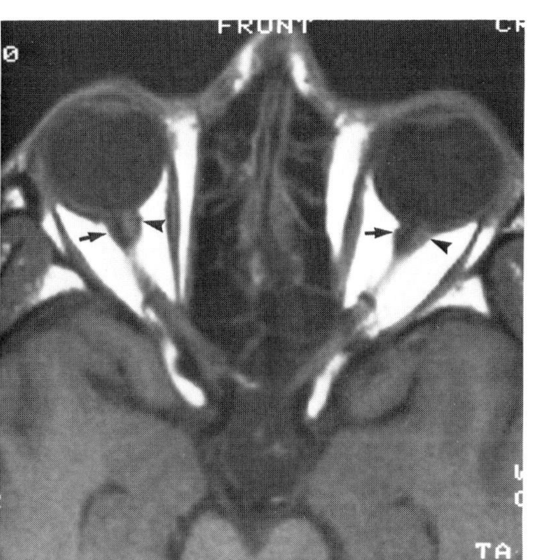

**FIGURE 17-13** Normal orbit. Axial $T_1$ (500/15) scan. Chemical shift artifact results in apparent widening of both optic nerve sheaths on patient's right (arrows) and narrowing on patient's left (arrowheads). Note intracanalicular optic nerves are well seen.

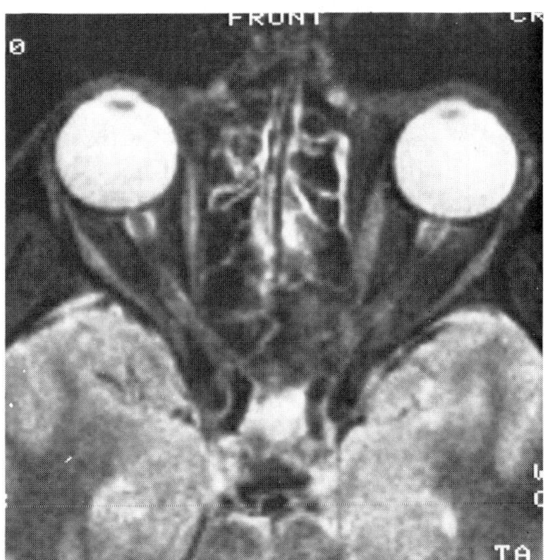

**FIGURE 17-14** Normal orbit. Axial STIR (2500/140/20) image. Optic nerves and muscles are visualized against hypointense fat. Hyperintense signal surrounding optic nerves represents cerebrospinal fluid.

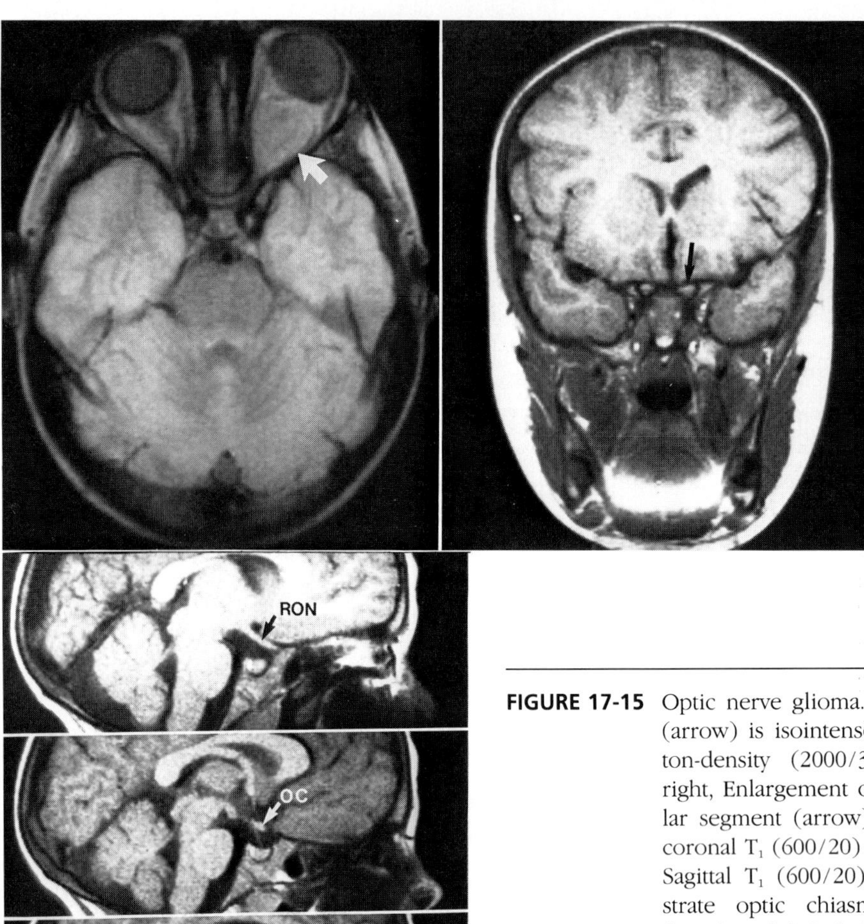

FIGURE 17-15 Optic nerve glioma. Top left, Mass (arrow) is isointense on axial proton-density (2000/30) scan. Top right, Enlargement of intracanalicular segment (arrow) is evident on coronal $T_1$ (600/20) image. Bottom, Sagittal $T_1$ (600/20) scans demonstrate optic chiasm (OC), right (RON) and left (LON) intracranial optic nerves are normal.

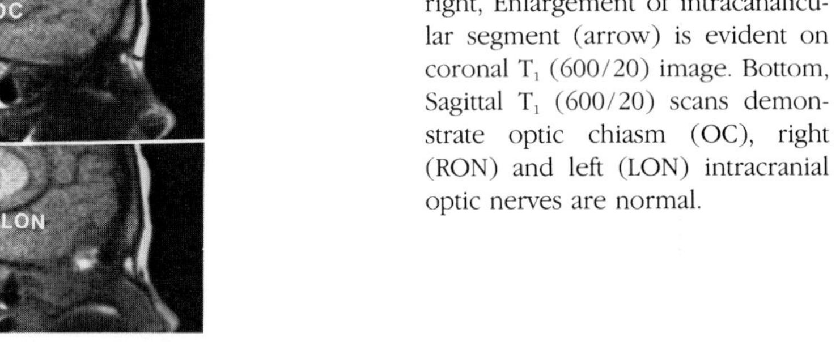

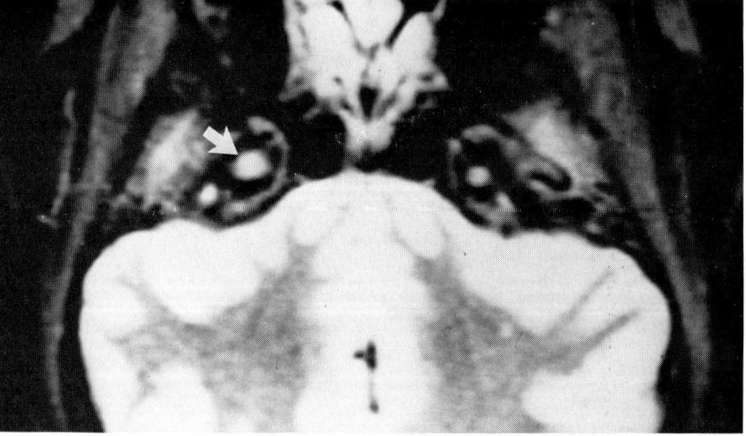

FIGURE 17-16 Optic neuritis. Coronal STIR (1800/140/30) image demonstrates enlarged left optic nerve (arrow) that is hyperintense relative to fat and extraocular muscles. *(Courtesy of William R. Scott, MD, Pensacola, Florida.)*

## Optic Nerve

MR affords visualization of the entire length of the optic nerve, from globe to chiasm. Because it is encased in bone, the intracanalicular segment of the optic nerve could be imaged only occasionally with CT, yet it is now routinely seen with MR. (See Figure 17-13.) As noted above, optic nerve/sheath meningiomas, often containing small calcifications, are better detected with CT (see Figure 17-10). However, MR is superior in detecting extension of optic nerve tumors beyond the orbit. A patient with a left optic nerve glioma is illustrated in Figure 17-15. Careful MR study revealed the glioma extending into the optic canal, but the intracranial portion of the optic nerve and the optic chiasm were not involved. Areas of optic nerve demyelination can also be detected with MR in patients with optic neuritis (Figure 17-16).[11]

## Optic Chiasm

Because visual loss is frequently caused by tumorous compression of the optic chiasm, careful neuroimaging of the perisellar area is essential. MR is now the modality of choice in studying the optic chiasm, consistently visualizing this structure axially, coronally, and sagittally.[12] Pituitary adenomas causing sellar enlargement and chiasmal compression are readily seen (Figure 17-17). Craniopharyngiomas may have solid and cystic areas with variable amounts of calcification. The calcifications are seen with CT, but not consistently with MR. However, MR visualizes the cysts well, because of their hyperintense signal on $T_1$- and $T_2$-weighted scans (Figure 17-18). Chiasmal gliomas are directly visualized with MR, and in patients with neurofibromatosis extension along the posterior visual pathways may be apparent.[13] The availability of a sagittal view with MR vividly depicts the empty sella syndrome and position of the optic chiasm (Figure 17-19).

## Cavernous Sinus

Less than a decade ago, CT was reported as the first technique to directly image the cavernous sinus. Yet MR has subsequently proved to be more effective than CT in delineating the cavernous sinus and disorders that affect it.[14] Like CT, MR delineates abnormalities in the size and shape of the cavernous sinus. In addition, MR is much more sensitive in detecting carotid artery compression and encasement, since the intracavernous carotid is seen as a flow void (Figure 17-20).[15] Cavernous sinus meningiomas are usually isointense with brain on $T_1$- and $T_2$-weighted images, but demonstrate hyperintense signal after intravenous gadolinium (Figure 17-20). Intracavernous carotid artery aneurysm is directly visualized with MR (Figure 17-21), and frequently eliminates the need for cerebral angiography for diagnostic purposes.

## Postchiasmal Visual Pathways

Visual field defects due to abnormalities of the optic tract, lateral geniculate nucleus, optic radiation or occipital cortex should be evaluated with MR. Tumor, vascular infarction (Figure 17-22), arteriovenous malformation, and demyelination

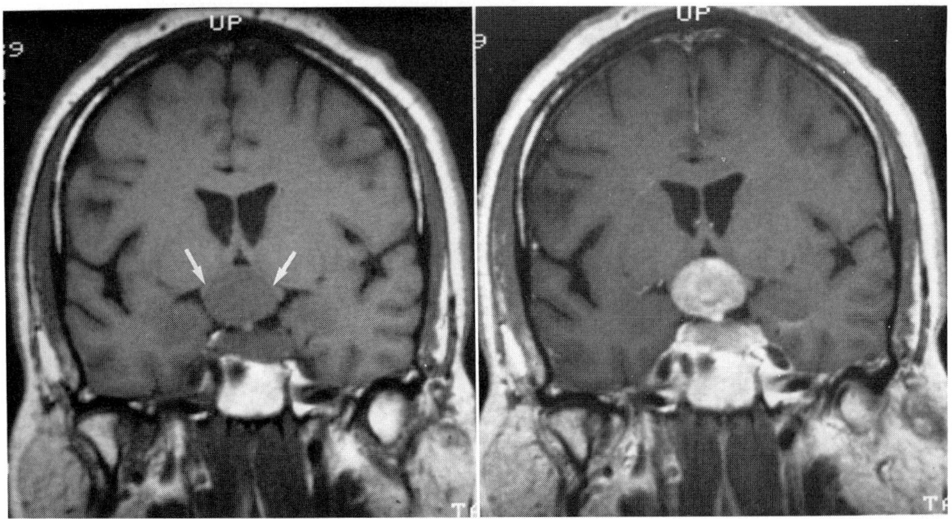

**FIGURE 17-17**  Pituitary adenoma. Left, Precontrast $T_1$ (500/15) image shows isointense sellar mass with suprasellar extension and compression of optic chiasm (arrows). Right, Enhancement of mass after intravenous gadolinium on coronal $T_1$ (500/15) scan.

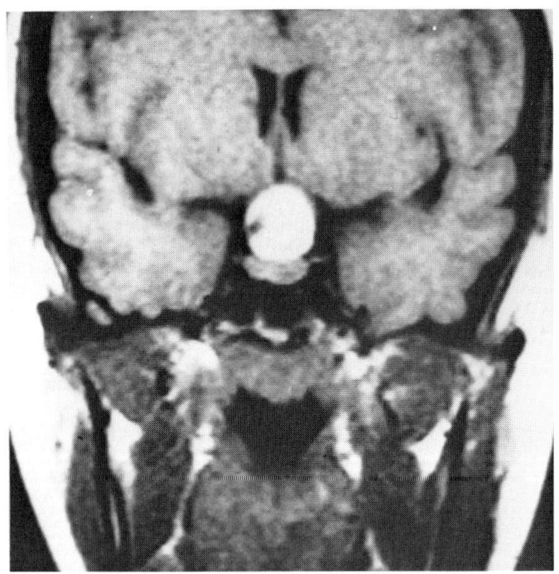

**FIGURE 17-18**  Craniopharyngioma. Coronal $T_1$ (600/20) image shows hyperintense suprasellar mass with compression of normal pituitary gland. *(Courtesy of Saunders Hupp, MD, Mobile, Alabama.)*

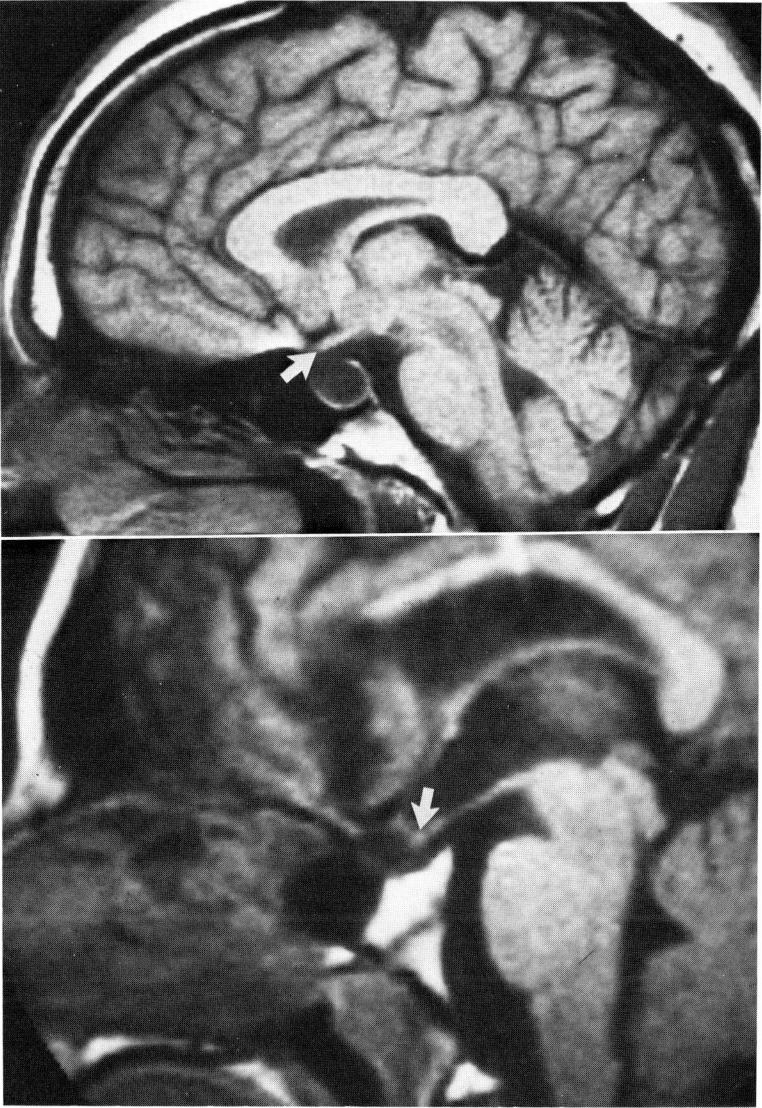

**FIGURE 17-19**  Empty sella syndrome. Top, Sagittal $T_1$ (600/20) image with chiasm (arrow) in normal position. Bottom, Sagittal $T_1$ (600/20) image of another patient reveals herniation of the optic chiasm (arrow) into the sella.

(Figure 17-23) can be visualized. MR can detect ischemic cerebral infarction at an earlier stage than can CT, but CT is more sensitive in detecting acute (less than 12 hours) hemorrhagic infarction.[16] As with CT, excellent correlation has been demonstrated between types and extent of visual field defect and MR findings.

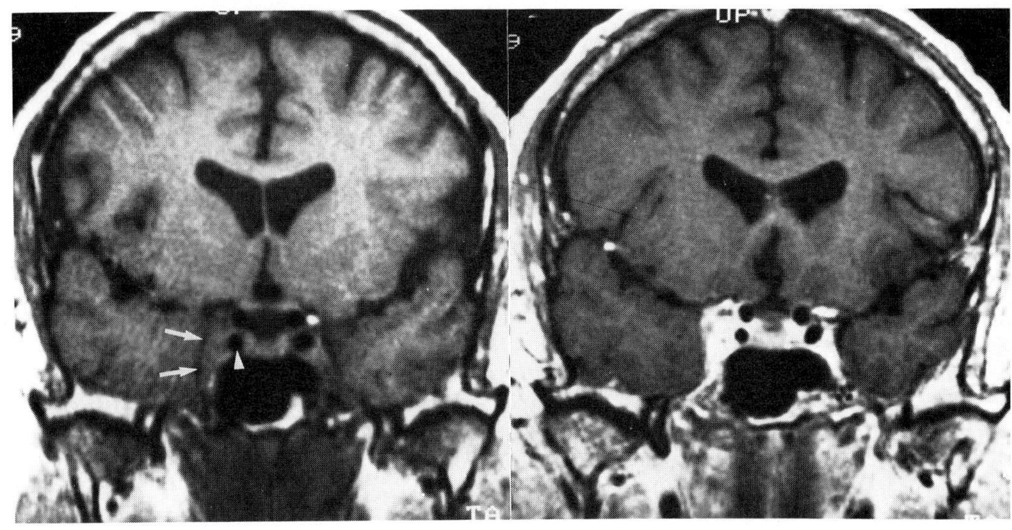

**FIGURE 17-20**  Cavernous sinus meningioma. Left, Coronal $T_1$ (500/15) scan. Isointense mass enlarges right cavernous sinus (arrows) and partially encases internal carotid artery (arrowhead). Right, Intense enhancement of mass following intravenous gadolinium on $T_1$ (500/15) image.

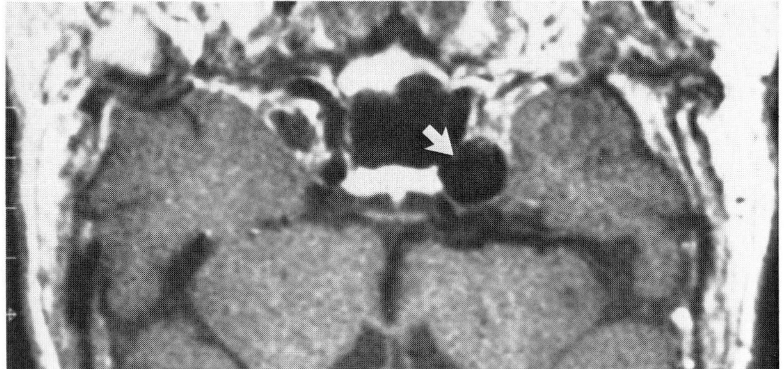

**FIGURE 17-21**  Intracavernous carotid artery aneurysm. Coronal, postcontrast $T_1$ (600/20) scan of hypointense aneurysm (arrow) demonstrating "flow void" phenomenon.

## Posterior Fossa

MR has clearly surpassed CT in the study of brain stem and cerebellum.[17] The beam-hardening artifacts of CT caused by the adjacent bones of the cranial vault are eliminated with MR. In particular, sagittal MR provides valuable anatomic detail of posterior fossa structures. Infarction, hemorrhage, and tumor (Figure 17-24) are easily visualized with MR. MR provides more precise anatomic information to

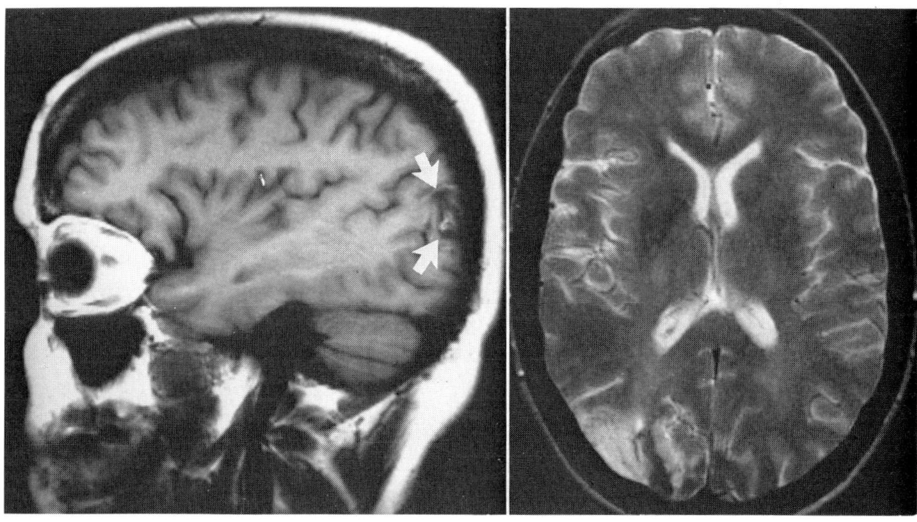

**FIGURE 17-22**  Hemorrhagic parieto-occipital infarction. Left, Sagittal $T_1$ (500/15) image reveals right occipital lobe hypointensity (arrows). Band of hyperintense signal represents subacute blood. Right, Axial $T_2$ (2200/90) image shows mixed signal intensity due to edema and hemorrhage in right parieto-occipital region.

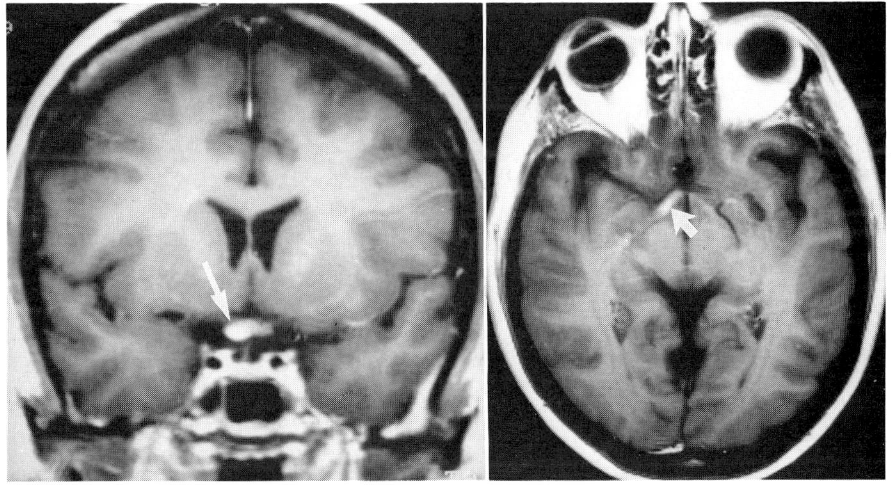

**FIGURE 17-23**  Multiple sclerosis. Postcontrast coronal (left) and axial (right) $T_1$ (500/15) images. Enhancing plaque (arrows) involving optic chiasm and right optic tract is demonstrated.

correlate with specific eye-movement disorders such as internuclear ophthalmoplegia, vertical and horizontal gaze palsies, and various forms of nystagmus.[18] MR visualization of feeding and draining vessels allows excellent evaluation and classification of arteriovenous malformations. Skull-base abnormalities are also clearly imaged. Arnold-Chiari I malformation, often leading to downbeat nystagmus, is one such example (Figure 17-25).

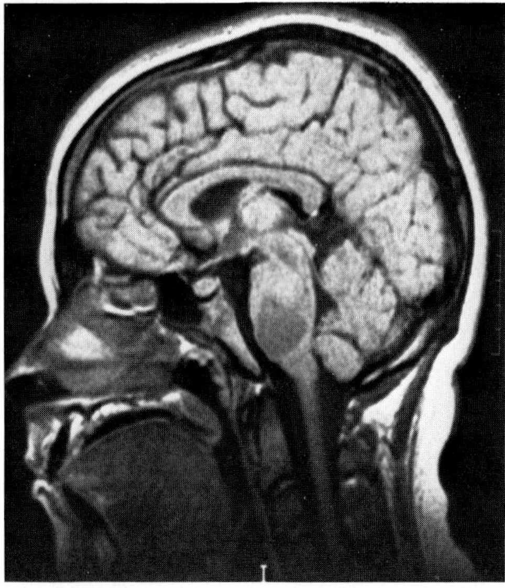

**FIGURE 17-24**  Brain stem glioma. Sagittal $T_1$ (600/30) scan shows hypointense mass involving pons and medulla.

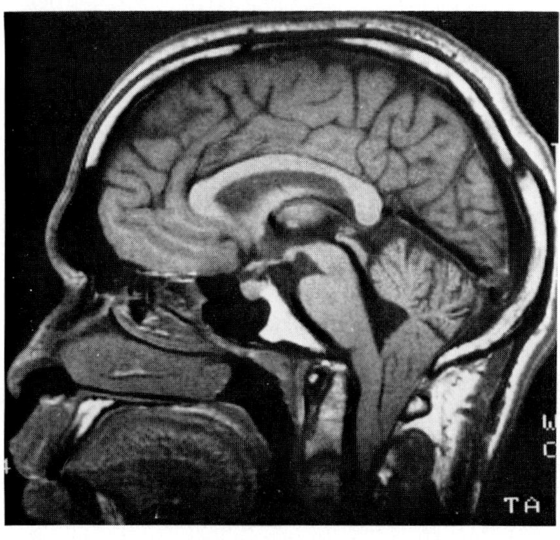

**FIGURE 17-25**  Arnold-Chiari I malformation. Extension of cerebellar tonsils through the foramen magnum is evident on sagittal $T_1$ (500/15) image.

## MR ANGIOGRAPHY

One recent development in MR that holds great promise as a noninvasive method of studying the cerebral circulation is MR angiography.[19] Several different techniques are available, resulting in blood appearing as increased signal intensity without injection of contrast medium (Figure 17-26). Computer reconstruction results in three-dimensional images that can be viewed in multiple projections.

In several small series, MR angiography has been used to evaluate aneurysms, arteriovenous malformations, infarctions, neoplasms, and the carotid bifurcation. Intracranial aneurysms have been detected with a high degree of accuracy, with the neck of the aneurysm readily demonstrated.[20] MR angiography is capable of showing small feeding vessels and draining veins of arteriovenous malformations.[21] In a study of the carotid bifurcation, MR correlated well with angiography

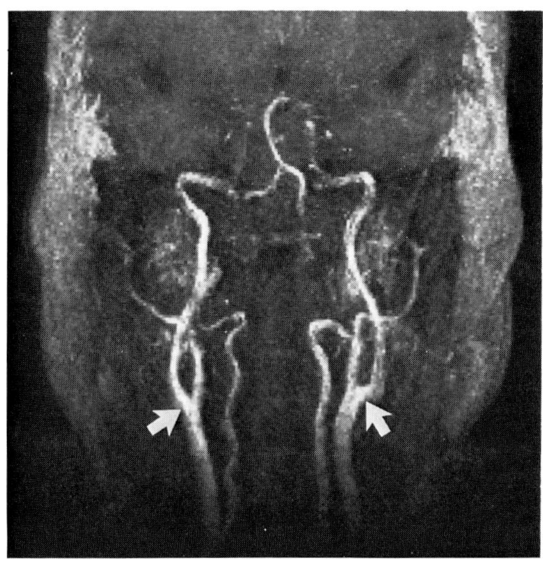

**FIGURE 17-26**  MR angiogram. Cerebral vasculature demonstrates hyperintense signal, yet no contrast is used. Note carotid bifurcations (arrows). *(Courtesy of Michael Mawad, MD, Houston, Texas.)*

in demonstrating carotid stenosis and ulceration.[22] With continued improvements in technique, MR angiography may replace invasive cerebral angiography in many cases.

## DISCUSSION

As we enter the 1990s, it appears that MR is clearly the imaging procedure of choice for the majority of ophthalmologic disorders. However, there are specific instances where CT is of great value:

- Detection of areas of calcification is important in certain ocular (e.g., retinoblastoma) orbital (e.g., optic nerve meningioma) and intracranial (e.g., craniopharyngioma) neoplasms.
- Bone changes, particularly if subtle, are imaged better with CT. This includes fractures, particularly of the skull base and orbit (e.g., blowout fracture), bone erosion (e.g., metastasis) and hyperostosis (e.g., meningioma).

MR has a number of artifacts and limitations.[23] Movement of the patient during scanning is the most common cause of image degradation. Another source of artifact is metallic dental appliances. Many are made of stainless steel that are ferromagnetic, causing distortion of the image in the plane of the metal. Dental amalgam does not cause artifacts, but metal used in root canal procedures does. While cobalt plaques used in ophthalmologic therapy are nonferromagnetic, they often cause distortion of the orbital images because of local magnetic field disturbance.

Patient selection is necessary before ordering an MR scan. Patients on certain types of life support systems or a respirator cannot be placed into a magnetic field. The metals of the monitoring devices and intravenous poles may be ferromagnetic and will be drawn into the magnet. Patient monitoring devices are also a source of noise in the MR image. Cardiac pacemakers and other monitoring devices can malfunction when exposed to a magnetic field. MR is contraindicated in patients with known or suspected foreign bodies, including intracranial ferromagnetic metallic aneurysm clips. Metallic foreign bodies can be displaced by the strong magnetic field. Any patient suspected of having any type of foreign body would be better evaluated with CT.

Despite the great advance MR represents in neuroimaging, a word of caution is in order. In part, the ability of MR to visualize the appropriate orbital or intracranial abnormality is a direct reflection of the diagnostic acumen of the referring clinician. Prior to ordering an MR scan, the specific area requiring examination should be identified. The radiologist should be supplied with as much clinical information as possible. The ophthalmologist must share in the responsibility when sending a patient for a neuroimaging study.

## References


1. Wolpert SM. Nuclear magnetic resonance vs. computed tomography. AJNR 1983: 996.
2. Stark DD, Bradley WR. Magnetic resonance imaging. St. Louis: CV Mosby 1988.
3. Simon J, Szumowski J, Totterman S, et al. Fat-suppression MR imaging of the orbit. AJNR 1988; 9:961-968.
4. Atlas SW, Grossman RI, Hackney DB, Goldberg H, Bilaniuk LT, Zimmerman RA. STIR MR imaging of the orbit. AJNR 1988; 9:969-974.
5. Bilaniuk LT, Schenck JF, Zimmerman RA, et al. Ocular and orbital lesions: surface coil MR imaging. Radiol 1985; 156:669-674.
6. Spencer G, Lufkin R, Simons K, Straatsma B, Foos R, Hanafee W. MR of a melanoma-simulating ocular neoplasm. AJNR 1987; 8:921-922.
7. Saint-Louis LA, Haik BG, Amster JL. Magnetic resonance imaging of the orbit and optic pathways. In Haik BG, ed, Advanced Imaging Techniques in Ophthalmology. Intl Ophthalmol Clin 1986; 26:169-185.
8. Kelly WM, Paglen PG, Pearson JA, San Diego AG, Solomon MA. Ferromagnetism of intraocular foreign body causes unilateral blindness after MR study. AJNR 1986; 7:243-245.
9. Albert DW, Olson KR, Parel JM, Hernandez E, Lee W, Quencer R. Magnetic resonance imaging and retinal tacks. Arch Ophthalmol 1990; 108:320-321.
10. Atlas SW, Bilaniuk LT, Zimmerman RA, Hackney DB, Goldberg HI, Grossman RI. Orbit: initial experience with surface coil spin-echo MR imaging at 1.5 T. Radiol 1987; 164:501-509.
11. Miller DH, Newton MR, van der Poel JC, et al. Magnetic resonance imaging of the optic nerve in optic neuritis. Neurology 1988; 38:175-179.
12. Daniels DL, Hefkins R, Gager WE, et al. Magnetic resonance imaging of the optic nerve and chiasm. Radiology 1984; 152:79-83.
13. Pomeranz SJ, Shelton JJ, Tobias J, Soila K, Altman D, Viammonte M. MR of visual pathways in patients with neurofibromatosis. AJNR 1987; 8:831-836.
14. Daniels DL, Pech P, Mark L, Pojunas K, Williams AL, Haughton VM. Magnetic resonance imaging of the cavernous sinus. AJR 1985; 144:1099-1114.
15. Yeakley JW, Kulkarni MV, McArdale CB, Haa FL, Tang RA. High-resolution MR imaging of juxtasellar meningiomas with CT and angiographic correlation. AJNR 1988; 9:279-285.
16. Zimmerman RD, Heier LA, Snow RB, Liu DPC, Kelly AB, Peck MDF. Acute intracranial hemorrhage: intensity changes on sequential MR scans at 0.5 T. AJR 1988; 150:651-661.
17. Lee BP, Kneeland JP, Deck MDF, Cahill PT. Posterior fossa lesions: magnetic resonance imaging. Radiology 1984; 153:137-143.
18. Atlas SW, Grossman RI, Savino PJ, et al. Internuclear ophthalmoplegia: MR-anatomic correlation. AJNR 1987; 8:243-247.
19. Edelman RR, Mattle HP, Atkinson DJ, Hoogewoud HM. MR angiography. AJR 1990; 154:937-946.
20. Masaryk TJ, Modic MT, Ross JS, et al. Intracranial circulation: preliminary clinical results with three-dimensional (volume) MR angiography. Radiol 1989; 171:793-799.
21. Edelman RR, Wentz KU, Mattle HP, et al. Intracerebral arteriovenous malformations: evaluation with selective MR angiography and venography. Radiol 1989; 173:831-837.
22. Masaryk TJ, Modic MT, Ruggieri PM, et al. Three-dimensional (volume) gradient-echo imaging of the carotid bifurcation: preliminary clinical experience. Radiol 1989; 171:801-806.
23. Saint-Louis LA, Haik BG. Magnetic resonance imaging of the globe. In Haik, BG, ed, Advanced Imaging Techniques in Ophthalmology. Intl Ophthal Clin 1986; 26:151-167.
24. Slamovits TL, Gardner TA. Neuroimaging in neuro-ophthalmology. Ophthalmol 1989; 96:555-568.

# 18 Topical Carbonic Anhydrase Inhibitors

Anne Louise Coleman, MD

**G**laucoma is an optic neuropathy with characteristic optic nerve and visual field changes. One of the risk factors for this optic neuropathy is elevated intraocular pressure,[1] a risk factor that can be manipulated with medications or surgery. Fortunately, the lowering of intraocular pressure 1-2 mmHg has been found to be associated with less glaucomatous optic nerve damage.[2] Clinicians have been using oral carbonic anhydrase inhibitors to lower intraocular pressure in humans since 1954.[3] Numerous systemic side effects have been reported from the use of oral carbonic anhydrase inhibitors since then, as shown in the box.[4]

The most serious side effect is a blood dyscrasia, idiosyncratic aplastic anemia. Over half the cases of aplastic anemia reported occur within 13 months of the initiation of therapy. Cases have also been reported as much as 5 to 6 years after the start of therapy;[4-6] and 30% of reported cases have been fatal.[5] If the occurrence of aplastic anemia is truly idiosyncratic, a reduction in the dose of carbonic anhydrase inhibitors may have no effect. However, if there is a dose response for aplastic anemia and carbonic anhydrase inhibitors, smaller doses, such as those used topically, will reduce the risk. Most of the other side effects from oral carbonic anhydrase inhibitors are thought to be dose related and should be less likely to occur with topical agents.[6] There has thus been extensive research on developing a topically active carbonic anhydrase inhibitor so that the beneficial pressure-lowering effect is not hampered by systemic side effects.

## HISTORY

The history and development of carbonic anhydrase inhibitors are closely linked to research on aqueous humor dynamics. In his 1950 Proctor Award Lecture, Friedenwald presented the idea that aqueous humor formation is an active process. He theorized that the oxidation of reduced cytochrome oxidase provided $OH^-$ that was buffered by $CO_2$ to create $HCO_3^-$.[7] In support of this theory, Kinsey reported years later that there was a large excess of bicarbonate and ascorbate in the posterior chambers of rabbits (compared to plasma); and Wistrand found carbonic anhydrase, the enzyme that catalyzes the formation of $HCO_3^-$ from $CO_2$ and $OH^-$, in the anterior uveas of rabbits.[9]

Carbonic anhydrase inhibitors were discovered in 1950 by Roblin and Clapp.[10] A few years later, Maren and coworkers reported on the pharmacology of the first marketed carbonic anhydrase inhibitor, acetazolamide (Figure 18-1).[11]

> ### Potential Systemic Side Effects of Oral Carbonic Anhydrase Inhibitors
>
> Metallic taste
> Paresthesias
> Renal calculi
> Malaise, fatigue
> Nausea, diarrhea
> Anorexia, weight loss
> Mental changes (depression, confusion, excitation)
> Loss of libido
> Alopecia, hirsutism
> Blood dyscrasias
> Fetal limb deformities

Becker had already reported that oral acetazolamide lowered intraocular pressure in humans.[3]

## PHARMACOLOGY AND PHYSIOLOGY

All carbonic anhydrase inhibitors have a free sulfonamide group ($-SO_2NH_2$) linked to an aromatic ring.[12] This free sulfonamide group competes for the active site of the carbonic anhydrase isoenzyme and thus blocks or slows the formation of $HCO_3^-$.[13] Decreased $HCO_3^-$ formation results in a reduction in the active secretion or accession rate of $HCO_3^-$ and $Na^+$ into the posterior chamber.[14,15] Since fluid flow is passively linked to the accession rate of $HCO_3^-$ and $Na^+$ into the posterior chamber, there is a concomitant reduction of aqueous formation when the accession rate of $HCO_3^-$ and $Na^+$ is reduced. Wistrand and coworkers[13] have reported that one of the three carbonic anhydrase isoenzymes, carbonic anhydrase isoenzyme II, is located in the pigmented and nonpigmented ciliary epithelium. X-ray crystallography has demonstrated the binding of acetazolamide to this isoenzyme.[16] Tonographic[3] and fluorophotometric studies[17,18] have confirmed that carbonic anhydrase inhibitors reduce aqueous secretion.

The effect of oral carbonic anhydrase inhibitors on intraocular pressure is unrelated to the effect of these substances as diuretics.[19,20] Although the pressure-lowering effect is unrelated to diuresis, metabolic and respiratory acidosis augment the reduction of intraocular pressure.[21,22] The finding of ipsilateral lowering of intraocular pressure after intracarotid injections of acetazolamide in cats supports the theory that carbonic anhydrase inhibitors exert a local effect on intraocular pressure.[23]

## TOPICAL CARBONIC ANHYDRASE INHIBITORS

Several investigators attempted to lower intraocular pressure in animals with topical or subconjunctival administration of acetazolamide, without success.[19,24-26] These experiments were unsuccessful because acetazolamide penetrates poorly through the cornea and sclera.[27] Maren and coworkers in 1983 established that

Compound        Chemical Structure

Aminozolamide

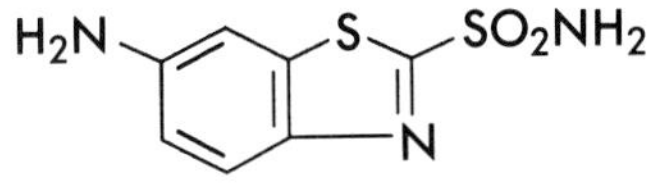

Acetazolamide

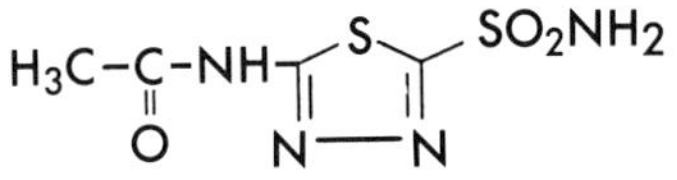

**FIGURE 18-1**    Note that both acetazolamide and aminozolamide have a free sulfonamide group ($-SO_2NH_2$) linked to an aromatic group. *(Courtesy of Erik Lippa, MD, PhD, Merck Sharp & Dohme.)*

an effective topical carbonic anhydrase inhibitor needs both lipid and water solubility.[27] Lipid solubility is essential for diffusion through tissue. Water solubility determines the amount of drug available for this diffusion.

New delivery systems[28,29] and new carbonic anhydrase inhibitors[30-36] have been created that are effective in lowering intraocular pressure in animals. They either have longer ocular contact time or greater lipid and water solubility. Not all of these compounds have been subjected to clinical trials because of either poor effectiveness or adverse reactions.

## Aminozolamide Gel

The first effective topical carbonic anhydrase inhibitor in humans was 3% aminozolamide gel (see Figure 18-1). Lewis and coworkers[29] in a double-masked study found a 26% reduction in intraocular pressure of treated eyes from predose baseline while untreated fellow eyes had a 6% reduction. None of the 18 patients had systemic side effects; however, 1 patient in the study group had conjunctival hyperemia. Another investigator[37] with fluorophotometry found a 9% reduction in aqueous flow between 2 and 7 hours after instillation of one dose of 3% aminozolamide gel in 21 normal volunteers. Ocular side effects were irritation, hyperemia, and blurred vision. Three of four volunteers had bulbar injection and follicular conjunctivitis after multiple doses.

## L-650,719

L-650,719 (6-hydroxybenzol[b]thiophene-2-sulfonamide) was effective and well tolerated in rabbits;[30] however, in a randomized, double-masked, placebo-controlled study, there was no significant effect on intraocular pressure after one week of twice-a-day dosing of 2% L-650,719 in 20 normal volunteers.[38]

## MK-927

MK-927 (5,6-dihydro-4-[2-methylpropyl]amino-4H-thieno[2,3-b]thiopyran-2-sulfonamide 7,7-dioxide hydrochloride) (Figure 18-2) has had significant intraocular pressure-lowering activity in several clinical trials. Lippa and coworkers[39] tested 3 drops of 2% MK-927 in 12 normal volunteers in a double-masked, placebo-

<table>
<tr><th>Compound</th><th>Chemical Structure</th></tr>
<tr><td>MK-927</td><td> 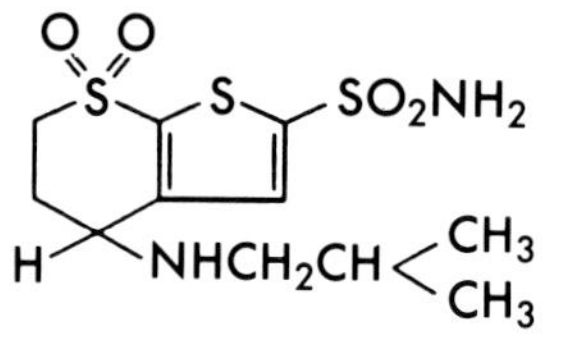</td></tr>
<tr><td>Sezolamide</td><td>S-Enantiomer of MK-927</td></tr>
<tr><td>MK-507</td><td> 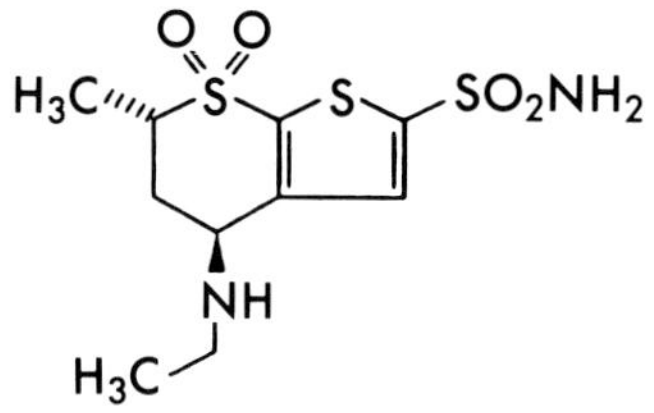</td></tr>
</table>

---

**FIGURE 18-2**    The free sulfonamide group in these topical carbonic anhydrase inhibitors competes for the active site of the carbonic anhydrase isoenzyme. *(Courtesy of Erik Lippa, MD, PhD, Merck Sharp & Dohme.)*

controlled study. Of the 10 subjects who received MK-927, 7 had a transient and mild conjunctival hyperemia. Four hours after the first dose, there was a 30% reduction in intraocular pressure in MK-927–treated eyes.

Bron and coworkers[40] reported a similar reduction in intraocular pressure from baseline (27%) 4 to 5 hours after 3 drops of 2% MK-927 in 25 patients. No contralateral effect due to MK-927 was noted. Only 1 of the 25 patients had transient hyperemia after MK-927 instillation. There were 4 patients who complained of transient burning after MK-927 instillation, compared to 2 who had the same complaint after placebo instillation. In another double-masked, placebo-controlled study,[41] intraocular pressure decreased 33% after 1 drop of 2% MK-927 in 24 patients. One patient, treated with MK-927 in one eye and a placebo in the other, had conjunctival hyperemia in both eyes.

In a single dose-response study,[42] Higgenbotham and coworkers treated 24 patients with 0.5% MK-927 in one eye and a placebo in the other and found that there was no significant difference between intraocular pressures. Maximum intraocular pressure reductions with 1% and 2% MK-927 were 21 and 25% respectively, and occurred six hours after drop instillation. There were no significant differences in ocular and systemic side effects between MK-927 and placebo treatment groups.

In another single dose-response study,[43] 0.125% and 0.5% MK-927 had no statistically significant effect on intraocular pressures of patients classified as "marked responders" to 2% MK-927. A patient was classified as a "marked responder" if the difference in peak intraocular pressure reduction was 6 mmHg or more between the MK-927–treated eye and the placebo-treated eye compared with the difference between the two eyes at baseline. Ten of 27 patients were "marked responders." The mean reduction of intraocular pressure 3 hours after 1 drop of 2% MK-927 (in the 27 patients) was 4.0 ± 0.8 mmHg. There was substantial variability in the amount of intraocular pressure lowering in individual patients. No ocular or systemic side effects were reported.

Fourteen days after twice-a-day dosing of 1% or 2% MK-927, mean intraocular pressure 2 hours after drop instillation was reduced from prestudy baseline 18% or 20%, respectively.[44] In both this and another study,[45] twice-a-day dosing of MK-927 had significant lowering of intraocular pressure 12 hours post-dose. However, this reduction was small, and thus, more frequent dosing of MK-927 may be needed in monotherapy of patients.

Serle and coworkers[46] found in a six-week study of 36 patients using 2% MK-927 or 0.5% timolol maleate twice-a-day that intraocular pressure reduction before the morning dose was 4.1 ± 0.9 mmHg for MK-927 and 6.3 ± 1.8 mmHg for timolol. No substantial ocular or systemic side effects were observed for 2% MK-927 during the six-week study.

## Sezolamide Hydrochloride (formerly MK-417)

Sezolamide hydrochloride, the S-enantiomer of MK-927 (see Figure 18-2), is the more active enantiomer in vitro and in vivo. In a crossover study in 27 patients, 1 drop of 1% sezolamide or 1% MK-927 lowered intraocular pressure 24% or 20%, respectively, 6 hours post-drop instillation.[47] In a parallel study in 48 patients,[48] 1.8% sezolamide and 2% MK-927 lowered intraocular pressure 20% and 19%, respectively. Both compounds caused statistically significant intraocular pressure reduction 12 hours post-drop instillation.

When thrice-a-day dosing of 1.8% sezolamide was compared to twice-a-day dosing of 0.5% timolol maleate in a four-day study,[49] both medications lowered intraocular pressure throughout the day. The larger effect was consistently seen with timolol, even though during the fourth day of treatment the amount of intraocular pressure lowering by sezolamide was greater than that observed during the first day of treatment.

## MK-507* (formerly L-671,152)

MK-507 (S,S-5,6-dihydro-4H-4-ethylamine-6-methylthieno-[2,3-b]-thiopyran-2-sulfonamide-7,7-dioxide HCL) (see Figure 18-2) is the newest topical carbonic anhydrase inhibitor and has more in vitro activity against carbonic anhydrase isoenzyme II than MK-927 and sezolamide.[50,51] In a parallel study in 24 volunteers, topical instillation of 2% MK-507 was without substantial side effects. Four and five hours post-MK-507 instillation, mean intraocular pressure was lowered 29% from baseline while in the placebo-treated fellow eyes it was lowered 13%.[52] In 18 patients using 2% MK-507 twice a day, Lippa and coworkers[53] reported that 2 hours after the third dose intraocular pressure was lowered 21% with 2% MK-507 and 11% with placebo.

In two clinical studies[54,55] comparing 1.8% sezolamide and 2% MK-507, there was not a statistically significant difference in intraocular pressure reduction between the two compounds with either twice-a-day or thrice-a-day dosing: 2% MK-

*Since this chapter was written, the name of MK-507 has been changed to Dorzolamide.

507 lowered intraocular pressure 26% and 1.8% sezolamide lowered it slightly less, 23%.[55]

## SUMMARY

So far, at least five topical carbonic anhydrase inhibitors have been tested for clinical efficacy. Four of the five lowered mean intraocular pressure approximately 20% to 30%; oral carbonic anhydrase inhibitors in a randomized, double-masked trial lowered mean intraocular pressure 21%.[18] This comparable effect on intraocular pressure by topical and oral carbonic anhydrase inhibitors is not associated with a comparable number of systemic side effects.

There have been no reports of systemic side effects from topical agents in these clinical trials. Ocular tolerance has been a problem for only one of the topically active agents, 3% aminozolamide gel. Mild, transient conjunctival hyperemia has been reported with MK-927, but it has not necessitated withdrawal of patients from clinical trials. Thus, of the five topical agents available for clinical use, only three (MK-927, sezolamide, and MK-507) are both efficacious and well tolerated locally. Although MK-927 and sezolamide are not as efficacious as timolol maleate in monotherapy of patients, all three compounds may be useful as adjunctive agents. Presently there will be clinical studies evaluating the additivity of these agents to beta-adrenergic antagonist therapy. If they are additive, they may replace oral carbonic anhydrase inhibitors in our armamentarium in the treatment of glaucomatous patients. Although no systemic side effects have been reported yet, clinicians should remember that systemic side effects from a topical agent are not always evident in early clinical trials. They eventually appear after the eye drop has come into widespread use, as happened with timolol maleate.

## References


1. Sommer A. Intraocular pressure and glaucoma. Am J Ophthalmol 1989; 107:186.
2. Kass MA, Gordon MO, Hoff MR, et al. Topical timolol administration reduces the incidence of glaucomatous damage in ocular hypertensive individuals: a randomized, double-masked, long-term clinical trial. Arch Ophthalmol 1989; 107:1590.
3. Becker B. Decrease in intraocular pressure in man by a carbonic anhydrase inhibitor, Diamox. Am J Ophthalmol 1954; 37:13.
4. Lichter PR, Newman LP, Wheeler NC, et al. Patient tolerance to carbonic anhydrase inhibitors. Am J Ophthalmol 1978; 39:885.
5. Fraunfelder FT, Meyer SM, Bagby GC, et al. Hematological reactions to carbonic anhydrase inhibitors. Am J Ophthalmol 1985; 100:79.
6. Lichter PR. Reducing side effects of carbonic anhydrase inhibitors. Ophthalmol 1981; 88:266.
7. Friedenwald JS. The formation of the intraocular fluid. Am J Ophthalmol 1949; 32:9.
8. Kinsey VE. Comparative chemistry of aqueous humor in posterior and anterior chambers of rabbit eye. Arch Ophthalmol 1953; 50:401.
9. Wistrand PJ. Carbonic anhydrase in the anterior uvea of the rabbit. Acta Physiol Scand 1951; 24:144.
10. Roblin RO, Clapp JW. The preparation of heterocyclic sulfonamides. J Am Chem Soc 1950; 72:4890.
11. Maren TH, Mayer E, Wadsworth B. Carbonic anhydrase inhibition. I. The pharmacology of Diamox 2-acetylamino-1,3,4-thiadiazole-5-sulfonamide. Bulletin of the Johns Hopkins Hospital 1954; 95:199.
12. Maren TH. Relations between structure and biological activity of sulfonamides. Ann Rev Pharmacol Toxicol 1976; 16:309.
13. Wistrand PJ, Schenholm M, Lonnerholm G. Carbonic anhydrase isoenzymes caI and caII in the human eye. Invest Ophthalmol Vis Sci 1986; 27:419.
14. Zimmerman TJ, Garg LC, Vogh BP, et al. The effect of acetazolamide on the movements of anions into the posterior chamber of the dog eye. J Pharmacol Exp Ther 1976; 196:510.

15. Zimmerman TJ, Garg LC, Vogh BP, et al. The effect of acetazolamide on the movement of sodium into the posterior chamber of the dog eye. J Pharmacol Exp Ther 1976; 199:510.

16. Kannark K. Structure and function of carbonic anhydrase: comparative studies of sulphonamide binding to human erythrocyte carbonic anhydrases B and C. In Roberts GCK ed, Drug action at the molecular level. Baltimore, 1977, University Park Press, p 73.

17. De Carvalho CA, Lawrence C, Stone HH. Acetazolamide (Diamox) therapy in chronic glaucoma. Arch Ophthalmol 1958; 59:840.

18. Dailey RA, Brubaker RF, Bourne WM. The effect of timolol maleate and acetazolamide on the rate of aqueous formation in normal human subjects. Am J Ophthalmol 1982; 93:232.

19. Becker B. The mechanism of the fall in intraocular pressure induced by the carbonic anhydrase inhibitor, Diamox. Am J Ophthalmol 1955; 39:177.

20. Friedman Z, Krupin T, Becker B. Ocular and systemic effects of acetazolamide in nephrectomized rabbits. Invest Ophthalmol Vis Sci 1982; 23:209.

21. Krupin T, Oestrich CJ, Bass J. Acidosis, alkalosis, and aqueous humor dynamics in rabbits. Invest Ophthalmol Vis Sci 1977; 16:997.

22. Maren TH, Haywood JR, Chapman SK, et al. The pharmacology of methazolamide in relation to the treatment of glaucoma. Invest Ophthalmol Vis Sci 1977; 16:730.

23. Kinsey VE, Reddy DVN. Turnover of total carbon dioxide in the aqueous humors and the effect thereon of acetazolamide. Arch Ophthalmol 1959; 62:78.

24. Green H, Leopold IH. Effects of locally administered Diamox. Am J Ophthalmol 1955; 40:137.

25. Foss RH. Local application of Diamox: an experimental study of its effect on the intraocular pressure. Am J Ophthalmol 1955; 39:336.

26. Gloster J, Perkins ES. Effect of the carbonic anhydrase inhibitor (Diamox) on intraocular pressure of rabbits and cats. Br J Ophthalmol 1955; 39:647.

27. Maren TH, Jankowska L, Sanyal G, et al. The transcorneal permeability of sulfonamide carbonic anhydrase inhibitors and their effect on aqueous humor secretion. Exp Eye Res 1983; 36:457.

28. Friedman Z, Allen RC, Ralph SM. Topical acetazolamide and methazolamide delivered by contact lens. Arch Ophthalmol 1985; 103:963.

29. Lewis RA, Schoenwald RD, Barfknecht CF, et al. Aminozolamide gel: a trial of a topical carbonic anhydrase inhibitor in ocular hypertension. Arch Ophthalmol 1986; 104:842.

30. Maren TH, Bar-Ilan A. The effect of 6-OH benzo[b]thiophene-2-sulfonamide, a new topical carbonic anhydrase inhibitor, on intraocular pressure in rabbits. Invest Ophthalmol Vis Sci 1987; 28(ARVO suppl):268.

31. Lotti VJ, Schmitt CJ, Gautheron PD. Topical ocular hypotensive activity and ocular penetration of dichlorphenamide sodium in rabbits. Graefes Arch Clin Exp Ophthalmol 1984; 222:13.

32. Maren TH, Bar-Ilan A, Castor KC, et al. Ocular pharmacology of methazolamide analogs: distribution in the eye and effects on pressure after topical application. J Pharm Exp Ther 1987; 241:56.

33. Stein A, Pinke R, Krupin T, et al. The effect of topically administered carbonic anhydrase inhibitors on aqueous humor dynamics in rabbits. Am J Ophthalmol 1983; 45:222.

34. Sugrue MF, Gautheron P, Schmitt CJ, et al. On the pharmacology of L-645,151: a topically effective ocular hypotensive carbonic anhydrase inhibitor. J Pharmacol Exp Ther 1985; 232:534.

35. Wang RF, Serle J, Podos S, et al. The ocular hypotensive effect of the topical carbonic anhydrase (ca) inhibitor MK-927 in glaucomatous monkeys. Invest Ophthalmol Vis Sci 1988; 29(ARVO suppl):16.

36. Wang RF, Serle JB, Podos SM, et al. The ocular hypotensive effect of the topical carbonic anhydrase inhibitor L-671,152 in glaucomatous monkeys. Arch Ophthalmol 1990; 108:511.

37. Kalina PH, Shetlar DJ, Lewis RA, et al. 6-Amino-2-benzothiazolesulfonamide: the effect of a topical carbonic anhydrase inhibitor on aqueous humor formation in the normal human eye. Ophthalmol 1988; 95:772.

38. Werner EB, Gerber DS, Yoder YJ. Effect of a topical carbonic anhydrase inhibitor, 6-hydroxy-benzo[b]thiophene-2-sulfonamide, on intraocular pressure in normotensive subjects. Can J Ophthalmol 1987; 22:316.

39. Lippa EA, Von Denffer HA, Hofmann HM, et al. Local tolerance and activity of MK-927, a novel topical carbonic anhydrase inhibitor. Arch Ophthalmol 1988; 106:1694.

40. Bron AM, Lippa EA, Hofmann HM, et al. MK-927: A topically effective carbonic anhydrase inhibitor in patients. Arch Ophthalmol 1989; 107:1143.

41. Pfeiffer P, Hennekes R, Lippa EA, et al. A single dose of the topical carbonic anhydrase inhibitor MK-927 decreases IOP in patients. Br J Ophthalmol 1990; 74:405.

42. Higgenbotham EJ, Kass MA, Lippa EA, et al. MK-927: A topical carbonic anhydrase inhibitor dose response and duration of action. Arch Ophthalmol 1990; 108:65.

43. Serle JB, Lustgarten JS, Lippa EA, et al. MK-927, a topical carbonic anhydrase inhibitor dose response and reproducibility. Arch Ophthalmol 1990; 108:838.

44. Tuulonen A, Hovding G, Gustad L, et al. Multiple-dose dose-response curve of the topical carbonic anhydrase inhibitor MK-927. Invest Ophthalmol Vis Sci 1989; 30(ARVO suppl):37.

45. Higgenbotham E, Kao SF, Kass M, et al. Once-daily and twice-daily treatment with the topical carbonic anhydrase inhibitor MK-927. Invest Ophthalmol Vis Sci 1989; 30(ARVO suppl):34.

46. Serle JB, Lustgarten JS, Lippa EA, et al. Six-week study of 2% MK-927 bid in ocular hypertensives. Paper presented at the meeting of the American Academy of Ophthalmology, Atlanta, Georgia, November 1, 1990.

47. Diestelhorst M, Bechetoille A, Lippa E, et al. Comparative potencies of the topical carbonic anhydrase inhibitors MK-417 and MK-927. Invest Ophthalmol Vis Sci 1989; 30(ARVO suppl):36.

48. George JL, Sirbet D, Lesure P, et al. MK-417 vs. MK-927: multiple-dose efficacy comparison of two carbonic anhydrase inhibitors. Invest Ophthalmol Vis Sci 1989; 30(ARVO suppl):4.

49. Lippa E, Sherwood M, Laibovitz R, et al. MK-417 vs timolol: comparative activity. Invst Ophthalmol Vis Sci 1990; 31(ARVO suppl):42.

50. Sugrue MF, Mallorga P, Schwam H, et al. The preclinical ocular hypotensive profile of the topical carbonic anhydrase inhibitor (cai) L-671,152. Invest Ophthalmol Vis Sci 1989; 30(ARVO suppl):99.

51. Baldwin JJ, Ponticello GS, Murcko M, et al. Three dimensional structure of the carbonic anhydrase inhibitor complex derived form human carbonic anhydrase II and the optical isomers of MK-927. Invest Ophthalmol Vis Sci 1989; 30(ARVO suppl):374.

52. Hoffman H, Lippa E, Feicht B, et al. L-671,152: local tolerability and activity of a new topical carbonic anhydrase inhibitor in normal volunteers. Paper presented at the Glaucoma Symposium, 26th International Congress of Ophthalmology, Singapore, March 17, 1990.

53. Lippa E, Laibovitz R, Clineschmidt C. L-671,152: a novel, active topical carbonic anhydrase inhibitor in patients. Paper presented at the Glauoma Symposium, 26th International Congress of Ophthalmology, Singapore, March 17, 1990.

54. Bourgeois H, Bron A, Lippa E, et al. 2% L-671,152: multiple-dose activity bid. Invest Ophthalmol Vis Sci 1990; 31(ARVO suppl):44.

55. Weinreb RN, Kass MA, Lippa EA, et al. MK-507 vs. MK-417: comparative efficacy of two topically active carbonic anhydrase inhibitors. Paper presented at the meeting of the American Academy of Ophthalmology, Atlanta, Georgia, November 1, 1990.

# 19 Management of Strabismus and Uncontrollable Facial Muscle Spasm with Botulinum A Toxin

Albert W. Biglan, MD

**B**otulinum A toxin is produced by the bacterium *Clostridium botulinum.* When this toxin is introduced into muscle tissue, it rapidly binds to the neuronal membrane at the motor end plate, and causes an irreversible blockade of motor transmission. After one or two days, a dose-related paralysis of striated muscle occurs.

The pioneering work of Alan B. Scott demonstrated that intramuscular injections of small concentrations of botulinum A toxin will cause a dose-related paralysis of the extraocular muscles for about 3 months.[1] Scott initially used this toxin, first in primates and later in humans, to develop an alternative method for correcting strabismus. Botulinum A toxin has subsequently been found useful for management of uncontrollable facial muscle spasm.

Botulinum A toxin has recently been released by the federal Food and Drug Administration (FDA) for treatment of strabismus in patients older than 12 years and for the treatment of patients with uncontrollable facial muscle spasm. Botulinum A toxin is commercially available in a freeze-dried form that is reconstituted with saline (Oculinum).

The principle upon which botulinum toxin treatment for strabismus is based is that a temporary paralysis of a relatively overacting extraocular muscle will cause an eye to assume a deviation opposite to that of the original deviation. Prolonged paralysis of the overacting muscle will cause an overcorrection of the strabismus and permit the antagonist muscle to develop a contracture. After 3 months, when the chemodenervation effect has resolved, the contracted antagonist muscle will prevent the eye from returning to the original deviation, and a lasting change in the ocular alignment will be effected.[1]

The boxes on p. 250 show some of the advantages and disadvantages of treatment of strabismus with botulinum A toxin and the categories of strabismus that respond either favorably or unfavorably to treatment with the toxin. Botulinum toxin has also been used with varying degrees of success to treat III cranial nerve palsy,[6] nystagmus,[7] strabismus in patients with thyroid disorders,[8] children with strabismus,[9] as a postoperative adjustment after strabismus surgery,[10] and as a supplement for extraocular muscle transposition procedures.[11]

### Treatment of Strabismus with Botulinum A Toxin

**Advantages**

Short office procedure
Only topical anesthesia is required
Low morbidity
Reduced scar and tissue reaction
Preserves the blood supply to the anterior segment
Cost effective

**Disadvantages**

Unpredictable hyperdeviation can be induced[2]
Prolonged overcorrection may be associated with diplopia
Repeat injections are often necessary
Delay in achieving the desired alignment
Not as precise as graded muscle repositioning procedures
Difficulty with reimbursement

### Categories of Strabismus

**With favorable response to treatment with botulinum A toxin**

Acute VI cranial nerve palsy[3, 4]
Overcorrected exotropia[5]
Sensory strabismus[5]
Malignant hyperthermia[5]
Small angle strabismus
Supplement to transposition procedures

**With unfavorable response to treatment with botulinum A toxin**

Restrictive strabismus
Strabismus and severe myopia
Strabismus with a large deviation
Exotropia
Vertical deviations
Dissociative vertical deviations

## Treatment Technique

Traditional diagnostic methods for evaluating ocular rotations and measuring the size of the deviation are used prior to treatment (Figure 19-1). After taking into consideration the magnitude and form of strabismus to be treated, the surgeon calculates the dose of botulinum A toxin that will be injected (Table 19-1).

The patient is placed in a recumbent position, and several drops of Proparacaine HCL are instilled in both eyes. After the toxin is reconstituted with non-

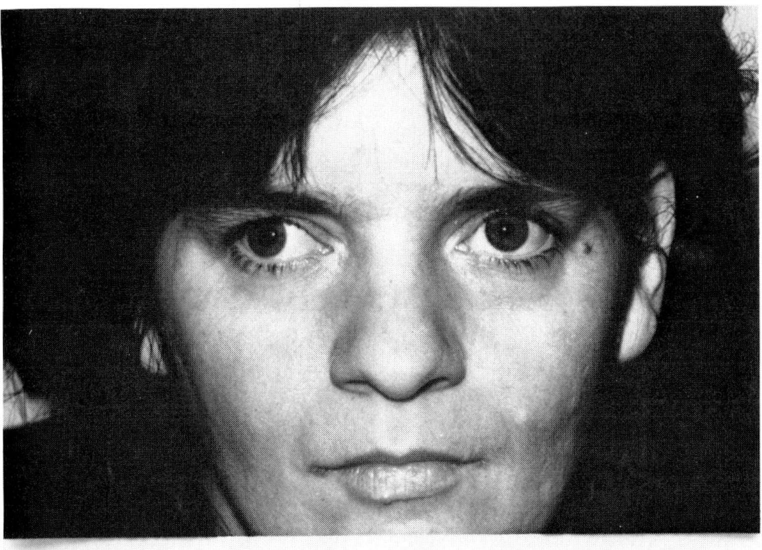

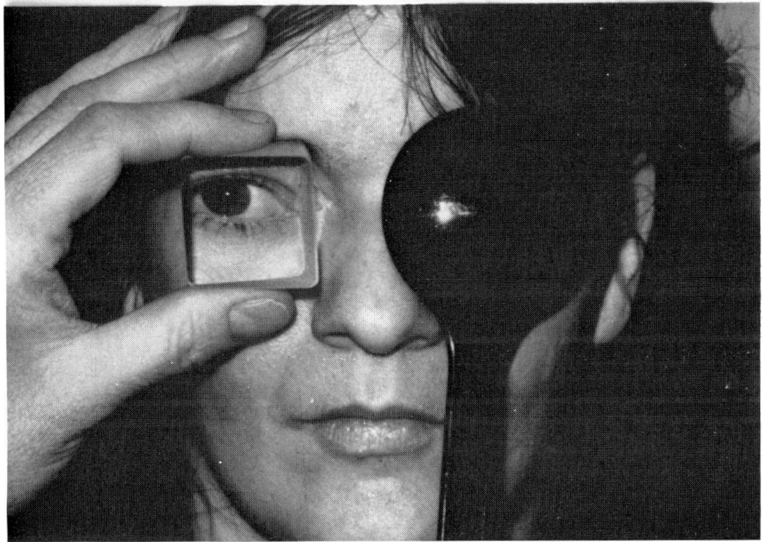

**FIGURE 19-1**    Top, A 30-year-old patient developed a persistent exotropia after a head injury. Bottom, The deviation measured 25 prism diopters.

**Table 19-1**    Suggested Dosages of Botulinum A Toxin for Treatment of Strabismus

| Deviation in prism diopters | Dose in units |
| --- | --- |
| Less than 20 prism diopters | 1.25-2.5 units |
| 20 or more prism diopters | 2.50-5.0 units |
| Sixth cranial nerve palsy | 2.50-5.0 units |

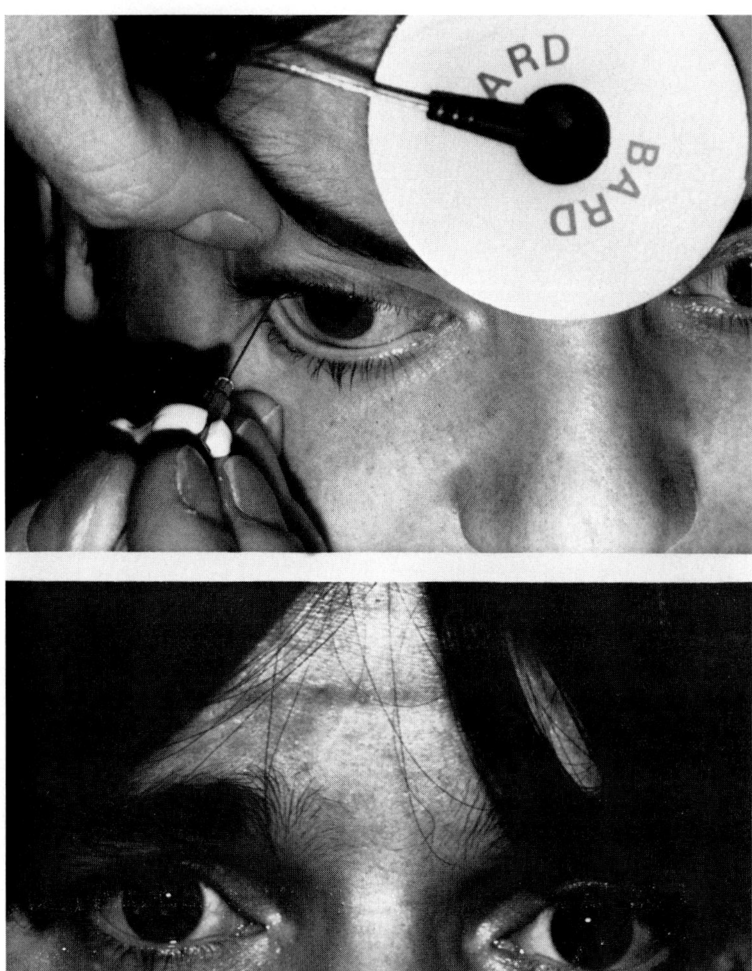

**FIGURE 19-2**   Top, The monopolar electrode needle is advanced into the muscle belly of the lateral rectus muscle under electromyographic control. Bottom, The maximum effect is seen 3 to 7 days after injection of the toxin.

preserved saline, the desired dose of botulinum A toxin is withdrawn using a tuberculin syringe. The volume of the drug to be injected should be 0.1 ml or less. The syringe containing the toxin is attached to a monopolar 25-gauge electrode needle, which is connected to a grounded electromyographic amplifier.

To insure patient cooperation during the procedure, the patient is asked to practice moving his or her eyes from left to right prior to injection. Excess toxin is then expressed from the tuberculin syringe so that the dose of toxin to be given is all that remains in the syringe. The monopolar electrode needle is carefully inserted in the conjunctiva overlying the muscle, and it is carefully advanced posteriorly over the muscle tendon (Figure 19-2). The electrode needle is advanced past the tendon until it enters the muscle belly (approximately 1.0 cm

---

### Complications Following Treatment of Strabismus with Botulinum A Toxin

Transient blepharoptosis[6]
Globe perforation[5]
Hypertropia[2]
Insufficient effect (undercorrection)[5]
Orbital hemorrhage[7]

---

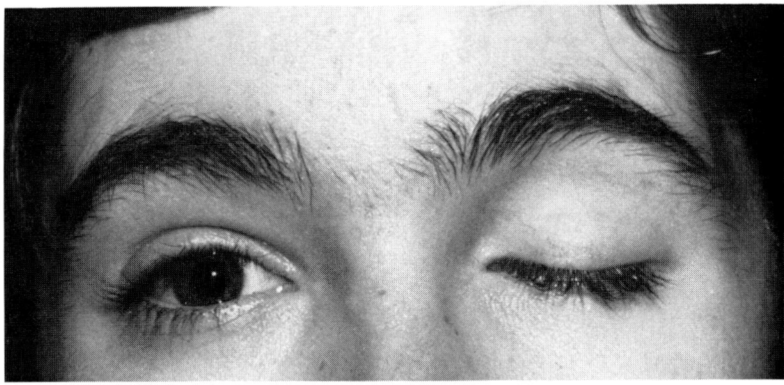

**FIGURE 19-3**    A complete ptosis of the left upper eyelid occurred 24 hours after injection of 5 units of botulinum toxin into the medial rectus muscle. The ptosis resolved after 8 weeks.

from the muscle insertion). When the muscle is located, the EMG will transmit the resting potential of the muscle. The patient is then instructed to look from right to left and the audible signal of the EMG will indicate the contraction and relaxation phases of the muscle that is to be injected. When the contraction phase is heard and the ophthalmologist is confident that the needle is within the muscle, the precalculated toxin dose is slowly injected into the muscle belly. The EMG noise will usually subside during the injection. Following this, the needle is carefully withdrawn.

After the treatment, the eye is not patched and antibiotics are not used. Within 24 to 48 hours, the effect of the drug can be observed. The maximum effect will occur one week following the injection (Figure 19-2), and the drug effect will usually last for 3 months.

The goal of the treatment is to achieve an overcorrection of the deviation by approximately 30% of the original deviation. Complications that can occur are listed in the box above. Complications result from improper placement of the electrode needle in the orbit or from the sensitivity of muscles in the orbit to this highly diffusable drug (Figure 19-3).

## SUMMARY

Injection of botulinum A toxin into the extraocular muscles offers the ophthalmolgoist an alternative method for producing a lasting change in the ocular alignment. The role of botulinum A toxin in the management of strabismus is beginning to become clear. With careful patient selection and good injection technique, the ophthalmologist can safely alter the ocular alignment in selected patients without the inconvenience of hospitalization.

## BOTULINUM A TOXIN TREATMENT OF UNCONTROLLABLE FACIAL MUSCLE SPASM

It is becoming evident that one of the more useful applications of botulinum A toxin is the control of facial muscle spasm in patients who are refractory to other forms of treatment or elect botulinum A toxin as the primary method of treatment. The three most common conditions that cause uncontrollable facial muscle spasm are essential blepharospasm, hemifacial spasm, and aberrant regeneration of the seventh cranial nerve.

### Essential Blepharospasm

Essential blepharospasm, which affects the obicularis oculi muscles, is characterized by episodes of involuntary, forceable closure of the eyelids. This condition typically afflicts females in the fifth and sixth decades of life; it is bilateral and has an unknown etiology. Symptoms are insidious in their onset, and the spasm usually increases progressively in both frequency and intensity.[14] Essential blepharospasm is exacerbated by bright light, by anxiety, and by watching television.

A less frequently occurring form of essential blepharospasm, Meige's syndrome, consists of uncontrollable eyelid closure and spasms of the lower facial musculature with involvement of speech and swallowing.[15]

The diagnosis of essential blepharospasm is established after a thorough history is taken and a complete ophthalmologic evaluation is made. The examination should be focused on excluding corneal disease, dry eye, or the presence of a corneal or conjunctival foreign body as the cause of the spasm.

Prior to botulinum toxin treatment, the management of essential blepharospasm consisted of sedation, biofeedback, seventh cranial nerve extirpation, and procedures that removed the affected facial muscles. Although some degrees of success have been achieved with these procedures and treatments, incomplete control or return of the spasm and of facial distortion are frequent recurring problems.

Control of essential blepharospasm was first attempted in 1983 by Allan Scott. He found that the injection of small quantities of botulinum A toxin into the periorbital muscles in patients with essential blepharospasm produced control of the spasm with few side effects. Since then, several investigators have expanded this experience, and botulinum A toxin can now be considered a primary method for control of the symptoms of essential blepharospasm.[16-22]

Prior to treatment, the face is carefully inspected for the location of the offending muscles, and the severity of the spasm is graded. If there is asymmetry

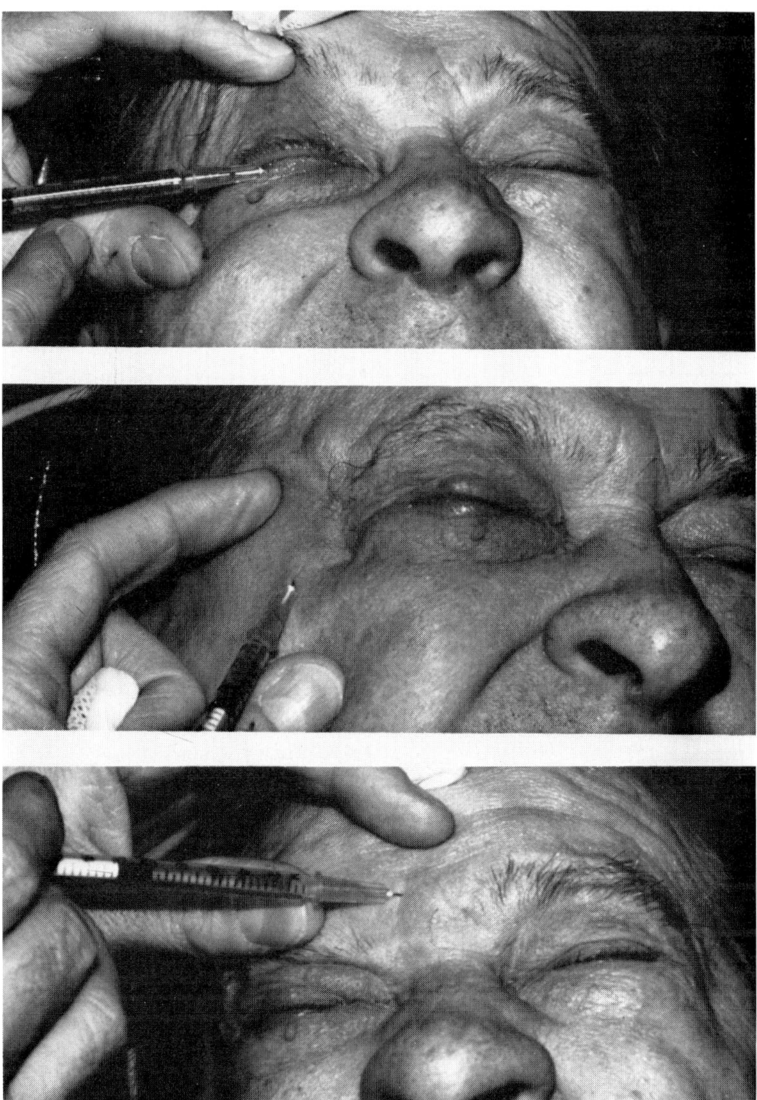

**FIGURE 19-4**  Treatment of essential blepharospasm requires injection of botulinum toxin into the pretarsal obicularis muscle (top), the lateral raphe area (middle), and the area of the procerus and corrugator muscles (bottom).

on one side or greater involvement on the other, a higher concentration of toxin may be administered to titrate the treatment of the involved orbicularis muscle. Each eyelid is treated with injections of botulinum A toxin into the pretarsal orbicularis muscles in the upper eyelid (7 units) and in the lower eyelid (3 units).

Additional injections of 25 to 30 units are given to the orbicularis muscle that is located posterior to the orbital rim. This is accomplished by injections into the upper, middle, and lower extensions of the orbicularis muscle near its raphe (Figure 19-4). Additional injections of 5 units each into the procerus, corugator, and nasalabialus muscles will help to control spasms involving the brow and the lateral aspect of the nose. The total dose of botulinum A toxin for a single treatment of essential blepharospasm will range from 50 to 100 units. When there is doubt about a patient's response to treatment, it is best to give less toxin. If the spasm continues at a disturbing intensity the patient can be retreated. If too much drug is administered, complications will occur.

Patients will usually experience relief of the blepharospasm within 24 to 48 hours and attain a maximum treatment response between 5 and 7 days. After 2.5 to 3 months, the blepharospasm will usually return, and the patient will seek retreatment.

## Hemifacial Spasm

Hemifacial spasm refers to unilateral involuntary paroxysms of contraction of the muscles innervated by the seventh cranial nerve. The spasm usually has a uniform distribution; but in some patients either the upper or the lower facial musculature may be more affected. Spasms are aggravated by fatigue and stress; they may persist at reduced levels during sleep. Between episodes of spasm, the facial musculature appears normal or even paretic.

The cause of hemifacial spasm is compression or irritation of the facial nerve by the posterior inferior cerebellar artery. Because a tumor may cause hemifacial spasm (1% of cases), patients with hemifacial spasm should receive appropriate neuro-imaging studies that examine the course of the seventh cranial nerve, especially where it exits from the brainstem.

Microsurgical decompression of the seventh cranial nerve (the Jannetta procedure) cures 90% of patients with hemifacial spasm. Some patients, however, may elect to forgo this neurosurgical procedure and choose periodic injections of botulinum toxin as an alternative method to control their spasms.[23,24]

The technique for treatment of hemifacial spasm is similar to the technique used in treating patients with blepharospasm. Along with treatment of the orbicularis muscle, additional injections of 5 units each may be given to the zygomaticus major and the mentalis muscle. Injections of 5 to 10 units into the platysma and the frontalis muscles will alleviate spasms in these muscle groups. Patients treated with botulinum A toxin injections usually will experience control of the spasm for 4 to 5 months.[24]

## Aberrant Regeneration of the Seventh Cranial Nerve

Following injury of the seventh cranial nerve or after Bell's palsy, nerve function may return with an aberrant regeneration pattern. For example, when a patient with an aberrant regeneration pattern smiles, the eyelids may close or the involved facial musculature may display other forms of synkinetic movement. Small doses (5 units) of botulinum toxin injected in the offending muscles will help to control these undesirable synkinetic muscle contractions.[25] With experience, treatment can be titrated so that the muscle can still function yet be weakened to such an extent that the undesirable synkinesis is reduced to an acceptable level.

## Complications

Other than mild bruising and oozing of blood at the injection sites, few complications result from treatment of the facial musculature.[18,24,26] When complications occur, they are transient and last for 2 to 3 months. They are usually well accepted by patients. Lagophthalmos occurs when excess drug is given to the pretarsal orbicularis muscle. The dry cornea is treated with wetting solutions during the day, and this is supplemented by use of ointments at night. In some patients, it may be necessary to close the eyelids with tape for a week or two.

If the toxin diffuses through the orbital septum, ptosis of the upper eyelid (8% to 10%) or palsy of an extraocular muscle (1% to 2%) may occur.[24] Complications usually subside after 4 to 6 weeks. These two complications are uncommon if care is taken to treat only the pretarsal portion of the orbicularis muscle. Effort is made to keep the injection of the drug as close to the lash margin of the eyelid as possible, then there will be less chance for diffusion of toxin through the orbital septum. If excess drug is given or the drug is improperly placed, there may be distortion of facial expression. If the zygomaticus major muscle group receives excess treatment, there will be a loss of the nasolabial crease, and the lateral aspect of the mouth may sag. Caution should be exercised in treating the muscles in the cheek or the perioral area. If these muscles become flaccid, patients may bite their cheeks or lips when chewing. In addition, treatment of the orbicularis oris muscle may weaken the watertight seal of the lips, and retention of liquids in the mouth may become difficult.

Other conditions amenable to treatment with botulinum A toxin, but not be yet approved by the FDA are spastic torticolis, spastic dysphonia, palatal myoclonus, and closure of the eyelids with a chemical tarsorrhaphy. A temporary (2- to 3-month) tarsorrhaphy can be achieved by injecting the levator palpebrae superiorus with a 5-unit dose of botulinum toxin. This may be helpful in the management of a corneal ulcer.

After several thousand treatments, with some patients receiving as many as 30 repeat injections, it appears that antibody production does not occur; or if it does, it is rare.[27]

## SUMMARY

Patients with uncontrollable facial muscle spasm can be satisfactorily controlled with periodic injections of botulinum A toxin. Repeat injections are required approximately every 3 months. Experience has demonstrated that patients can have satisfactory long-term (3- to 4-month) control of their facial muscle spasm, even after 28-30 treatments.

## References

1. Scott AB. Botulinum toxin injection of eye muscles to correct strabismus. Trans Amer Ophthalmol Soc 1981; 79:734-770.

2. Shippman S, Weseley AC, Cohen KR, and Wang F. Secondary vertical deviations after Oculinum injection. Am Orthop J 1986; 36:120-123.

3. Scott AB, Kraft SP. Botulinum toxin injection in management of lateral rectus paresis. Ophthalmol 1985; 92:677-683.

4. Wagner RS, Frohman LP. Long-term results: botulinum for sixth-nerve palsy. J. Pediatr Ophthalmol Strabismus 26:106-108, 1989.

5. Biglan AW, Burnstine RA, Rogers GL, Saunders RA. Management of strabismus with botulinum A toxin. Ophthalmol 1989; 96:935-943.

6. Metz HS, Snell L: Botulinum toxin for the treatment of strabismus. Am Orthopt J 1985; 35: 42-47.

7. Helveston EM, Pogrebniak AE. Treatment of acquired nystagmus with botulinum A toxin. Am J Ophthalmol 1988; 106:584-586.

8. Dunn WJ, Arnold AC, O'Connor PS. Botulinum toxin for the treatment of dysthyroid ocular myopathy. Ophthalmol 1986; 93:470-475.

9. Magoon EH, Scott AB. Botulinum toxin chemodenervation in infants and children: an alternative to incisional strabismus surgery. J Pediatr. Ophthalmol Strabismus 1987; 110:719-722.

10. McNeer KW. An investigation of the clinical use of botulinum A toxin as a postoperative adjustment procedure in the therapy of strabismus. J Pediatr Ophthalmol Strabismus 1990; 27:3-9.

11. Rosenbaum AL, Kushner BJ, Kirschen D. Vertical rectus muscle transposition and botulinum toxin (Oculinum) to medial rectus for abducens palsy. Arch Ophthalmol 1989; 107:820-823.

12. Burns CL, Gammon JA, Gemmill MC. Ptosis associated with botulinum treatment of strabismus and blepharospasm. Ophthalmol 1986; 93:1621-1627.

13. Lingua RW. Sequelae of botulinum toxin injection: Am J Ophthalmol 1985; 100:305-307.

14. Jankovic J, Ford J. Blepharospasm and orofacial-cervical dystonia. Clinical and pharmacological findings in 100 patients. Ann Neurol 1983; 13:402-411.

15. Tolosa ES. Clinical features of Meige's disease (ideopathic orofacial dystonia): a report of 17 cases. Arch Neurol 1981; 38:147-151.

16. Frueh BR, Felt DP, Wojno TH, Musch DC. Treatment of blepharospasm with botulinum toxin: a preliminary report. Arch Ophthalmol 1984; 102:1464-1468.

17. Shorr N, Seiff SR, Kopelman J. The use of botulinum toxin in blepharospasm. Am J Ophthalmol 1985; 99:542-546.

18. Frueh BR, Musch DC. Treatment of facial spasm with botulinum toxin. Ophthalmol 1986; 93:917-923.

19. Scott AB. Botulinum treatment for blepharospasm. In Smith BC, Della Rocca R, Nesi FA, Lisman RD, eds, Ophthalmic plastic and reconstructive surgery. St Louis, CV Mosby, 1987; 609-613.

20. Dutton JJ, Buckley E. Long-term results and complications of botulinum A toxin in the treatment of blepharospasm. Ophthalmol 1988; 95:1529-1534.

21. Jankovic J, Orman J. Botulinum A toxin for cranio-cervical dystonia: a double-blind, placebo-controlled study. Neurol 1987; 37:616-623.

22. Blitzer A, Brin MF, Fahn S, Lovelace RE. Localized injection of botulinum toxin for the treatment of facial laryngeal dystonia (spastic dysphonia). Laryngoscope 1988; 98:193-197.

23. Gonnering RS. Treatment of hemifacial spasm with botulinum A toxin. Ophthalmic Plastic Recon Surg 1986; 2:143-146.

24. Biglan AW, May M, Bowers RA. Management of facial spasm with *Clostridium* botulinum toxin, type A (Oculinum), Arch Otolaryngol Head Neck Surg. 1988; 114:1407-1412.

25. Putterman AM. Botulinum toxin injections in the treatment of seventh-nerve misdirection. Am J Ophthalmol 1990; 110:205-206.

26. Kalra HU, Magoon EH. Side effects of the use of botulinum toxin for treatment of benign essential blepharospasm and hemifacial spasm. Ophthalmic Surg 1990; 21:335-338.

27. Biglan AW, Gonnering RS, Lockhart LB, Rabin BL. Absence of antibody production in patients treated with botulinum A toxin. Am J Ophthalmol 1986; 101:232-235.

# 20 State of the Art: Cyclosporine

Benjamin Rubin, MD
Robert B. Nussenblatt, MD

Over the last 10 years, the ophthalmic community has evaluated the use of cyclosporine (CsA) for the treatment of ocular disease. Cyclosporine, which entered the arena of immunosuppressives as a reinforcement in the battle against organ transplant rejection, has become a mainstay drug used by many organ transplant surgeons. Beneficial effects of cyclosporine have been reported in literature on patients with severe sight-threatening uveitis, who either failed a trial of steroids or could not tolerate the side effects of steroids or cytotoxic agents. Early usage of this medication demonstrated that it was steroid sparing and a relatively specific immunosuppressive but that its use resulted in a great deal of toxicity because of the high daily dose being used (10 to 15 mg/kg). This chapter provides a summary of the uses and side effects of cyclosporine for the ophthalmologist, who can then work in conjunction with an internist when recommending cyclosporine as a treatment for inflammatory diseases.

Randomized clinical trials in Israel, Japan, and Turkey have shown that cyclosporine is an effective drug in active Behçets disease.[1,2,3,4] CsA therapy effectively abrogated the acute phase of the ocular attack and either totally prevented, or markedly reduced, the recurrences of these attacks.[5] Diseases that have responded to treatment with cyclosporine include pars planitis, intermediate uveitis of the non–pars planitis type, and Vogt-Koyanagi-Harada syndrome (VKH).[6] We have found cyclosporine ineffective in treating serpiginous choroiditis.

## HISTORY

During vacation in Norway in 1969, a Sandoz pharmacist collected soil samples later to be analyzed for new strains of antibiotic-producing fungi. In 1972, J. Borel and his associates discovered the immunosuppressive properties of this cyclic peptide (molecular weight 1202), and in 1978 clinical trials in renal transplant patients started. As of June 1988, nearly 5,000 patients suffering from many autoimmune diseases had been treated with this medication. Since 1983, more than 8,000 articles on cyclosporine have been published.

Work on cyclosporine published by Nussenblatt and colleagues early in the 1980s showed that it was steroid sparing and a specific immunosuppressive in ocular disease. At the National Eye Institute, cyclosporine, because of its relative lack of bone marrow toxicity, has become a mainstay drug treatment for recalcitrant uveitis. Early usage of this medication, however, resulted in much toxicity because of the high daily dose that was being used (10 to 15 mg/kg). With lower doses, combination therapy with other immunosuppressive agents, and attentive monitoring of patients, toxicity has been minimized.

## CLINICAL USAGE

Cyclosporine is an effective medication in many uveitic conditions that are resistant to other medications. In general we elect not to treat unless there is a significant decline in visual acuity (<20/40 on the ETDRS chart) and bilateral activity. In the patient with unilateral disease, we usually observe the patient who has had just one attack. If vision is decreased or if intervention is indicated we begin treatment with periocular steroids. Behçet patients with bilateral disease experiencing their first attack are treated with oral steroids. If reactivation occurs, cyclosporine is added after a slow taper of oral steroids. For bilaterally active, recurrent sight-threatening complications of Behcet's disease, cyclosporine is our drug of first choice. In other inflammatory conditions and in corneal transplants, it is a drug that can be used in patients who have failed prior therapy with corticosteroids or who have responded to, but cannot tolerate the side effects of, either moderate-dose or high-dose steroids or cytotoxics. We have found that patients who had responded poorly to steroids, either periocular or oral, demonstrated an improved response to steroid treatment when on a maintenance dose of cyclosporine. The drug does not induce long-lasting tolerance, and therefore patients who miss doses and allow falls in their whole blood levels may experience flare-ups of their disease. Cyclosporine is not an effective drug for the treatment of an acute flare-up (see immunology section), which is best treated with steroids. How long one should treat a patient with cyclosporine is not known. An extended therapeutic regimen is indicated in most patients since a lasting immune-tolerant state does not occur with this medication. We have discontinued treatment in many patients without recurrence and believe that in these patients the disease process has run its course.

Cyclosporine is a nephrotoxic drug, and it is therefore incumbent upon the treating physician to take a careful history and to suggest a renal evaluation of the patient if indicated. Important questions should include any history of pyelonephritis, urinary tract infection, obstructive uropathy, drug use, and sexual activity. When conducting the drug history, it is important specifically to name analgesics by trade name (e.g., Ibuprofen, Motrin, Advil, Naprosyn, Phenergan, Aspirin, Tylenol, Acetomenophin, Pandolol, Feldene, Goody powder). Non-steroidal anti-inflammatory drugs potentiate the renal toxic effects of cyclosporine. Patients over 60, long-standing diabetics, and hypertensive patients often have intrinsic renal disease. A complete physical examination should be done. In women a cervical smear and breast examination are performed. In our clinic the presence of carcinoma is an exclusionary criterion for treatment with CsA. Tests should include serum creatinine, urinalysis, and creatinine clearance.

We typically test the glomerular filtration rate (GFR) and renal blood flow (RBF) utilizing $^{99m}$-Tc and $^{131}$-I respectively before commencement of therapy because normal serum creatinine values can be found in patients with abnormal GFRs and RBFs.[7] If any abnormality is encountered, a nephrologist is consulted for further evaluation. We recommend that cyclosporine *be used only* in patients with a GFR (corrected for body surface area) greater than 89 cc/min/1.73 m$^2$

(young normal men average 125 ml/min/1.73 m² ± 15 ml/min, young normal women average 105 ml/min/1.73 m² ± 15 ml/min). Women are advised to use contraception since there is insufficient human data to warrant the safety of cyclosporine during pregnancy and lactation.[7]

Once the patient is deemed acceptable, we begin with 5 mg per kilogram per day in a divided dose (some of the patients and physicians opt for once a day dosage). Low-dose steroids are maintained between 5 mg and 20 mg per day or every other day. Periodic ocular, physical, and laboratory examinations are made. If there is improvement in two months, the medication is maintained. Otherwise, the drug is discontinued. Hepatic function is monitored by liver-function tests (Figure 20-1). Renal function is monitored by blood urea nitrogen, creatinine, potassium and magnesium levels, CBC, urinalysis, 24-hour urine creatinine and magnesium levels, and creatinine clearance (see Figure 20-1). Periodic

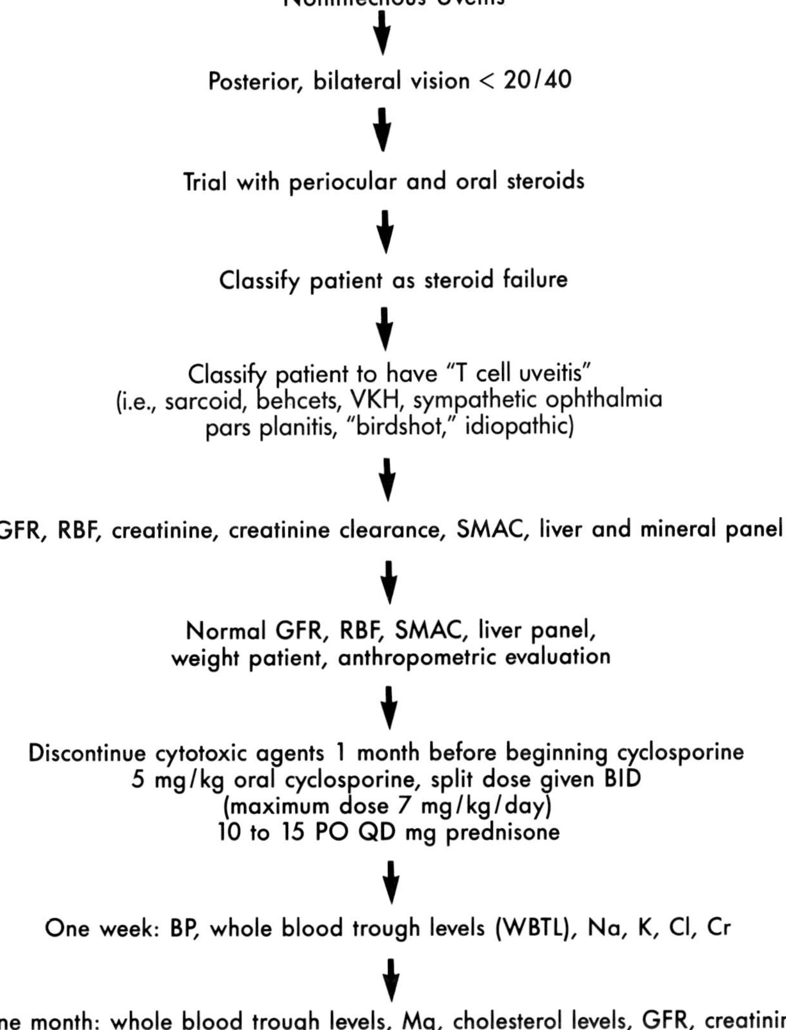


**FIGURE 20-1**   Algorithm for therapy.          *Continued.*

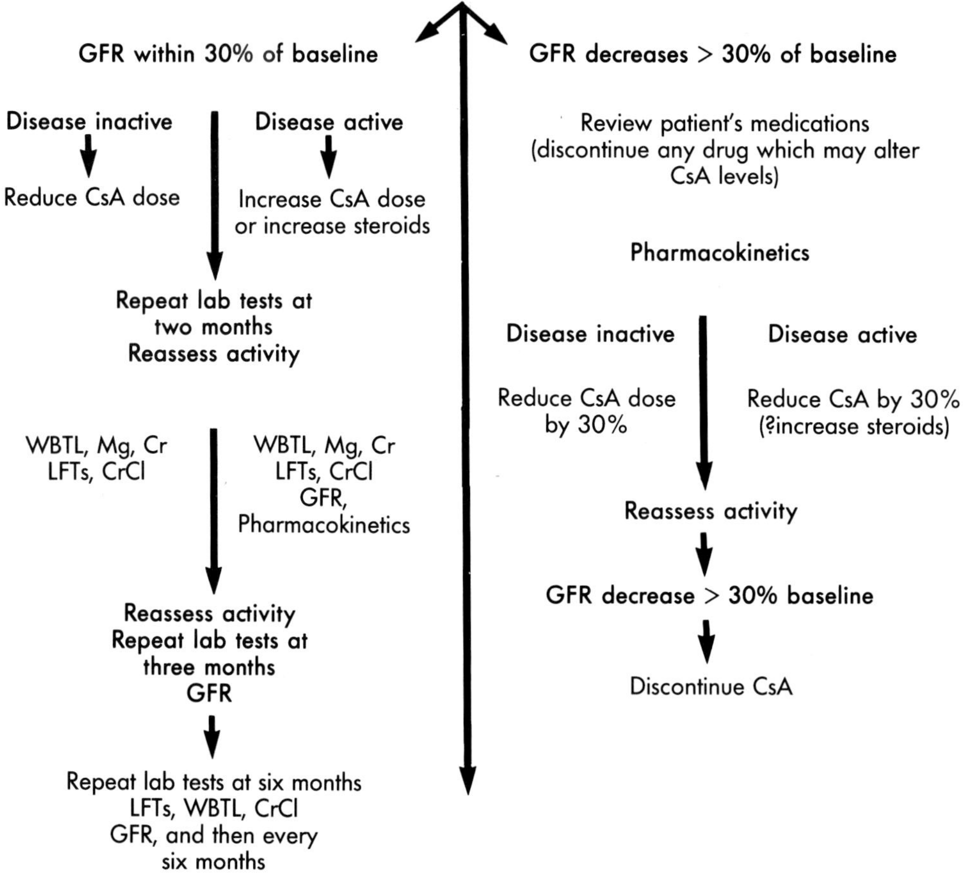



**FIGURE 20-1, cont'd.**    Algorithm for therapy.

radio-nucleotide tests to monitor GFR and RBF are performed (see Figure 20-1). Even though creatinine levels may be stable, we have seen as much as a 20% reduction in GFR and RBF. The dosage is modified, depending on these results. If the serum creatinine increases by 50% or the GFR decreases by 30%, the dose should be decreased by 30%. Except in a small number of cases, renal dysfunction has reversed itself if the dose is reduced promptly after the identification of compromised renal function.

## IMMUNOLOGY

Cyclosporine does not suppress the entire immune system, rather it selectively affects clonal expansion of cytotoxic T lymphocytes (Figure 20-2). It has a reversible direct effect on T helper cell activation, sparing T suppressor cells, resulting in suppression of cell-mediated immune responses.[8] Neither chemotactic nor phagocytic activity of neutrophils is inhibited. It does not directly affect B cells, but it inhibits immune system activation, blocking delivery of important secondary signals for T and B cell maturation.[9] There is little effect on already-activated, antibody-producing B cells, and macrophage and granulocyte function

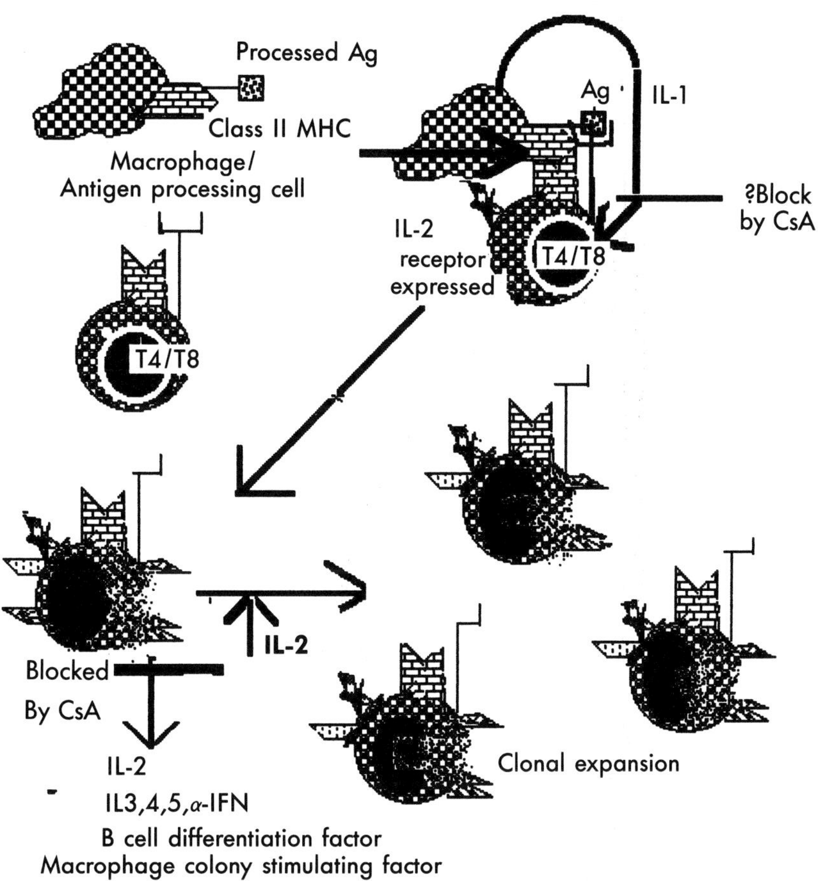


**FIGURE 20-2**   Immune response requires antigen presentation and the expression of class II major histo-compatability complex products on the membrane of the antigen presenting cell (APC). Interleuken-1 (IL-1) is secreted by the APC, stimulating the cytotoxic T cell precursor to express its IL-2 receptor. IL-2 is secreted by these cells, along with interleukens 3, 4, 5, and gamma interferon, resulting in clonal expansion and activation and recruitment of B cells, macrophages, and granulocytes. Cyclosporine blocks IL-2 production. With the blockage of this and other cytokines, inflammatory induction and effector mechanisms are inhibited.

are unaffected.[10] For these reasons, cyclosporine depresses chronic inflammation but is not very effective during the acute inflammatory event.

The mechanism of cyclosporine is uncertain, but it has been postulated that cyclosporine binds cyclophilin, an intracellular protein, diminishing the T cell response to interleuken one and dampening the production of interleukins 2, 3, 4, 5, gamma interferon, and granulocyte macrophage colony stimulating factor.[11]

## TOXICITY

The adverse effects of cyclosporine are summarized in the box on p. 264. **Gastrointestinal** symptoms are manifest in 20% of patients, beginning with the first dose of cyclosporine. Nausea and gastric distress are the two main complaints, but in our clinic, this rarely prevents patients from continuing therapy. Diarrhea,

---

### Summary of Adverse Effects of Cyclosporine

| Gastrointestinal | Endocrine | Hepatotoxicity | Nephrotoxicity | Neurotoxicity | General |
|---|---|---|---|---|---|
| Nausea, vomiting, gastric distress | Hyperglycemia (nonketotic) | Cholestasis | Fluid retention | Tremor | Normochromic normocytic anemia |
| Bloating | ↑ Skeletal alkaline phosphatase | ↑ Bilirubin | Dependent edema | Muscle cramps | ↑ Facial-body hair, epidermal cysts, pilar keratosis, acne folliculitis, sebaceous hyperplasia |
| Anorexia | | ↑ SGOT, SGPT | Hypertension | Convulsions with intravenous dose | |
| Abdominal pain, diarrhea, colitis | | | ↑ Serum creatinine | Headache | |
| Gingival hypertrophy | | | Hyperchloremic hyperkalemic metabolic acidosis | Parasthesia, temperature sensitivity | |

↑  = increased

---

abdominal pain, and colitis have also been reported in patients with very high trough whole blood levels.[12] The reason for withdrawal from cyclosporine most frequently found in the literature is gastrointestinal symptoms.[13] These adverse reactions are reduced with a decrease in the dose or with the use of split dosing (one-half the daily dose given b.i.d.). Dose-related hepatotoxicity is manifest by early and/or late mild elevations of serum transaminases (SGOT, SGPT) and serum bilirubin. Early onset elevations often respond to cyclosporine reduction, whereas late elevations may necessitate termination of treatment with cyclosporine. Gingival hyperplasia similar to that seen with phenytoin therapy has been noted in 25% of the patients. This condition is exacerbated by poor oral hygiene and peridontal disease.

**Nephrotoxicity** is frequently the limiting factor in the usage of this drug. Some studies have suggested that cyclosporine-induced renal dysfunction is due to the initial dosage during early therapy and is reversible after dosage reduction. Other authors have reported development of end-stage disease, presumably due to chronic cyclosporine kidney injury.[14,15] These reports are from kidney, liver, and heart transplant centers where other factors may be involved, and higher doses (10-15 mg/kg) are utilized to induce allograft tolerance.[16] The clinical syndrome of cyclosporine nephrotoxicity is related to changes in the vessels induced by cyclosporine. Renal toxicity occurs in three forms: 1) acute reversible decrease in GFR with parallel reduction in renal perfusion, 2) acute microvascular disease with thrombotic microangiopathy, and 3) chronic irreversible disease.[17] The chronic nephrotoxic injury seen in patients treated by the ophthalmologist is due mainly to a mixture of arteriolar vasospasm and/or mesangial cell contraction resulting in ischemia.[18] The toxic effects of vasospasm occur at the arteriole, glomerulus and proximal tubule.[19] Alterations in the production of thromboxane A$^2$ have also been implicated.[20] Information gathered and published by our group revealed that in 73 patients (in whom there was an absence of hypertension, allograft rejection, other nephrotoxic drugs, or evidence of renal disease) treated initially at a starting dose of 10 mg/kg, 27 patients were observed to have a 50% elevation of serum creatinine within three months of starting cyclosporine A.[21] Of the 73 patients who had been treated for an average of two years, 17 had some degree of interstitial fibrosis, tubular atrophy, or both.[22] Chronic pathologic changes were seen even in the patients with normal renal function and cyclosporine plasma levels within the recommended norms. The extent of chronic histologic change was not strongly related to the clinical assessments of the glomerular filtration rate at the time of the renal biopsy.[22] Repeat biopsies demonstrated progression of parenchymal injury in some cases, in spite of cyclosporine reduction and stable renal function. A reduced creatinine clearance with elevated serum creatinine, decreased glomerular filtration rate, hyperkalemia, hypertension, and tubular dysfunction (hyperuricemia and hyperkalemic hyperchloremic type IV renal tubular acidosis with preserved sodium reabsorption) could be demonstrated when patients were on cyclosporine for a prolonged period.[19,23] Several authors have reported reversibility of renal dysfunction after withdrawal of cyclosporine in patients with elevated serum creatinine for several months.

**Systemic hypertension** has been noted in 25% of patients treated with cyclosporine and in a greater proportion of those with alterations in renal function.[24] Patients treated with cyclosporine and steroids have a higher incidence or greater severity of hypertension than those treated with azathioprine and steroids.[25] The hypertension appears to be more easily controlled at lower doses of cyclosporine. Prior to treating the hypertension, we often assess renal function for toxicity and adjust the dose of cyclosporine accordingly. We generally begin therapy with a sodium-restricted diet and then Methyldopa, 250 mg b.i.d. and tend to use no diuretics since cyclosporine-induced prerenal azotemia can be aggrevated by overdiuresis, resulting in an increase in blood pressure.[26] Beta blockers, alpha adrenergic antagonists, direct arterial vasodilators, and centrally acting agents often need to be used if the hypertension does not respond to dose reduction or if dose reduction is inappropriate. The exact mechanism of CsA hypertension is unknown, but it appears to be dose related. Clinical researchers have not confirmed an increase in plasma renin activity, thereby challenging animal studies which postulate that cyclosporine hypertension is due to an effect on the renin-angiotensin-aldosterone system.[25] Patients on both cyclosporine and steroids appear to have an extracellular, volume-dependent, associated hypertension. The hypertension usually affects both systolic and diastolic pressures, although the diastolic pressures can be more resistant to lowering by medication.[27]

Some patients on cyclosporine have developed increased facial hair, body hirsutism, epidermal cysts, pilar keratosis, acne folliculitis, and sebaceous hyperplasia. Women are usually more troubled by these side effects. Balding men may report an increase in hair growth on their head.

Paresthesia and temperature sensitivity occur in 90% of the patients within several days of starting cyclosporine and often remit on their own. This sensitivity may be related to an induced hypomagnesemia.[28] A fine tremor has also been noted to occur and frequently abates during therapy. Headache, confusion, and seizures have been reported in the organ transplant patients treated with intravenous cyclosporine.[29]

Normochromic normocytic anemia is found in 25% of patients, with the hematocrit rarely falling below 30%. Leukopenia is not seen, and the mechanism of the anemia is presumed to be the inhibition of lymphokines regulating erythropoiesis.[13] An evaluation of the anemia should be made to rule out other causes. The erythrocyte sedimentation rate is also increased in 40% of the patients despite a clinical improvement in their disease. This can confuse therapeutic intervention if erythrocyte sedimentation rate is used as a barometer of disease. In the organ transplant literature, venous thromboembolic complications have been reported to be associated with the cyclosporine-prednisone combination but not with azathioprine-prednisone. We have not documented this complication in our patient population.

Secondary lymphomas and opportunistic infections have not been of clinical concern. At the National Eye Institute our patients have not experienced an increased incidence of Herpes or CMV viral infections that have been reported in some patients treated with cyclosporine.[30] A review of 5,000 transplant recipients (on CsA and steroids) showed that the incidence of lymphoma was no higher in patients on cyclosporine than in patients receiving other immunosuppressive regimens. Most of the lymphomas developed early on in the treatment and regressed with discontinuation of the immunosuppression.[31]

A reversible cyclosporine myopathy, which consisted of severe muscle pain, cramps, and increased creatinine kinase levels, has been described in a female with Graves ophthalmopathy.[32]

## DRUG INTERACTIONS

Since cyclosporine appears to be metabolized through the P-450 microsomal enzyme system, drugs that affect hepatic clearance will effectively alter cyclosporine metabolism. Renal failure does not alter cyclosporine elimination. In children, clearance is reported to be 40% higher than in adults.[10] A number of our patients have had acceleration of renal-function deterioration or have not reversed their functional abormality if they were concurrently being treated with nonsteroidal antiinflammatory drugs. These drugs have been shown to alter renal blood flow and perfusion by inhibiting prostaglandin E2 mediated vasodilation.[19] The nonsteroidal antiinflammatory drugs potentiate the renal toxic effects of cyclosporine by potentiating the decrease in renal blood flow reduction. In the animal model, this combination decreases renal blood flow and increases renal toxicity and morbidity.[33] Aminoglycoside antibiotics, even at low doses, can also potentiate the renal toxicity of cyclosporine.[34]

**Table 20-1**  Summary of Cyclosporine Drug Interactions

| Drug[43,44,45] | Cyclosporine blood level | Metabolic pathway |
|---|---|---|
| Phenytoin | decreases | increases hepatic P450 |
| Phenobarbital | decreases | increases hepatic P450 |
| Rifampin | decreases | increases hepatic P450 |
| Isoniazid | decreases | increases hepatic P450 |
| ?Nafcillin | decreases | increases hepatic P450 |
| Ketaconazole | increases | decreases hepatic P450 and/or excretion of cyclosporine and may also enhance enterohepatic recirculation |
| Erythromycin | increases | enzyme inhibition |
| Danazol, Norethindrol | increases | mechanism unclear |
| Methylprednisilone (High Dose) | increases | mechanism unclear |
| Melphalan | increases | mechanism unclear |
| Diltiazem > Nicardipine, or Verapamil | increases | |
| Nifedipine | no effect | mechanism unclear |
| Metaclopramide | increases | enhance enterohepatic recirculation |
| Cimetidine, Ranitidine | ?increases | mechanism unclear |
| IV Sulfamethoxazole & Trimethoprim (not oral) | ?increases | |

*Sources:* Kahan BD. Cyclosporine. N Engl J Med 1989; 321:1725; Bos JD, Joust TV, Powles AV, Meinardi MMHM, Heule F, Fry L. Use of cyclosporine in psoriasis. Lancet 1989; 1500; Hansten PD, Horn JR. Drug Interactions Newsletter 1985; 5:113; 1987; 7(7):2; 7(8)35; 7(9):39.

Digoxin toxicity due to elevated digoxin levels can occur when cyclosporine is added. Bidirectional ventricular tachycardia and AV block with accelerated junctional rhythm are a manifestation of digoxin toxicity. Interaction between cyclosporine and digoxin results in a decreased volume distribution and plasma clearance of digoxin.[35]

Drugs in which synergistic renal toxicity occurs with cyclosporine include furosemide, nonsteroidal antiinflammatory drugs, sulfamethoxazole-trimethoprim, amphotericin B, melphalan, and aminoglycoside antibiotics. Table 20-1 provides a summary of cyclosporine drug interactions.

## MONITORING THE PATIENT

It is difficult to ascertain which assay provides the best reflection of adequate levels since it is difficult to provide a universal therapeutic range for CsA (Table 20-2). Each physician must set his own range and criteria. Toxic concentrations of CsA occur when complications of toxicity appear. If they occur, we decrease cyclosporine even if the activity of disease occurs. Blood is collected in EDTA tubes. We utilize whole blood levels in conjunction with the other lab values (renal and liver function tests, creatinine clearance, GFR to titrate dosage schedules). Trough levels are measured of patients taking either daily or bi-daily regimens. Due to incomplete and variable intrapatient absorption, periodic monitoring should be performed. Initial oral absorption may be erratic. Bioavailability of cyclosporine in the posttransplant patient is reported to increase with time after transplant.[36] Ideally, trough levels should be less than 250 ng/ml. At present we allow a 30% increase in serum creatinine. If possible, the dosage is tapered,

**Table 20-2**   Summary of Cyclosporine Monitoring Systems

| Method/maximum level | Measures | Expense |
|---|---|---|
| HPLC: whole blood <200 ng/ml (Whole blood levels may be effected by hematocrit, and leukocyte level) | CsA specific | Large sample Labor intensive (6 hrs) Expensive |
| RIA, polyclonal: whole blood <500 ng/ml serum <100 ng/ml | CsA, metabolites | Small sample Less labor and expense |
| Estimates of in vivo CsA concentration by polyclonal RIA are 2-4 times greater than HPLC results. | | |
| RIA, monoclonal: whole blood <200 ng/ml serum <50 ng/ml | CsA specific, some metabolites | Small sample Less labor (2 hours) and expense |

HPLC = High pressure liquid chromotography   RIA = Radioactive immune assay

with vision, frequency, and quality of inflammatory exacerbations monitored as the titration indicators. Unfortunately, because of the low therapeutic index, mainly due to nephrotoxicity and hypertension, the full potential of this drug can not always be obtained.

## SUMMARY

Patients with preexisting renal impairment should be excluded from treatment, and those with preexisting hypertension should be regarded as high risk patients. Concomitant therapy with nephrotoxic drugs should be avoided. Toxicity seems to be greater both in very thin patients and in patients who are greater than 20% over ideal body weight. Initial dose of CsA should generally not exceed 5 mg/kg and should be used in conjunction with low dose corticosteroids. Cyclosporine is used only in cases of bilateral posterior uveitis in which vitreal haze and/or cystoid macular edema is associated with vision less than 20/40. The dose of cyclosporine should be adjusted in accordance with renal function tests. Finally, physicians who treat patients with cyclosporine should be experienced in the use of immunosuppressive agents. Ophthalmologists who do not routinely use this drug should employ the assistance of a general physician who is familiar with managing these patients and has adequate laboratory and supportive medical resources.

## PHARMACOKINETICS

Cyclosporine is a highly stable, 11-amino-acid cyclic polypeptide.[31] Due to its lipophilic nature, cyclosporine has low oral bioavailability (20% to 50%).[37] Bioavailability is reported to increase with continued therapy.[38] The drug is dissolved in olive oil and diluted with chocolate milk or orange juice for consumption. The effect of foods and diet on the absorption of cyclosporine is not clearly delineated. Cyclosporine is absorbed in the upper small intestine.[39] Most of cyclosporine in the blood is bound to either erythrocytes or plasma lipoproteins (high, low, and very low density lipoproteins).[40] Cyclosporine's volume of distribution is large, with the highest concentrations in the liver, kidneys, adipose tissue, and endocrine

**Absorbtion of Cyclosporine after Oral Administration[42]**

| | |
|---|---|
| Time it takes to absorb | 0.5 hour |
| Time to peak plasma concentration | 2-4 hours |
| Peak plasma concentration | 1.0 ng/mL/mg of dose |
| Peak blood concentration | ranges from 1.4 ng/mL/mg to 2.7 ng/mL/mg for low and high doses |

glands.[41] Removal by hemodialysis is very difficult. The cytochrome P-450 liver microsomal enzyme system is believed to be the major pathway for cyclosporine metabolism, resulting in approximately 15 metabolites. The primary route of elimination of cyclosporine and its metabolites is the biliary system. A small fraction (6%) is excreted in the urine. The half-life of oral cyclosporine in patients with normal renal function follows a two-compartment model; the second half-life ranges from 10 to 27 hours, with 87% of the drug excreted within 96 hours (see box above).[27,38]

*Factors that decrease cyclosporine absorption* include liver failure, external bile drainage (T tube), ileus, cholestasis, steatorrhea, slow gastric emptying, increased gastrointestinal motility (diarrhea), pancreatic disease (reduced exocrine secretion), and cystic fibrosis.[38,42]

---

# References



1. Masuda K, Urayama A, Kogure M, Nakajima A, Nakae K, Goro I. Double-masked trial of cyclosporine versus colchicine and long-term open study of cyclosporin in Behçet's disease. Lancet 1989; 1093.
2. Masuda K, Nakajima A. A double-masked study of ciclosporin treatment in Behçets disease. In Schindler R, ed, Ciclosporin in autoimmune diseases. Berlin, 1985, Springer-Verlag, pp 162-164.
3. BenEzra D, Cohen E, Chajek T, et al. Evaluation of conventional therapy versus cyclosporine A in Behçet's syndrome. Transplant Proc 1988; 20(3 Suppl 4):136-143.
4. Assuman Ü, Müftüoglu H, Pazarli S, et al. Treatment of ocular involvement in Behçet's disease with ciclosporin A (preliminary report). In Schindler R, ed, Ciclosporin in autoimmune diseases. Berlin, 1985, Springer-Verlag, pp 147-151.
5. Nussenblatt RB, Palestine AG, Chan CC, Mochizuki M, Yancey K. Effectiveness of cyclosporin therapy for Behçet's disease. Arthritis Rheum 1985; 28:671-679.
6. Nussenblatt RB, Palestine AG, Chan CC. Cyclosporine therapy for uveitis: long-term followup. J Ocul Pharmacol 1985; 1:369.
7. Bos JD, Joost TV, Powles AV, Meinardi MMHM, Heule F, Fry L. Use of cyclosporine in psoriasis. Lancet 1989; 1500.
8. Nussenblatt RB, Palestine AG, Chan CC. Cyclosporine A therapy in the treatment of intraocular inflammatory disease resistant to systemic corticosteroids or cytotoxic agents. Am J Ophthalmol 1983; 96:275.
9. Kahan B. Pharmacokinetics and pharmacology of cyclosporine. Transplant Proc. 1989; 21(3):9.
10. Von Graffenried B. Sandimmun (ciclosporin) in autoimmune diseases. Am J Nephro 1989; 9(1):51.
11. Kim J, Perfect JR. Infection and cyclosporine. Rev Infect Dis 1989; 11:677.
12. Innes A, Rowe PA, Foster MC, Steiger MJ, Morgan AG. Cyclosporin toxicity and colitis. Lancet 1988; 1:957.
13. Von Graffenried B, Friend D, Shand N, Schiess W, Timonen P. Sandimmun in autoimmune disorders, Basle, Switzerland, 1990. Clinical Research Sandoz Ltd. CH-4002.
14. Meyers BD. Cyclosporine nephrotoxicity. Kidney Int 1986; 30:964.
15. Myer BD, Sibley R, Newton L, et al. The long term course of cyclosporine associated chronic nephropathy. Kidney Int 1988; 33:590.

16. Kahan BD, Van Buren, Widerman CA, et al. N Engl J Med 1985; 312:48.

17. Remuzzi G, Bertani T. Renal vascular and thrombotic effects of cyclosporine. Am J Kidney Diseases 1989; 13(4):261.

18. Bennet WM, Norman DJ. Action and toxicity of cyclosporine. Ann Rev Med 1986; 37:215.

19. Kahan, BD. Cyclosporine nephrotoxicity: pathogenesis, prophylaxis, therapy, and prognosis. Am J Kidney Dis 1986; 8(5):323.

20. Rossini M, Belloni A, Perico N, Remuzzi G. Thromboxane receptor antagonist attenuates renal function deterioration in isolated rats given cytclosporine. Kidney Int. 1989; 35:508.

21. Austin HA III, Palestine A, Sabnis S, et al. Evolution of cyclosporine nephrotoxicity in patients treated for autoimmune uveitis. Am J Nephrol 1989; 9:392.

22. Palestine AG, Austin HA III, Barlow JE, et al. Renal histopathologic alterations in patients treated with cyclosporine for uveitis. N Engl J Med 1986; 314:1293.

23. Palestine AG, Austin HA III, Nussenblatt RB. Cyclosporine induced nephrotoxicity in patients with autoimmune uveitis. Transplant Proc 1985; 17:209.

24. Palestine AG, Nussenblatt AG, Chan CC. Side effects of systemic cyclosporine in patients not undergoing transplantation. Am J Med 1984; 77:652.

25. Weidle PJ, Vlasses PH. Systemic hypertension associated with cyclosporine: a review. Drug Int Clin Pharm 1988; 22:443.

26. Bennet WM, Porter GA. Cyclosporine associated hypertension. Am J Med 1988; 85:131.

27. Scott JP, Higenbottam TW. Adverse reactions and interactions of cyclosporine. Med Toxicol 1988; 3:107.

28. Palestine AP, Austin HA, Nussenblatt RB. Renal tubular function in cyclosporine treated patients. Am J Med 1986; 81:419.

29. Atkinson K, Biggs J, Darveniza P, Boland J, Concannon A, Dodds A. Cyclosporine associated central nervous system toxicity agter allogenic bone marrow transplantation. N Engl J Med. 1984; 310:527.

30. Abramowicz M. Cyclosporine: a new immunosuppressive agent. The Medical Letter 1983; 25:77.

31. Nussenblatt RN, Palestine, AG. Cyclosporine: immunology, pharmacology the therapeutic uses. Surv Ophthalmol 1986; 31:159.

32. de Groen PC. Cyclosporine: a review and its specific use in liver transplantation. Mayo Clin Proc 1989; 64(6):680.

33. Williamson HE. Interaction of cyclosporine and indomethacin in the rat. Res Commun Chem Pathol Pharmacol 1988; 61(1):141.

34. Morales JM, Andres A, Prieto C, Diaz Rolon JA, Rodicio JL. Reversible acute renal toxicity sinergic effect between gentamicn and cyclosporine. Clin Neph 1988; 29(5):272.

35. Dorian P, Strauss M, Cardella C, et al. Digoxin cyclosporine interaction: severe digitalis toxicity after cyclosporine treatment. Clin Invest Med 1988; 11(2):108.

36. Kahan BD, Reid M, Newburger J. Pharmacokinetics of cyclosporine in human in renal transplantation. Trans Proc. 1988; 15:446.

37. Cockburn ITR, Krupp P. An appraisal of drug interactions with sandimmun. Trans Proc 1989; 21:3845.

38. Kahan BD. Cyclosporine: a powerful addition to the immunosuppressive armeamentarium. Am J Kidney Dis 1984; 3:444.

39. Kahan, BD. Cyclosporine. N Engl J Med. 1989; 321:1725.

40. Niederberger W, Lemaire M, Maurer G, Nussbaumer K, Wagner O. Distribution and binding of cyclosporine in blood and tissues. Trans Proc 1983; 15 Suppl 1:203.

41. de Groen PC. Cyclosporine, low density lipoprotein, and cholesterol. Mayo Clinic Proc 1988; 63(10):1012.

42. Vine W, Bowers LD. Cyclosporine: structure, pharmacokinetics and therapeutic drug monitoring. Crit Rev Clin Lab Sci 1987; 25(4):275.

# 21 Pathology for the Practicing Ophthalmologist

Jan M. McDonnell, MD

In most departments of ophthalmology, the importance of pathology is based largely on its teaching function. Clinicopathologic correlations, important in many ocular diseases, are emphasized during residency training and on the ophthalmology boards. Once residency is completed, pathology assumes additional importance because of its role in patient care, which hinges upon accurate and timely diagnosis of tissue or laboratory specimens. A clinician needs at least occasionally to rely on the pathologist as a clinical colleague and collaborator to provide the patient with the best possible care. The following is intended to help the ophthalmologist obtain the most from this interaction.

## PREPARATION OF TISSUE SPECIMENS

Crucial to the pathologist's ability to render an accurate diagnosis on a specimen is the way in which the specimen was treated by the clinician who obtained it. Most specimens obtained in ophthalmic practice are small biopsies, but similar rules apply to enucleated globes and even to exenteration specimens. A major element in preparation of tissue specimens is the technique by which they are obtained. Small specimens are easily crushed, rendering them useless for diagnosis (Figure 21-1). Likewise, cautery causes irreversible changes at the cauterized edges of tissue that may render a very small specimen unreadable or may compromise the pathologist's ability to analyze a margin. Gentle treatment is essential, and a minimum of gentle handling maximizes the clinician's chances of learning something from the excised tissues. The routine procedure for specimen preparation involves five features:

1. Use of a container of appropriate size. Most fixatives exert their effect by cross-linking proteins and other cellular elements, and the speed of the reaction is based on the volume of tissue to be fixed in relation to the volume of fixative available. To avoid autolysis, an adequate volume of fixative is necessary, and the more fixative the better. Ideally, the container should be large enough to hold the specimen plus at least 3 to 4 times its volume in fixative.

2. Selection of an appropriate fixative. A standard, all-purpose fixative is 10% neutral buffered formalin, available in small lots from many companies. Some distributors also sell packaged fixative-containing specimen bottles that are large enough for most ocular specimens. Formalin does not

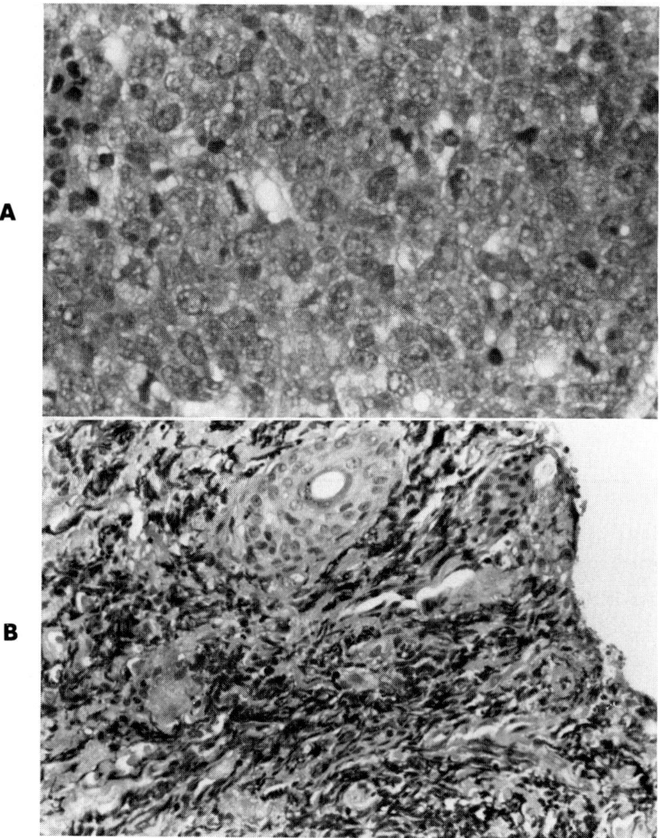



**FIGURE 21-1** Two biopsies from an orbital lymphoid lesion demonstrate the distortion caused by crushing cells. **A,** Uncrushed cells. **B,** Crushed lymphoid cells have a dark, streaked appearance and may be mistaken for fungal hyphae by the inexperienced. They cannot be studied for cell type even by the experienced (hematoxlyin and eosin, A 400×, B 200×).

deteriorate, so it can be stored in an office or operative site for several years. The fixative should be clearly labeled, as most are highly toxic.

3. Immediate fixation. A specimen must not be allowed to dry out on gauze or on a tongue depressor. The specimen container and fixative should be at hand when the biopsy is obtained. For very small biopsies, the time it takes to locate and open the bottle of fixative may be enough to let the biopsy dry out and become unreadable. If a brief delay is necessary, wrapping the specimen in saline-soaked gauze can prevent drying.

4. Accurate labeling of bottle and orientation of specimen. The specimen bottle should be labeled immediately with the patient's name and chart number, the date of the procedure, and the source of the specimen, all marked with a permanent marker that will not dissolve in water or organic solvents. If it is important that specific areas of the specimen be identified (for example, in biopsy or resection of a possible tumor), the specimen should be marked so the pathologist can properly orient the tissue and identify the deep and the lateral margins (see orientation section). Tissues such as conjunctiva may need to be pinned out to maintain their orien-

tation. One container should be used for each specimen if samples are taken from more than one area.

5. Expeditious and careful transport of specimen. The pathologist should be consulted about the best way to send the tissue or slides.

## CULTURES

All cultures for organisms, and most assays for antigen or antibody (ELISA, etc.), require fresh, sterile material. Once the specimen has been put in fixative or touched in nonsterile fashion, cultures and other studies may be unreliable. Some cultures, such as those used for anaerobes, require special containers. In a large clinic with its own laboratory or in some hospitals, the laboratory may take care of these matters so that the clinician need only supply a big enough piece of fresh, sterile tissue in a sterile container, with instructions about what organisms are to be ruled out. This is becoming a much less common practice, however, and such service is certainly not available in a small or solo-practice office. In that case, the clinician is responsible for obtaining the appropriate tubes, plates, and other materials.

An excellent review details the latest diagnostic methods in ophthalmic microbiology.[1] Special materials are needed for mycobacteria, anaerobes, amoeba, gonorrhea, and others, and it may not be cost-effective to keep these materials on hand in the office, since most of them have a limited shelf life. Some state or commercial pathology laboratories may be willing to stock an office with these items in a rotating fashion, provided they are under contract to perform the cultures on a fee-for-service basis. Another alternative is to send sterile tissue to a local university or reference laboratory, strictly following instructions about how to process and ship specimens. The instructions for transport will be based on what the clinician expects to recover. The majority of microbiology laboratories see few, if any, ocular specimens. An ophthalmologist must be explicit in instructions about which organisms to culture. Acanthamoeba, in particular, requires culture methods seldom used by most laboratories.[2] Finding a good laboratory may entail a certain amount of searching. A university-affiliated ophthalmology or diagnostic pathology department may be able to identify the appropriate laboratory.

## ORIENTATION

Specimens should be oriented any time that this might possibly matter. For example, any time a tumor is even a remote possibility, it is important that the specimen be oriented and processed in an orderly fashion. Enough places on the specimen should be marked to permit the pathologist to identify the superior, inferior, nasal, temporal, etc. areas. Larger specimens can be marked with different-colored sutures (e.g., blue nasal, black superior), different numbers of suture, different lengths of ties, and so on. The Davidson Marking System (Bradley Products, Inc., Bloomington, Minn.) provides five different colors of indelible ink that can be placed on fresh specimens without causing tissue damage. We have found this to be valuable in orienting specimens. Specimens such as conjunctiva can also be pinned out on a saline-soaked wooden tongue depressor, a picture can be drawn right on the wood, and the whole thing can then be placed in a jar of fixative. However the specimen is marked, it is crucial that the orientation be communicated to the pathologist with a map or drawing. With very small specimens, it may also be necessary to specify which areas are of greatest concern; on the basis of size of the specimen, all margins may not be amenable to sampling.

In some cases, for example, primary acquired melanosis or probable basal cell carcinomas in sun-exposed skin, biopsies can be taken from multiple sites during one operative procedure. Each specimen should be placed in a different specimen bottle and carefully labeled. It may be extremely helpful to draw a map of the conjunctiva or face to show the locations of the different specimens (Figure 21-2).

## PREPARATION OF SMEARS

Smears are usually performed for one of two reasons: to look at cytologic details or to look for microorganisms. Optimum evaluation requires a different method of preparation for each of these goals.

### Smears for Cytologic Detail

Smears to be examined for the presence of abnormal cells, such as keratinized or dysplastic cells, should be fixed *immediately*. To prepare the smears, the following must be at hand:

- A screw-top jar filled to the height of the slide with 95% ethanol. Coplin jars have slots that allow placement of many slides in a single jar without the slides touching each other, but any bottle big enough to hold a slide upright will do as well for a few smears at a time. Ethanol will be subject to federal tax unless the clinician has a license to purchase it, as do most hospitals and large laboratories.
- A Kimura spatula or whatever instrument is to be used to obtain the material.
- Clean, dry, glass slides, already labeled. Frosted slides may easily be labeled with the patient's name using a soft lead pencil. Because standard ball point ink dissolves in the fixatives, such a pen should not be used, nor should gummed labels, which can become loosened in the fixative. If frosted slides are not used, a diamond pencil can be used to scratch the patient's name onto one end of the slide. Frosted and unfrosted slides, diamond pencils, and Coplin jars are available from a variety of vendors of histopathology supplies.

To obtain the smear, follow this procedure:

- Open the jar of fixative.
- Obtain the material and smear it near the middle of the labeled slide or slides. Do not place material too close to the end of the slide, as it tends to be difficult to place a coverslip over the stained material and information may be lost.
- Place *immediately* in fixative. Do *not* wave the slide around in the air. Although there is a myth that material will adhere to a slide better if allowed to air dry, this is only a myth. Air drying does not make more material adhere to the slide, it just dries the cells out so they are harder

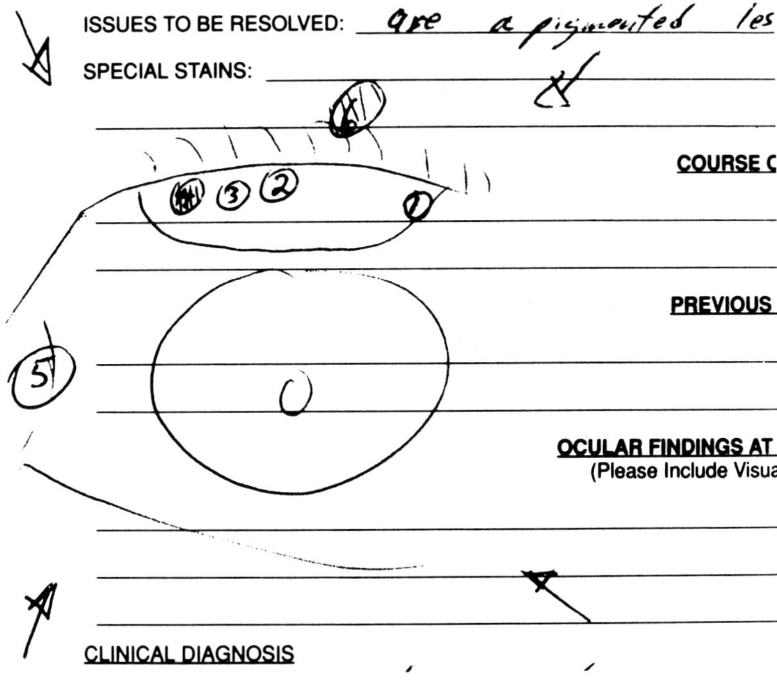


**FIGURE 21-2**  Pathology sheet submitted with a series of biopsies from a 38-year-old woman with multiple recurrences of conjunctival melanoma. The map clearly shows the site of each of the biopsies, and the surgeon numbered the individual specimen jars to correspond to the drawing. Such a map lets the surgeon know exactly what is going on in each location.

to evaluate (Figure 21-3). Once the specimen is in the fixative, close the jar (vapors can be irritating). If more than one slide is being prepared and a Coplin jar is not used, two slides may be placed back to back in the same bottle without disturbing the smears. When slides have fixed for 20 minutes, they can be placed in a folder and allowed to dry.

An alternative fixative is standard nonaerosolized cytopathology fixative, available from medical supply houses. Nonaerosolized hair spray will serve in a pinch, but it is not recommended because the formulation may be changed without notice. The procedure with spray fixative is much the same: obtain the material, smear it on an already labeled slide, and *immediately* spray. The slide can then be placed in a folder and allowed to air dry.[3]

## Smears for Identification of Microorganisms

Many microorganisms are easily identified on alcohol-fixed smears. The Papanicolaou stain, standard for decades in cytopathology, will stain fungi, chlamydial inclusions, herpetic inclusions, and a variety of other organisms. However, the gram stain for bacteria is best performed on air-dried smears. In that case, air drying and quick heating of the smeared slide will result in maximum yield. As a general rule, smears should be air dried only when a gram stain to look for bacteria is planned, or if a Giemsa stain to look for chlamydia inclusions is to be performed.

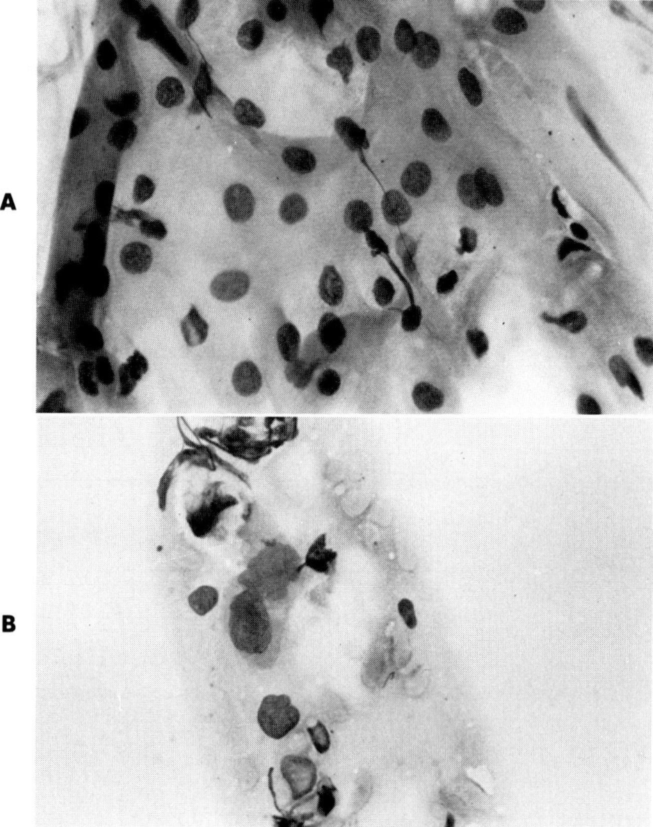

**FIGURE 21-3**    Different areas from a conjunctival smear demonstrating the cellular distortions brought about by air drying. **A** is from a well-fixed area. Nuclei in **B,** the air-dried area of the specimen, appear larger and less distinct, and cytoplasm also appears indistinct. Although air-dried smears can often be read, cellular details are much more easily evaluated on specimens that have been fixed immediately after smearing (hematoxylin and eosin, 400×).

## ASPIRATES

Aspirates from the anterior chamber or vitreous are a valuable diagnostic tool with applications similar to those for smears: identification of cellular elements and of microorganisms. Many such aspirations are performed in order to culture for organisms, and leftover material is then sent to an anatomic pathology laboratory for additional evaluation. When such a specimen is obtained, the order in which the material is allocated is important.

- Culture first, keeping the specimen sterile. Also, set aside some material for ELISA, ACE, or other analyses that require fresh material if such analyses are to be done.
- Smear for gram stain and air dry if this is preferred.
- Smear unconcentrated material for cytology; fix *immediately* as described earlier.
- Mix the remainder of the liquid specimen with an equal volume of 95% ethanol for cytology techniques that make use of larger volumes of fixed cellular material. If 95% ethanol is not available, the specimen should be

delivered immediately to pathology for processing. However, the specimen should be handed to someone personally, rather than placed in a specimen box; autolysis happens quickly. If it is after hours, or if there is neither alcohol nor access to pathology services, the unfixed specimen may be placed in a refrigerator to retard autolysis. Again, the goal is maximum fixation.

- If leukemia or lymphoma is suspected, the pathology or hematopathology laboratory should be informed before the aspirate is obtained. Air-dried, non heat-fixed smears of leukemia or lymphoma cells may be preferred by some pathologists, while others may want to have the material fixed for other analyses.

## NEEDLE ASPIRATION OF INTRAOCULAR TUMORS

Intraocular tumors may be amenable to sampling via needle aspiration of involved aqueous or vitreous, or of the tumor itself. These procedures may permit tissue diagnosis without resort to more invasive biopsy techniques or even enucleation. Aspirates are treated in the manner described earlier. Solid tumor masses have been successfully sampled in cases of intraocular lymphoma, metastatic or primary melanoma, and metastatic carcinoma.[4,5] Needle aspirates of solid intraocular masses may be treated in a manner slightly different from the technique used with liquid material, and the pathologist should be consulted in advance as to how to submit the sample. Filter preparations, cytospin, smears, and cell blocks (individually or in combination) can be prepared from the samples. Fixation methods vary with the types of evaluations to be performed, which in turn depend on the volume of material obtained and the type of lesion suspected in the patient.

## IMPRESSION CYTOLOGY

Impression cytology is a process whereby cellulose acetate filter paper is applied to the conjunctival surface, then gently pressed and removed. Superficial conjunctival epithelial cells that adhere to the paper can then be stained and evaluated. The technique is useful in evaluating patients with dry eyes, whose samples are examined for the presence or absence of goblet cells and the extent of cellular change reflecting squamous metaplasia.[6,7] This specialized technique so far has been used primarily by ophthalmologists rather than by pathologists.

## MOHS' HISTOGRAPHIC SURGERY

Mohs first described his technique of cutaneous cancer excision almost 50 years ago. It has been called chemosurgery, micrographic surgery, histographic surgery, and Mohs' surgery.[9,10] The terms refer to the mapping out of the margins of the excised lesion and the examination of all margins of the tissue by frozen section at the time of the surgical procedure. Entire margins are embedded and fully cut through, generating scores of slides from all levels of the tissue and ensuring that no tumor is present anywhere in the specimen. If tumor is identified, the original mapping permits a precise localization of the positive margins. Additional tissue, taken only from the positive regions, is subjected to complete histopathologic evaluation, again using frozen sections. Excision and examination of a large tumor can take many hours to complete, but the technique permits more extensive tissue-saving than might occur with standard excision. According to Mohs, the histopathologic evaluation is done by the surgeon, and reconstruction should not be performed; rather, the lesions should be allowed to heal by formation of granulation tissue.[9] If reconstruction is done, it can add several additional hours to the surgery.[10] Most physicians who use the technique are specially trained in dermatologic or plastic surgery and in Mohs' technique. This technique requires a substantial expenditure of time and materials, as well as expertise on the part of the person embedding the tissue, cutting the blocks, and reading the slides. Many general pathology departments do not evaluate tissues using the Mohs technique. An ophthalmologist interested in learning about Mohs' surgery should contact local experts in plastic surgery or dermatoplastics.

## THE PATHOLOGY CONSULTATION

In certain cases it may be advisable to contact the pathologist in person before obtaining a specimen (see the box below). This should be considered in the following situations:

1. Whenever there is the possibility that frozen sections might be wanted, even if this is not yet certain. *Frozen sections* are intraoperative pathology consultations during which the pathologist immediately examines specimens that have been prepared by cutting the frozen tissue, placing it on a microscope slide, and staining and reading it in the usual manner. Frozen sections can be extremely useful in planning the extent of surgery, especially for excisions of tumor. However, they do have limitations, and it is advisable to contact the pathologist in advance of a case during which frozen section analysis may be indicated. There are several reasons for doing so. The pathologist can help plan a strategy for obtaining tissue that is optimal for frozen sections. A recent, frustrating case involved excision of a sebaceous carcinoma. By the time the surgeon had sampled the margins, near the end of the excision, the surface epithelium had been completely denuded and the status of the margins could not be determined (Figure 21-4). In this case, evaluation of smears taken preoperatively or of intraoperative smears or biopsies preceding the main excision would have been much more informative than were the frozen sections.

---

**Circumstances When Preoperative Pathology Consultation is Suggested**

1. Frozen sections are contemplated
2. Operative margins must be evaluated
3. The clinician is not sure how to preserve the specimen
4. The patient may have sarcoma, lymphoma, or leukemia
5. The ophthalmologist is performing definitive surgery based on a previous biopsy
6. There are special concerns or time constraints

The pathologist may suggest that frozen sections will be counterproductive. Although the immediacy of a successful frozen section diagnosis is appealing to surgeon, pathologist, and patient, some difficult histopathologic diagnoses, such as the diagnosis of primary acquired melanosis, melanoma, or lymphoma, are best performed on optimally fixed, paraffin-embedded sections. In the case of a small lesion or small biopsy, the artifacts introduced by freezing may well obscure the details, so that a definitive diagnosis cannot be rendered.

The pathologist needs to know what the clinician thinks the lesion is in order to know how best to evaluate the frozen sections. The intraoperative frozen section is probably not the best item to submit to see how well the pathologist can do with an "unknown."

A final, very important reason to contact a pathology department before requesting a frozen section is to make sure that someone is available to prepare and read frozen sections. Not all hospitals offer this as a daily service. If the surgery will be done in an office or clinic, there are pathologists, usually members of private practice groups, who travel from place to place to do frozen sections. They, too, require advance appointments.

2. When margins are a concern, regardless of whether frozen sections are contemplated. The pathologist may be able to suggest ways to orient the specimen.
3. When the clinician is not sure what to do with a specimen, wondering whether it should be frozen, smeared, plated, or placed in formalin or ethanol.

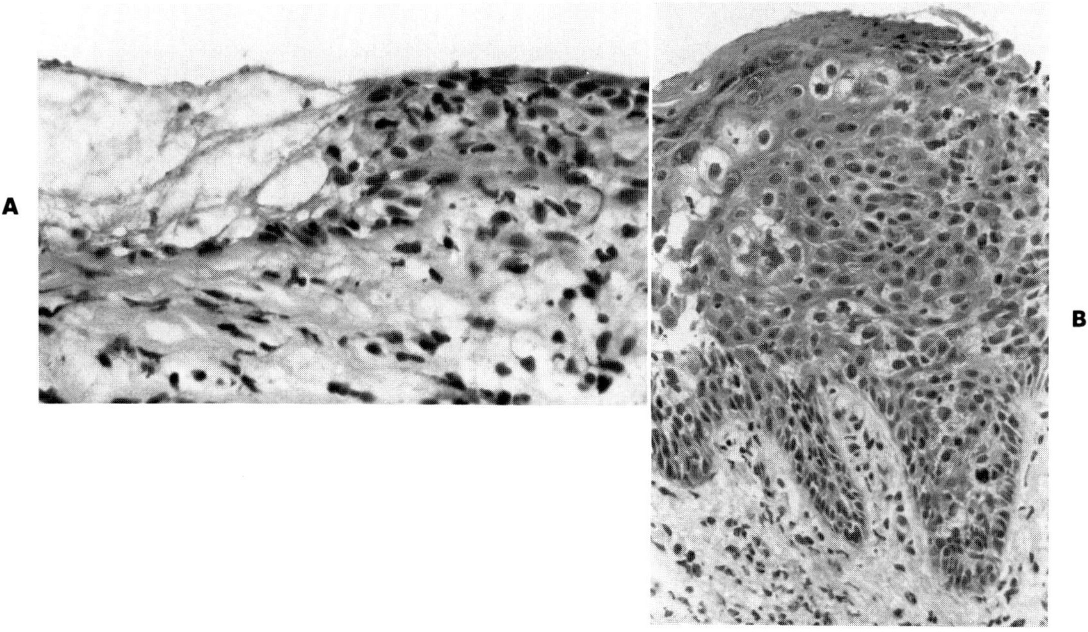

**FIGURE 21-4**   Frozen section from the margin of a conjunctival excision for sebaceous carcinoma. There is no epithelium remaining on the tissue, and a thin layer of fibrinous material shows where epithelium has recently been eroded away, **A. B** illustrates the appearance of sebaceous carcinoma exhibiting pagetoid spread elsewhere on the patient's conjunctiva (hemotoxylin and eosin, 200×) (**A** and **B**).

4. *Any* case in which lymphoma or sarcoma is to be ruled out. These tissues often require special preparation to establish the diagnosis. In the case of a possible lymphoma, fresh-frozen tissue is essential for lymphocyte marker studies and immunoglobulin gene rearrangement studies. Results of these studies often determine whether a lymphoid proliferation represents atypical hyperplasia or lymphoma. The easiest way to determine whether material needs to be stored fresh-frozen is to have the pathologist present for an intraoperative frozen section. The pathologist can then decide whether or not the lesion is suspicious for lymphoma and can process the tissue accordingly.

   A similar situation exists for cases of possible sarcoma. Although most ophthalmologists rarely come across a patient with sarcoma, the orbit is the single most common location in the body for rhabdomyosarcoma in children, and osteosarcoma as a second tumor in patients with heritable retinoblastoma often occurs in the orbital bones. We have recently seen several patients with von Recklinghausen's neurofibromatosis who developed neurogenic sarcoma of the orbit. Thus it may be that the ophthalmologist is the first physician to evaluate a patient with a sarcoma. In undifferentiated sarcomas, special studies are often necessary to determine what cell type is present. Both tissue for electron microscopy and frozen tissue should be obtained if the biopsy is large enough. This practice, like that of storing frozen portions of lymphoid lesions, is now standard practice in most pathology departments, not only because determining cell type assists oncologists in planning the best treatment regimen but also because it may assist in determining the value of additional surgery.

5. The pathologist should be consulted when the surgery is based on a previous biopsy. The pathologist should review all previous biopsies to confirm the diagnosis, even if the original biopsy was read in the same laboratory, and especially if it was read elsewhere. If additional surgery is to be done in a hospital, the hospital will probably not allow additional treatment unless the tissue establishing the patient's diagnosis has been reviewed by its pathologist. If slides from a patient's biopsy are on file elsewhere, representative sections should be requested for the pathologist or the pathology division of the hospital where the surgery will be performed. This has prevented unnecessary or even mutilating surgery based on misdiagnosis more than a few times.

6. The pathologist should be called in advance of surgery when these are special concerns or time constraints. For example, if the patient will be returning to have sutures removed on Wednesday, the pathologist should know that at least a preliminary report is needed for review with the patient by then, if possible.

## RECENT ADVANCES IN PATHOLOGY
### Immunohistochemistry

Immunohistochemical analysis is the technique whereby predominantly monoclonal antibodies for specific cellular components or microorganisms are applied to tissue sections or smears. If the component is present, antibodies form a complex with it. The bound antibodies are then identified through a variety of techniques, including fluorescent tags or secondary antibodies with other labels.[11,12] Immunohistochemistry can no longer be referred to as a recent advance, but there is a continual parade of new diagnostic antibodies on the market. Their value to the diagnostic pathologist is the subject of many articles in the pathology literature. Some of the most reliable antibodies in use are detailed in Table 21-1. Although it is not worth the clinician's effort to learn all of the antibodies and their purposes, it is important to recall that no single antibody, in and of itself, is diagnostic of a disease or lesion. Most diagnoses using immunohistochemistry are based on the appearance of the lesion as stained with hematoxylin and eosin, combined with the results of a panel of antibody-stained sections. The ophthalmologist's clinical input may be essential in selecting the antibodies to be used.[11,12]

One application of immunohistochemical studies is in the identification of cell markers of hematologic proliferations. Most ocular lymphoid processes involve B cells, and evaluation of the percentage of cells bearing kappa or lambda light chains is extremely helpful in distinguishing between polyclonal, presumably benign processes, and monoclonal, malignant ones. Many of the studies of lymphoid lesions must be performed on fresh-frozen specimens.

## In Situ Hybridization

In situ hybridization is a process using labeled complementary nucleic acid probes by which target nucleic acids in tissues or smears are identified. Usually, both target and probe are DNA, although messenger RNA can also be the target to look for evidence of cellular expression of specific genes, for example, oncogenes. Most in situ hybridization is done at present for research purposes, but the process is perceived as a diagnostic technique for the future, especially in microbiology.

In situ hybridization can also be performed on nylon or cellulose membranes to which specimen DNA has been affixed. The DNA is usually transferred to the membrane after it has been processed and separated on a gel. The transferred nucleic acid can be used as the substrate for in situ hybridization to look for target sequences. Such analyses, termed Southern analyses, may be done for diagnostic purposes to look for specific abnormal genes, such as that responsible for retinoblastoma.[13] One analysis with potential value for ophthalmologic specimens is the study of immunoglobulin genes in lymphoid proliferations, a technique known as immunoglobulin gene rearrangement studies.

**Table 21-1**　Commonly Used Diagnostic Antibodies

| Antibody | Positive Identification of |
| --- | --- |
| Cytokeratins | Epithelial cells, subclassification of carcinomas |
| Glial fibrillary acidic protein | Astrocytes, neoplastic ependyma, choroid plexus |
| Vimentin | Mesenchymal cells: muscle, fat, nerve sheath |
| Leukocyte common antigen | Hematopioetic cells |
| S-100 | Melanocytes, cartilage, nerve sheath, others |
| HMB-45 | Melanocytes |
| Desmin | Smooth, skeletal, or cardiac muscle |

Source: Corwin DG, Gowan AM. Review of selected lineage-directed antibodies useful in routinely processed tissues. Arch Path Lab Med 1989; 113:645-652.

## Gene Rearrangement Studies

In each clone of mature B or T lymphocytes, the immunoglobulin genes or T-cell receptor genes, respectively, have become irreversibly and uniquely rearranged in the heavy and light chain regions. By analyzing the DNA to determine the number of different rearrangements present, it is possible to identify a monoclonal, and presumably malignant, clone even if the cells account for only 10% of a total specimen. This analysis has become a powerful tool in the analysis of B and T cell lymphomas,[8,14] and in ophthalmology it could be particularly useful in distinguishing atypical lymphoid hyperplasia from lymphoma in the conjunctiva or orbit. The analysis does require forethought, however, because tissues must be fresh-frozen; it is also expensive and time consuming.

## Gene Amplification

One of the most recent advances in molecular pathology has been the simplification of techniques to amplify specific target DNA sequences in such a way that they can be detected in samples where they may be present in very low copy number.[15,16] The method by which the DNA is amplified is known as the polymerase chain reaction (PCR). PCR has been found useful in the identification of human genes, such as that for sickle cell anemia,[15] and the DNA of microorganisms such as herpes simplex[16] and human papillomavirus.[17] As this is written, PCR has not been approved as a diagnostic test, but approval will probably be granted soon for some tests, such as Human Immunodeficiency Virus (HIV). Current HIV tests are based on the presence of antibodies and may be negative several months after infection. HIV tests using PCR are immediately positive.

## Electron Microscopy

The "recent" news about electron microscopy (EM) as a diagnostic technique is that its limitations are becoming more and more apparent over time. Because EM permits objects to be enlarged tens of thousands of times, as opposed to the maximum 1000 X magnification of most light microscopes, it was hoped that cells would show ultrastructural features that would enable pathologists to tell at a (highly magnified) glance whether a process was benign or malignant. Although there are numerous papers describing the ultrastructural details of benign ocular processes versus those of malignant, the designations are, in all cases, based on light microscopy and clinical behavior. EM is not generally helpful for diagnosis is this respect. It is, however, invaluable in identifying the phenotypic structural aspects of individual cells. By analysis of EM features, it is possible to distinguish epithelial cells from smooth muscle from melanocytes from skeletal muscle, and so on. EM as a diagnostic tool is most valuable in distinguishing the cell type in malignancies that appear undifferentiated by light microscopy.

Another role for EM is in the diagnosis of viral infection, particularly in small biopsies such as retinal biopsies. EM is usually used in this setting to confirm an impression based on hematoxylin- and eosin-stained sections, but it may also be a primary diagnostic modality. EM is expensive and is usually available only in a university or large hospital setting. In a limited number of instances, EM may be invaluable, although it may soon be replaced by PCR in the diagnosis of viral infections.

## HOW TO SELECT OR EVALUATE A PATHOLOGIST

An ophthalmologist may not need to consult with a pathologist very often, but when this becomes necessary, it is important that the pathologist be a good one. Here are some important questions to ask yourself about the pathologist:

- Does the pathologist have any training in or knowledge of the eye? Someone who will diagnose "sebaceous hyperplasia" on a full-thickness lid resection, not knowing that sebaceous glands are normally present in the lid, while missing a squamous dysplasia of the conjunctiva is obviously unacceptable. Such a case was recently referred to our laboratory. Likewise, the corneal dystrophies, which require precise diagnosis because of what they mean for the patient and family, are not included in the training of the vast majority of general anatomic pathologists. It is critical to make sure specimens are being read by someone who knows how to read them. The converse also applies: the person who ultimately signs the report must be board-certified in pathology. Because the Joint Commission on Accreditation of Healthcare Organizations strongly suggests that a person running an anatomic pathology laboratory and signing pathology reports be board certified in anatomic pathology, this should not pose a problem.
- Does the pathologist provide basic, high-quality service?
  - Is the turn-around time for a telephoned report reasonable? Once the specimen arrives in the laboratory, a verbal report should be available in 1 or 2 business days for a biopsy, 3 business days for a major tumor specimen. Written reports may take longer.
  - Does the pathologist call personally when the diagnosis is unusual, unexpected, or if it might drastically alter the clinician's management plans? This courtesy would certainly be expected from an ophthalmologic consultant, and the same should be true of the pathologist.
  - Will the pathologist reconsider a diagnosis and reexamine the slides if her or his diagnosis does not fit the clinical picture? A good pathologist will diagnose only what is on a slide and will not alter what is present in the specimen, but an ophthalmologist also needs to deal with someone who is receptive to input and willing to reexamine the material.
  - Does the pathologist call personally if the permanent sections reveal that the frozen-section diagnosis was in error? Since doctor and patient probably consider what has just been done to be a definitive procedure, it is important that the pathologist call immediately if review of the permanent sections shows that an alternate diagnosis is more likely. The matter can then be discussed immediately with the patient to reconsider the treatment options.
  - Is the pathologist gracious about sending specimens or slides elsewhere for a second opinion if requested?
  - Is the pathologist available for frozen sections, given notice, at times convenient to the clinician?
  - What are the billing policies? Will the pathologist or group bill the

clinician, and expect him or her to bill the patient, or will they bill the patient, in which case the patient should be warned that a pathologist's bill is coming? Frozen sections, in particular, are very costly, and most pathologists charge per specimen, so it is a good idea to look into details before contracting with a group.

- Does the pathologist provide references from the literature when they are requested? While the ophthalmologist is evaluating the pathologist, he or she may, in turn, be under scrutiny. It is advisable to return the favor of passing on references or clinical photographs pertaining to shared cases if asked.

- Is the pathologist willing to review slides with the clinician? Does the pathologist ever openly look something up or utter the words "I don't know"? Someone who knows his or her limits and admits them is generally to be preferred.

Most ophthalmology training programs tend to underemphasize the practical aspects of pathology in favor of its obvious importance in teaching. Many practicing ophthalmologists, who seldom require the expertise of a pathologist, are unprepared to evaluate the strengths and limitations of the pathologist when they need one. I have provided guidelines, both concrete and philosophical, to assist in interactions with pathologists. Their ultimate goal is to enable the clinician to provide patients with the best possible care.

---

## References


1. Rao NA. A laboratory approach to rapid diagnosis of ocular infections and prospects for the future. Am J Ophthalmol 1989; 107:283-291.

2. Auran JD, Starr MB, Jakobiec FA. Acanthamoeba keratitis: a review of the literature. Cornea 1987; 6:2-26.

3. Keebler CM, Reagan JW: A manual of cytotechnology, ed 6, Chicago, 1983, American Society of Clinical Pathologists Press, pp 319-349.

4. Green WR. Diagnostic cytopathology of ocular fluid specimens. Ophthalmol 1984; 91:726-749.

5. Augsburger JJ, Shields JA. Fine needle aspiration biopsy of solid intraocular tumors: indications, instrumentation and techniques. Ophthalmic Surg 1984; 15:34-40.

6. Egbert PR, Lauber S, Maurice DM. A simple conjunctival biopsy. Am J Ophthalmol 1977; 84:798-801.

7. Pflugfelder SC, Huang AJW, Feuer W, Chuchovski PT, Pereira IC, Tseng SCG. Conjunctival cytologic features of primary Sjögren's syndrome. Ophthalmol 1990; 97:985-991.

8. Korsmeyer SJ, Hieter PA, Ravetch JV, Poplack DG, Waldmann TA, Leder P. Developmental hierarchy of immunoglobulin gene rearrangements in human leukemic pre-B cells. Proc Natl Acad Sci USA 1981; 78:7096-7100.

9. Mohs FE. Micrographic surgery for the microscopically controlled excision of eyelid cancers. Arch Ophthalmol 1986; 104:901-909.

10. Anderson RL. Mohs' micrographic technique. Arch Ophthalmol 1986; 104:818-819 (editorial).

11. Taylor CR: Immunomicroscopy: a diagnostic tool for the surgical pathologist, Philadelphia, 1986, WB Saunders Co.

12. Corwin DG, Gown AM. Review of selected lineage-directed antibodies useful in routinely processed tissues. Arch Pathol Lab Med 1989; 113:645-652.

13. Cavenee WK, Murphree AL, Shull MM, et al. Prediction of familial predisposition to retinoblastoma. N Engl J Med 1986; 314:1201-1207.

14. Kamat D, Laszewski MJ, Kemp JD, et al. The diagnostic utility of immunophenotyping and immunogenotyping in the pathologic evaluation of lymphoid proliferations. Mod Pathol 1990; 3:105-112.

15. Saiki RK, Gelfand DH, Stoffel S, et al. Primer-directed enzymatic amplification of DNA with a thermostable DNA polymerase. Science 1988; 239:487-491.

16. Crouse CA, Pflugfelder SC, Pereira IE, Rabinowitz SS, Levine JA, Atherton SS. Diagnosis of herpetic ocular disease using PCR. Invest Ophthalmol Vis Sci 1990; 31(Suppl):221.

17. McDonnell JM, Mayr AJ, Martin WJ. DNA of human papillomavirus type 16 in dysplastic and malignant lesions of the conjunctiva and cornea. N Engl J Med 1989; 320:1442-1446.

# 22 Evaluation of the Patient with Narrow Anterior Chamber Angles

Paul Palmberg, MD, PhD

Our ability to manage patients with narrow anterior chamber angles has improved steadily over the past few decades. First of all, we now have a better understanding of the mechanisms underlying the different types of angle closure glaucoma, along with better recognition of the distinguishing clinical features of each. We also have long-term clinical experience with different modes of treatment for each type, so that at least a rough consensus has emerged as to how each type should be managed. Finally, we have much safer and more effective treatments, including potent new pharmacological agents and lasers, so that the outcome of most cases is satisfactory.[1,2]

Unfortunately, actual practice in the management of patients with narrow anterior chamber angles has lagged behind developments in the field. Many important aspects of gonioscopic technique are not widely appreciated, resulting in inaccurate decisions as to whether or not angle closure is present.[3] In addition, lack of familiarity with the relatively rare nonpupillary block types of angle closure can result in failure to consider them or to look for their hallmarks when they are indeed present. We will illustrate some of the nuances of the management of patients with narrow angles by presenting and discussing 4 cases.

## Case 1

*A 62-year-old woman was seen for a change in her hyperopic correction. Upon slit lamp examination, she was noted to have a shallow peripheral chamber angle. Gonioscopy revealed asymptomatic closure of the superior half of the angle in each eye. However, because the patient denied symptoms of angle closure (episodes of ocular pain, blurred vision, colored halos around lights) and had tensions of 13 mm Hg OU, evidently it was decided that the patient was at low risk, and no action was taken.*

*Four months later, when the patient was hospitalized for a laminectomy, she received preoperative atropine intramuscularly and noted bilateral ocular pain for the remaining 7 days of her hospitalization. Upon discharge, she saw her ophthalmologist and was referred for management of bilateral acute angle closure glaucoma. The tensions were OD 44 mm Hg and OS 42 mm Hg. After argon laser iridotomy OU (1.5 watts, 0.02 seconds, 50 u spot), about ⅔ of the angle was sealed by PAS in each eye, and full medical therapy was needed to control her pressures at 18 mm Hg OU.*

"

## Discussion

This case introduces the dilemma of what should be done with an asymptomatic patient with a normal intraocular pressure who has partial closure of the angle due to some degree of pupillary block. Had the intraocular pressure been elevated or had the patient reported typical angle closure symptoms, the first ophthalmologist would have performed a laser iridotomy, and the subsequent pharmacologically induced attack would not have occurred. Perhaps he could not reconcile a tension of 13 mm Hg with the presence of genuine angle closure and doubted his observation.

What should have been done? First, the initial examination should have been completed by the performance of indentation gonioscopy.[3] Indentation gonioscopy not only allows a distinction to be made between appositional and synechial angle closure but also allows the examiner to confirm that the functional (pigmented) meshwork is indeed covered by iris. During indentation, the examiner sees the angle open, disclosing the pigmented meshwork, and during the release of the indenting force watches the iris cover the meshwork again.

Most glaucoma specialists would advise iridotomy if any part of the angle is synechially closed, and the majority would advise iridotomy if a quarter or more of the angle were even appositionally closed. Those of us who advocate iridotomy for even appositional closure argue that the function of the trabecular meshwork is harmed by depriving it of the nutrient aqueous, as evidenced by the observation of secondary open-angle glaucoma in patients after relief of long-standing pupillary block.

Had the angles been narrowly open rather than closed, the patient should have been warned of the symptoms of angle closure and scheduled for a followup examination to watch for the development of angle closure. The risk of a spontaneous attack of angle closure would have been low enough to warrant a choice of observation rather than iridotomy. Had a forewarned patient gone on to have a pharmacologically induced attack, presumably she and her orthopedic surgeon would have recognized the symptoms and sought ophthalmologic consultation promptly, with a better outcome. Under unusual circumstances, an iridotomy might even be recommended for very narrow but open angles, as when there is a family history of severe angle-closure glaucoma or when the person at risk might not be capable of seeking medical attention because of senility, living in a remote location, or extreme anxiety about the risk of an attack.

### Case 2

*A 70-year-old woman presented with a 2 week history of blurred vision without pain in the left eye. Mild corneal edema was present OS, and the tensions were OD 14 mm Hg and OS 42 mm Hg. Gonioscopy revealed angle closure in the left eye and a YAG iridotomy was performed. However, the pressure rose again to OS 40 mm Hg by the next day, and the patient was treated with apraclonidine and methazolamide and referred.*

*On examination, the Va was OD 20/50 with +4.00 + 0.75 × 140 and OS 20/ 25 with +1.00 + 0.75 × 50. The central anterior chamber was 3 corneal thicknesses deep OD and only 2 corneal thicknesses deep OS. Mild iris bombe was present OD but not OS, and there was a patent iridotomy OS. There was slight nuclear sclerosis OU and no phakodonesis. The tensions were OD 14 mm Hg and OS 17 mm Hg, and gonioscopy revealed OD: appositional closure above and slit-I angles below; OS: PAS for 180 degrees above and appositional closure below, which with indentation gonioscopy could be pressed open with firm pressure to grade II. The last roll of the iris appeared prominent, and diagnoses of plateau iris syndrome and aqueous misdirection (ciliary block) glaucoma were considered. An undilated fundus view revealed OD: cup/disc 0.2; and OS: cup/disc 0.5, suggesting a chronic glaucoma. A laser iridoplasty was performed in the inferior half of the angle OS in a modified form of the technique of Ritch[4] (18 spots of 500 u at 0.3 watts in a blue iris and 1.0 s duration, delivered through an Abraham lens), with no resulting opening of the angle. Upon reconsideration, tropicamide 1% was administered, with a deepening of the central chamber depth to 2½ corneal thicknesses and opening of the inferior angle to grade I. Advancement to hyoscine 0.25% deepened the central anterior chamber to 3 corneal thicknesses and the inferior half of the angle to grade II. Thereafter the patient did well on chronic cycloplegia OU.*

## Discussion

Spontaneous aqueous misdirection (ciliary block) glaucoma[5] is a rather uncommon condition but one that can and must be recognized in order to be properly treated. The hallmark of this condition is a foreward movement of the lens-iris diaphragm, with a shallower central anterior chamber depth on the affected side, in the absence of such alternative causes of forward movement of the lens-iris diaphragm as choroidal swelling, phacodonesis, or lens intumescence. When the lens-iris diaphragm is displaced forward, it is best to begin therapy with a mild cycloplegic and to observe the resultant effect on chamber depth and angle configuration. A positive response helps to support the diagnosis and gives the ophthalmologist the courage to administer a potent, long-lasting cycloplegic agent. In this case, both the referring ophthalmologist and glaucoma subspecialist suspected ciliary block glaucoma but hedged their bets by taking steps to treat possible pupillary block and plateau iris syndrome mechanisms. Such unnecessary actions might have increased ciliary congestion and compromised the response to the appropriate treatment. Detection of otherwise unexplained asymmetry (e.g., no unilateral myopia, lens swelling, or phakodonesis) in central anterior chamber depth should have suggested administering a mild cycloplegic agent as the first therapy.

---

### Case 3

*A 68-year-old woman underwent a dilated fundus examination for age-related macular degeneration. The predilation tensions were normal OU. That night she noted severe ocular pain OS, and she presented in the early morning hours with a normal tension in her pseudophakic OD and tension of 70 mm Hg in her phakic OS. After treatment with timolol, apraclonidine, pilocarpine, and 4 ounces of oral glycerine reduced her tension to 40 mm Hg, a YAG laser iridotomy was performed, but the angle did not open. The patient was referred.*

*The patient had 3+ corneal epithelial edema, ciliary flush, a patent iridotomy, tension OS: 40 mm Hg, and appositionally closed angles OS that could be pressed open with indentation gonioscopy. During indentation gonioscopy, the imprint of the ciliary processes could be seen in the peripheral iris, creating a prominent last roll of the iris. After partial clearing of the corneal edema with topical anhydrous glycerine, iridoplasty was performed, with 14 applications of a 500 u argon spot at 0.3 watts, 1.0 second duration. The first few spots were placed in the mid-iris to heat-shrink and retract the iris further from the cornea, so that a furrow was created that could be advanced to and around the peripheral iris without injuring the corneal endothelium (Figure 22-1). The tension fell immediately to OS: 10 mm Hg, and the angle opened to grade II. The angle remained open and pressure normal at followup examinations.*

## Discussion

This case illustrates that the intense ocular congestion of an acute attack of angle-closure glaucoma can induce a superimposed second mechanism of closure. Thus, a pharmacologically induced pupillary block angle-closure attack led to ciliary-choroidal swelling, with a forward rotation of the ciliary body processes, pressing the iris against the angle. The key to proper management in this case was the performance of repeat gonioscopy after pupillary block had been eliminated by laser iridotomy. That gonioscopy revealed that angle closure was still present, that the closure was appositional rather than synechial, and that upon indentation gonioscopy the imprint of underlying ciliary body processes could be seen in the peripheral iris, just as in plateau iris syndrome. The treatment employed was just that which we would use to treat plateau iris syndrome, peripheral iridoplasty. It creates heat shrinkage of the iris and forces the underlying ciliary processes to move posteriorly, opening the angle. However, since the underlying ciliary congestion was likely to resolve once the ocular pressure was reduced, we used fewer than the 36 laser applications recommended by Ritch for spontaneous plateau iris syndrome.

---

### Case 4

*A 63-year-old latin male who saw his ophthalmologist for a recurrent papilloma of the left caruncle noted to have tensions of OD: 18 mm Hg and OS: 45 mm Hg. Upon referral, the patient was asymptomatic with regard to the pressure elevation, had Va OU 20/20, central chamber depths that were normal and equal, tensions of OD: 18 on no medication and OS: 20 on timolol, and OD grade II angles and OS 270 degrees of appositional angle closure. An argon laser iridotomy was performed, and the angle opened to grade I, with a prominent last roll of the iris still present.*

*During the next 3 years, the angles in both eyes were noted to narrow steadily, until there was appositional angle closure present for most of the angle in each eye and tensions of OD: 26 mm Hg and OS: 32 mm Hg. Pilocarpine 1% opened the angle OS to grade I-II, but 1 week later the superior angle was closed even on pilocarpine and a laser iridoplasty was performed (Figure 22-2, A-D). An argon laser iridotomy was performed in the right eye. Both eyes remain open at grade II some 4 years later.*

## Discussion

This case illustrates the occurrence of a delayed onset of plateau iris syndrome. As noted several years ago by Robert Ritch, patients with angle-closure glaucoma must be followed after performance of iridotomy, since some of them will re-develop angle closure in the presence of a patent iridotomy. Over a 7-year period in our institution in which 1724 iridotomies were performed, at least 40 eyes of 27 patients had or developed plateau iris syndrome. Of the 24 patients for whom useful records were available, 54% presented with classic plateau iris syndrome, but 33% developed delayed plateau iris syndrome, and 13% had asymptomatic

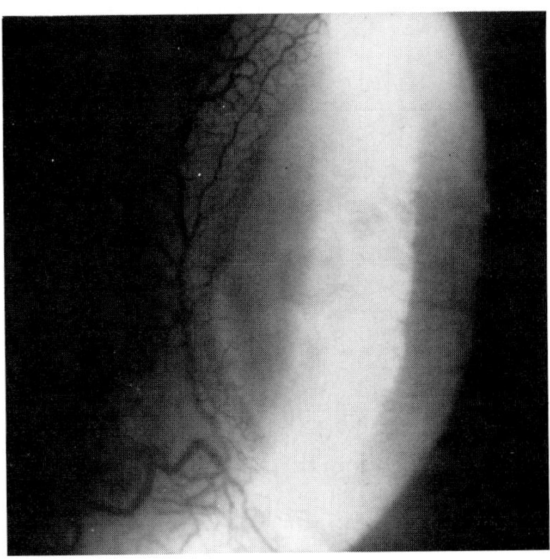

**FIGURE 22-1**  Laser iridoplasty burns in a patient with angle closure due to ciliary congestion.

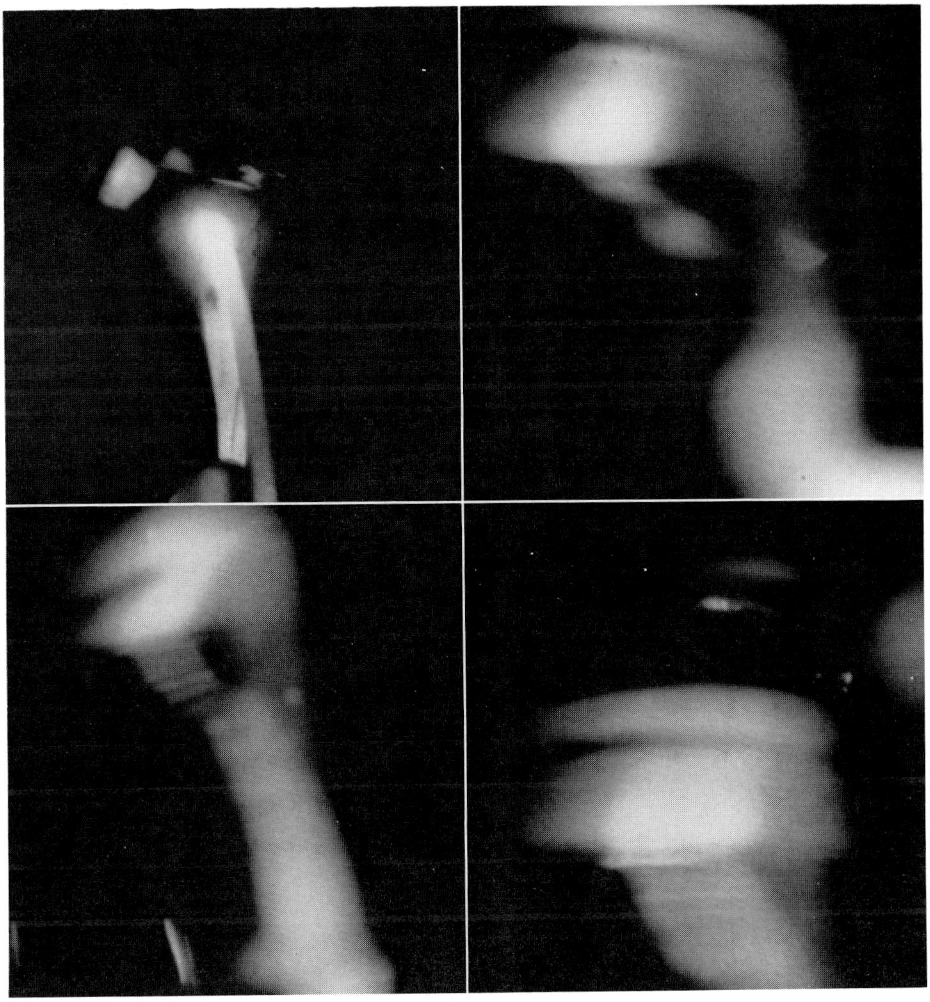

**FIGURE 22-2**  Plateau iris syndrome. **A,** Patent iridotomy. **B,** Appositional angle closure. **C,** Indentation gonioscopy opens the angle. **D,** Open angle following laser iridoplasty.

**Table 22-1**  The Differential Diagnosis and Treatment of Angle-Closure Glaucoma

|  | Hallmark | Occurrence | Treatment |
|---|---|---|---|
| Primary angle closure | Iris bombe | Common | Iridotomy |
| Plateau iris syndrome | Prominent last roll of iris | 1:43 vs primary | Iridoplasty |
| Aqueous misdirection | Asymmetric central AC depth | 1:500 vs primary | Cycloplegia |

appositional angle closure in a previously iridectomized eye. Thus we estimate that a minimum of 1 in 43 cases of angle closure has or will develop plateau iris syndrome, a condition best treated with iridoplasty.[6]

## SUMMARY

The keys to the proper management of patients with narrow chamber angles are skillfully performed gonioscopy and recognition of the mechanisms underlying angle closure. Gonioscopy is best performed with a Zeiss-type lens, since this allows the performance of indentation gonioscopy, with care to avoid artifacts that open closed angles.[3] While pupillary block is by far the most common mechanism underlying angle closure, consideration must also be given to detecting angle closure due to plateau iris syndrome, aqueous misdirection (ciliary block), ciliochoroidal congestion, lens swelling or dislocation, uveitis, or neovascularization. Thereafter, treatment is directed to correcting or offsetting the underlying mechanism, and followup gonioscopy is required to assess resolution of the problem. Table 22-1 summarizes the differential diagnosis and treatment.

## References

1. Lowe RF, Ritch R, Reyes A. Angle closure glaucoma. In Ritch R, Shields B, Krupin T, eds, The glaucomas, St Louis, 1989, Mosby–Year Book, pp 825-864.
2. Anderson DR. Angle closure glaucoma. In Lichter PR, Anderson DR, eds, Discussions on glaucoma, New York, 1977, Grune & Stratton.
3. Palmberg P. Gonioscopy. In Ritch R, Shields B, Krupin T, eds, The glaucomas, St Louis, 1989, Mosby–Year Book, pp 345-360.
4. Ritch R, Liebmann J, Soloman IS. Laser iridectomy and iridoplasty. In Ritch R, Shields B, Krupin T, eds, The glaucomas, St Louis, 1989, Mosby–Year Book, p 597.
5. Schwartz AL, Anderson DR. "Malignant glaucoma" in an eye with no antecedent operation or miotics. Arch Ophthalmol 1975; 93:379-381.
6. Moolchandani J, Jin CC, Palmberg P. A retrospective study of laser iridoplasty for plateau iris syndrome. Paper presented at meeting of the American Academy of Ophthalmology, Atlanta, October 1990.

# THE EVOLUTION OF CURRENT PRACTICE—THEN AND NOW

# 23

# Phacoemulsification Then and Now

Charles D. Kelman, MD

According to some commentators, cataract surgery had reached the zenith of perfection in the 1960s. Derrick Vail stated in 1965 that extracapsular cataract surgery had become as "extinct as the buffalo."

Somewhat later, some of our most respected ophthalmic surgeons railed against phacoemulsification as though it had been conceived by Satan himself.

Confronted with the results of a 1990 poll which show phacoemulsifications as the preferred method of cataract extraction by 52% of ophthalmic surgeons interviewed, one can only be wary of speaking in absolutes where removal of the crystalline lens is concerned.

I began performing phacoemulsification in the posterior chamber. To teach the technique more easily, I went to the anterior chamber and still believe this to be the safest version of the technique. Certainly, it is the only method I recommend for those beginning phacoemulsification. The ease of conversion to standard extracapsular procedure when the nucleus is in the anterior chamber insures a successful completion of the extraction with a technique the surgeon has already mastered.

While my views on anterior chamber phacoemulsification are well known, I have never maintained that there is only one correct way to perform phacoemulsification any more than I would claim that phaco itself is the end point in the evolution of cataract extraction techniques.

The work of Gimbel and Neuhann in the area of continuous circular capsulorhexis in 1984 and 1985 piqued my curiosity. Hydrodissection and nucleofractus drew my interest posteriorly, especially in cases of endothelial disease or very soft, difficult-to-prolapse nuclei. Greater sophistication in all parameters (flow, vacuum, etc.) with the newest phacoemulsification machines has given surgeons better control in the posterior chamber. My own efforts in developing curved phacoemulsification tips augur well for the future of emulsification in the posterior chamber.

Though my early (and admittedly less sophisticated) versions of hydrodissection and nucleofractus are documented in the AJO and in my personal records of 1967 and 1968, I am considered, with some justification, a proponent of phacoemulsification in the anterior chamber. Yet it was not until 1972 after working in the posterior chamber since 1967 that I perfected a technique to bring the nucleus into the anterior chamber.

Prolapse of a firm nucleus through an adequately dilated pupil is relatively simple with the seesaw technique. The potential risks to the iris and posterior capsule with posterior chamber phaco are avoided; a visco-elastic substance is used to protect the corneal endothelium.

## ANTERIOR CHAMBER TECHNIQUE

The technique is as follows: After anterior capsulotomy (in my case, a Christmas-tree opening achieved with 3 or more tears using the Kelman double cystotome) a cystotome placed against a relatively hard nucleus can exert a force on the lens mass and move it. By using the side of the cystotome blade rather than its cutting edge to displace the nucleus, it is often possible to prolapse the lens first from the 3 o'clock or 9 o'clock position, and then from the opposite pole. This maneuver is carried out with anterior chamber irrigation using the incision as a fulcrum. I place the cystotome 3 mm from the center of the lens and, without deforming the incision, I push it gently to the side until the nasal or temporal edge is brought halfway across the pupil and out of the capsular bag. (A lens pushed less than half-way will snap back into the bag.) When one pole of the lens is forward of the iris plane, I release the cystotome and place it 3 mm toward the opposite edge behind the iris. I press down on this area and move the engaged lens across the pupil and over the iris in the other direction to bring the second edge out of the capsule. At this point I irrigate and the lens floats free in the anterior chamber.

If the edge of the nucleus cannot be brought easily above the iris plane as described above (pupil too small, nucleus too soft, etc.) I use viscoelastic to facilitate the prolapse. After displacing the lens with the cystotome until one edge is visible, I push the iris back by injecting viscoelastic at the nuclear edge. I then move the cannula to the opposite nuclear pole and push the nucleus toward the area of viscoelastic-depressed iris. Once an edge of the nucleus has been brought into the anterior chamber the tip of the cannula can be used to rotate the nucleus into position forward of the iris plane.

I prefer to begin anterior chamber phaco with a 15-degree tip, bevel up, engaging the posterior surface of the nucleus at the superior pole. Being careful not to create a tunnel in which the phaco tip might get stuck, I sculpt the center of the nucleus to produce a croissant shape. I aim for a wide central cavity and, as I reach the inferior pole of the nucleus, I decrease phacoemulsification power so as not to break through suddenly and engage the iris. As nuclear fragments become smaller I reduce the power further to avoid anterior chamber chatter with attendant endothelial damage.

To remove cortical material, my choice is a .5 tip, port kept upward, on a Kelman Cavitron 9000 or 10000 machine. I begin inferiorly engaging cortex and tugging longitudinally in a piston-like fashion toward the incision. The maneuver is repeated for 360 degrees to clear all cortex from the capsular fornices.

The most important points to keep in mind for anterior chamber phaco are that the emulsifying tip should always point toward the scleral spur, never posteriorly in the direction of vitreous; the emulsification should be a piston-like, in-and-out motion so that lens material disappears in front of the tip and the lens is not pushed against the endothelium. Finally, emulsifying from back to front keeps the tip pointed toward the scleral spur and avoids pushing the lens back toward the posterior chamber.

I stand by my recommendation that all beginning phacoemulsification surgeons should use the anterior chamber method. Its ease and safety (with rapid conversion to traditional extracapsular extraction) have withstood the test of time.

Today with improved phacoemulsification machinery and more certain means of maintaining pupillary dilation, I am returning, so to speak, to my roots with posterior chamber phacoemulsification.

## POSTERIOR CHAMBER TECHNIQUE

My posterior chamber protocol has been evolving with the assimilation of new techniques and technology as well as the reincorporation of the hydrodissection and nuclear fracturing maneuvers I used in the late sixties.

I begin by creating a fornix based conjunctival flap 0.5 mm from the limbus using sharp Wescott scissors. Hemostasis is achieved using a wet-field eraser. With a lamellar knife such as a Beaver 6600 or an angulated Alcon crescent knife, a groove is made approximately 3 mm posterior to the vascular arcade. A scleral tunnel is then created utilizing the same lamellar knife. (The width of this tunnel is dependent upon the incision size required for IOL implantation.) Care is taken to insure that the dissection is carried forward into clear cornea.

The anterior chamber is entered with a 3.2-mm angulated keratome held parallel to the iris. The keratome is carefully advanced until the point of the blade is visible just anterior to the vascular arcade. The point of the knife is tipped posteriorly so that a small dimple is seen and the knife is carefully advanced, adjusting the angle of the blade so that a straight line is visible on its anterior surface as Decemet's is incised. This assures the successful creation of a self sealing flap valve.

A viscoelastic is instilled and a double cystostome is used to create a small inverted V-shaped tear in the inferior portion of the anterior capsule. A Utrata forceps is utilized to complete a continuous tear capsulorhexis in a manner similar to that described by Howard Gimbel and Thomas Neuhann in the mid-1980s.

I prefer to use a 30-gauge cannula on a syringe for hydrodissection of the nucleus. The nucleus is rotated to assure that hydrodissection has adequately cleaved cortical adherences. A deep groove is made in the lens to ¾ depth with a curved high efficiency phaco tip (10% smaller in diameter than a standard tip) using moderate power and low vacuum. I use the phaco tip to rotate the nucleus 90 degrees and sculpt an additional groove bisecting the inferior half. This additional groove facilitates the fracture, vacuum-bonding and phacoemulsification of the first quadrant to be emulsified. Viscoelastics are again instilled into the eye to deepen the chamber.

With a Ringberg forceps the lens is split in half inferiorly and superiorly. With a channel dissected away in the middle of the lens, it is now easy to introduce the phacoemulsifier into each portion of the lens. Emulsification begins using low power and high vacuum to draw one quarter of the lens towards the center of the pupil. Following the emulsification of the first pie-shaped quarter of nucleus, the remaining quarter and half of the nucleus are very simply and easily vacuum-bonded and emulsified in similar fashion.

My irrigation/aspiration is performed using an angulated I&A tip with a 0.3mm or 0.5mm port. In some cases I will use ultrasonic I&A to facilitate cortical aspiration. I like a blunt, flattened cannula on a bulb irrigator for capsule polishing. The incision is enlarged using the appropriate angulated blunted keratome. Under viscoelastic the intraocular lens is placed into the capsular bag through the capsulorhexis. The IOL is checked for proper centration and Miochol is instilled. I aspirate the remaining viscoelastic with the irrigation/aspiration handpiece of the phacoemulsifier.

Although I construct a potentially sutureless wound which I believe to be a great advantage in the event of an intraoperative complication, I elect, in most cases to close the wound with a single 9-0 nylon suture. The conjunctival flap is drawn up and subconjunctival Garamycin and Solu-Medrol is injected.

# 24

# Argon-Laser Trabeculoplasty

Arthur L. Schwartz, MD, FACS

During the last decade, argon laser trabeculoplasty has become the primary initial surgical treatment for uncontrolled open-angle glaucoma *unresponsive to medical therapy*. Its acceptance around the world has revolutionized the management of glaucoma. During these past 10 years, we have refined the indications for laser trabeculoplasty, modified the surgical technique to reduce complications, and learned about the long-term results and the role of retreatment. The precise mechanism of action of argon laser trabeculoplasty is still under investigation, as is its role as the initial treatment for newly diagnosed glaucomas. This chapter attempts to put the evolving role of argon laser trabeculoplasty into perspective for the practicing ophthalmologist.

Krasnov first used laser treatment of the trabecular meshwork for the management of open angle glaucoma in 1973.[1] This author used a high-powered ruby laser to make microscopic punctures through the trabecular meshwork and into Schlemm's canal.[1] This original surgical procedure produced an excellent intraocular pressure-lowering effect, but the response lasted only a few months, and retreatment was required to sustain the effect.

David Worthen and Gary Wickham were the first to report on treating part of the angle with the argon laser.[2] They reported an average IOP reduction of 9.6 mm Hg in 20 patients with a short followup. They were appropriately cautious in their recommendations, partially because of Gaasterland and Kupfer's 1974 report on the production of glaucoma experimentally in monkeys by heavy, repeated treatment of the angle with argon laser energy.[3] This report raised the possibility that laser therapy could aggravate rather than help glaucoma in some situations, and thus served to dampen the enthusiasm for this treatment modality.

In 1977, Bruce Bleiman, a second-year resident, and I initiated some early studies on argon-laser treatment of part of the angle using an informed-consent protocol at the Washington Hospital Center. In view of the limited and somewhat conflicting data in the literature, we initially used this technique on a few patients with end-stage open-angle glaucoma, and the results were not encouraging.

At the 1978 Wilmer meeting, James Wise presented a pilot study in which he reported a greater than 90% success rate with a mean IOP decrease of 10 mm Hg in argon-laser–treated phakic eyes with open angle glaucoma. His technique differed from that described in Worthen's report in that all 360 degrees of the angle were treated. Wise's excellent results with 360-degree laser trabecular treatment rekindled our interest, and we modified our laser protocol to follow his treatment regimen. In the spring of 1978, we reported 360-degree treatment on our first 6 patients. They had previously had seven failed surgical procedures

**Table 24-1**  Mean Change in Pressures (mm Hg) from Baseline in Eyes Treated with Argon-Laser Trabeculoplasty

| Time | No. of Eyes | Mean mm Hg | P | % IOP Reduction |
|---|---|---|---|---|
| 2 months | 76 | −9.7 | <0.0001 | −37.8 |
| 6 months | 78 | −9.0 | <0.0001 | −35.1 |
| 12 months | 66 | −7.8 | <0.0001 | −30.1 |
| 24 months | 32 | −7.3 | <0.0001 | −29.7 |
| 36 months | 20 | −6.8 | <0.0001 | −28.0 |
| 42 months | 10 | −5.9 | <0.0028 | −24.2 |

among them. All were successfully treated, with an average drop in pressure of 10 mm Hg at six months after treatment. Our enthusiasm for the procedure increased, and by November of 1978 we offered laser trabecular surgery to all patients as an alternative to standard filtering surgery.

Our initial report dealt with 35 phakic eyes with clinically uncontrolled open-angle glaucoma which underwent 360-degree treatment to the trabecular meshwork.[4] We utilized the intraocular pressure in the untreated eye as a control. The mean pressure change in the treated eye at four months was 10 mm Hg, and this drop was maintained throughout the initial 18-month followup period. We also reported a statistically significant increase in outflow for the first six months after treatment. Our major complication was the formation of peripheral anterior synechiae, a finding that David Worthen mentioned in his initial report.

At the 1980 American Academy of Ophthalmology meeting, three independent reports by Wise,[5] Wilensky,[6] and ourselves[4] all confirmed the efficacy of 360-degree argon-laser treatment to the trabecular meshwork. Since 1980, argon-laser trabeculoplasty (ALT) has been the primary initial surgical treatment for uncontrolled open-angle glaucoma. Its acceptance around the world has revolutionized the management of the glaucoma patient.

Our early results were very exciting. However, at the 1982 meeting of the academy we reported a decrease from our initial success rate of 97% to 70%, with a mean followup of 24 months.[7] We also began to see a decrease in pressure-lowering effect in successfully treated patients with longer followup. The peak intraocular pressure-lowering effect was seen at 2 months, but at 42 months the pressure-lowering effect was decreased to 5.9 mm Hg (Table 24-1).

Specific patient characteristics significantly influenced our success rate. A diagnosis of exfoliation syndrome or open-angle glaucoma, an age greater than 60, and a baseline pressure of less than 26 mm Hg were each associated with higher success rate. Patients with uveitis and angle recession glaucoma were almost uniformly unresponsive. We also found that the outcome in the first eye appeared to be predictive of the outcome in the fellow eye.

In 1985 we reported our long-term followup in the initial 82 phakic eyes that underwent 360-degree laser trabeculoplasty.[8] After five years of observation, the success rate decreased from 77% to 46%. In addition, there was a decrease in pressure lowering in successfully treated eyes from 9.8 to 4.9 mm Hg. Figure 24-1 graphically shows pressure change over time in the treated eye. Our clinical population was unique in that the majority of our patients were black. Initially,

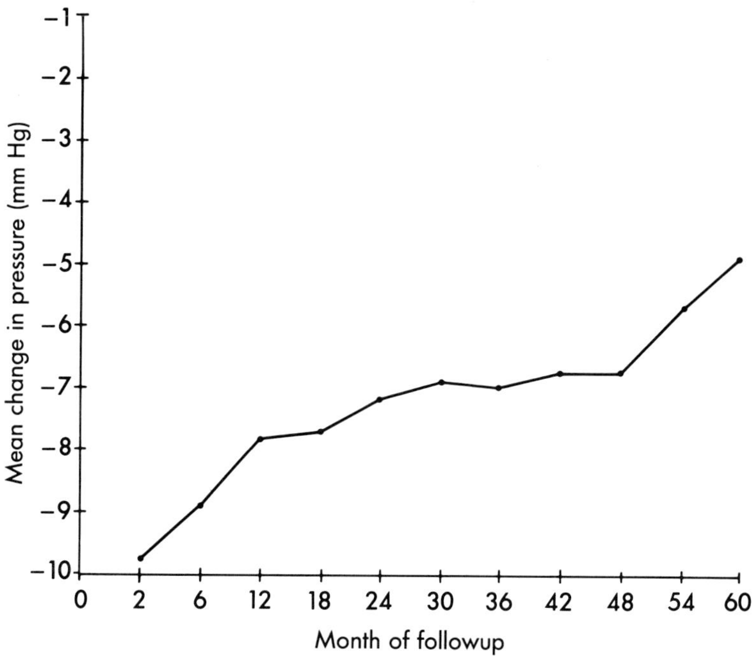

**FIGURE 24-1**    Average intraocular pressure change vs. time. *(Reproduced with permission from Archives of Ophthalmology, 1985; 103:1483. Copyright 1985, American Medical Association.)*

race did not appear to influence our success rate, but it became an important factor with long-term followup. Five years after treatment, only 32% of cases involving black patients were successful. Although the reasons for this difference are not known, it is possible that blacks had more advanced disease at the time of laser surgery and were therefore more likely to fail with time. Exfoliation syndrome initially had the highest success rate, but between 1½ and 4 years, the success rate decreased markedly. Significantly, Shingleton et al[9] and Wise[10] also found a decreasing success rate with time on long-term followup. Failure seems to occur at the rate of 9% to 15% per year.

These long-term results have served to refine my present indications for laser trabeculoplasty. Initially, ALT was offered only to patients with end-stage glaucoma. However, it is currently the standard of care for all patients with un-controlled, open-angle type glaucoma despite maximally tolerated medical therapy in whom the procedure is likely to be successful. I do not recommend it for patients with juvenile glaucoma, glaucoma secondary to uveitis, or angle recession. ALT is very unlikely to provide patients under 45 years of age with a lifetime cure. A filtering procedure is a more appropriate initial surgical choice for these patients. If patients have significant compliance problems or pressures that are above 40 mm Hg, I also usually recommend initial filtering surgery except for patients who have exfoliation syndrome.

The increasing experience with argon-laser trabeculoplasty has caused me to redefine maximally tolerated medical therapy. Prior to the advent of argon-laser trabeculoplasty, the side effects of medical therapies had to be endured because the major alternative was filterering surgery with its known complications. The risk–benefit ratio of argon-laser trabeculoplasty has made it an attractive early therapy, since increased experience and modification of the technique have reduced the complication of a sustained early pressure elevation.

Many patients no longer need to suffer with the side effects of medical therapy. Patients with an IOP causing progressive visual field loss are placed on full medical therapy, including a beta blocker, miotic, and a short-term trial of a carbonic anhydrase inhibitor (C.A.I.) if not contraindicated. I then schedule a pressure check and possible laser trabeculoplasty two weeks after initiating carbonic anhydrase inhibitor treatment. If the intraocular pressure has responded and the patient is tolerating the C.A.I., I do not perform argon-laser trabeculoplasty. However, if the IOP has not responded or the patient is not tolerating the C.A.I., ALT is performed. Carbonic anhydrase inhibitors are not prescribed for long-term use by patients with unilateral glaucoma, a history of kidney stones, a sulfa allergy, or multiple medical problems requiring diuretics or for patients who appear frail or weakened. Argon-laser trabeculoplasty is employed as a primary treatment modality if topical therapy is not sufficient for these patients.

I do not recommend argon-laser trabeculoplasty in patients who have elevated pressure without any signs of damage to visual function (disc or field changes) or in patients whose pressures are well controlled with tolerated medical therapy. About 1% of the patients will be made worse by argon-laser trabeculoplasty, with pressures higher than they were at baseline; and with time, the success rate of argon-laser trabeculoplasty diminishes. Therefore, I do not want a patient with normal visual function to be at risk of having to undergo filtering surgery because of an untoward effect from premature argon-laser trabeculoplasty.

## SURGICAL TECHNIQUES

Just as the indications have changed during the last twelve years so have the surgical techniques. However, a few important aspects of the technique have not changed, and I feel it is worthwhile to reemphasize them.

Argon trabeculoplasty is performed as an oupatient procedure under topical anesthesia. I prefer the gonioscopic mirror of an antireflected coated 3-mirror lens with a knurled ring. Occasionally I treat a patient with a small palpebral aperture who requires a single-mirror gonioscopic lens. Before initiating treatment, it is critical to identify the angle landmarks: Schwalbe's line, the trabecular meshwork, and the scleral spur. I always start with the gonioscopic mirror at the 12 o'clock position viewing the inferior angle because the inferior angle tends to be the most open and more heavily pigmented, this makes the angle structures easier to define.

In patients with a high iris roll and a prominent Sampaolesi's line (pigment deposition anterior to Schwalbe's line associated with exfoliation syndrome), one can either mistake Sampaolesi's line for the pigmented trabecular meshwork and treat the wrong part of the angle or not recognize an angle closure component. On a few occasions, I have started out planning to do an argon-laser trabeculoplasty; but after more careful study of the angle, I found areas of peripheral anterior synechia or such a narrow approach that I concluded that treating the trabecular meshwork would be difficult. In these eyes, a laser iridectomy is initially performed to treat the narrow angle component or to facilitate a future laser trabeculoplasty. I usually prefer to assess the effect of the iridectomy on intraocular pressure and angle configuration before proceeding with trabeculoplasty.

In patients in whom only a small area of the angle is obscured because of a high iris role, a gonioplasty, as popularized by Simmons is performed.[11] Treatment is directed to the peripheral hump of iris, causing the iris to retract and open.

Some glaucomatologists still advocate treating 360 degrees in one treatment. Initially I treated 360 degrees, but for the last eight years, I have treated 180 degrees and waited 4 weeks before deciding whether to treat the second half. I have found it helpful to use a standardized treatment technique starting with the mirror at the 12 o'clock position and rotating it clockwise. In the right eye I always treat the temporal 180 degrees initially and in the left eye the nasal 180 degrees. If I do not achieve a significant clinical response (i.e., about a 25% lowering of the intraocular pressure in patients with baselines above 20 mm Hg, or a 20% pressure lowering in those with baselines less than 20 mm of Hg) I proceed with the second half of the treatment. Patients are advised that more than 75% of them will require the second half of the treatment at some future point. However, if there are transportation or medical problems and followup visits are difficult, I will treat 270 degrees or 360 degrees at the outset.

In patients with low-tension glaucoma in whom I am trying to maximize the pressure lowering, I sometimes will also treat 360 degrees. In patients with exfoliation, 180-degree treatment often gives an excellent initial clinical response, and offers the opportunity for retreatment if the pressure starts to rise between 1½ and 4 years later. This repeat treatment will often be effective for another period of time.

A continuous-wave argon-laser blue/green light is used, with a 50-micron spot size, $-0.1$ second exposure time, and a power setting between 700 and 1,000 milliwatts (average 850 milliwatts). A power setting is chosen that produces blanching of the pigmented trabecular meshwork or vaporization bubbles at the point of impact. Since our initial report, we have moved the application of the laser energy more anteriorly. Previously we aimed at the center of the pigmented trabecular meshwork band, but now we aim at the anterior border of the junction of the pigmented and nonpigmented trabecular meshwork. This is preferable because Thomas et al reported that the more posterior the treatment, the greater the incidence of pressure elevations.[12] Traverso et al reported that peripheral anterior synechia (PAS) developed in 43% of eyes treated posteriorly but in only 12% of eyes treated anteriorly.[13]

Precise focus of the aiming beam is critical. The aiming beam should be small and round. If the trabecular meshwork cannot be visualized easily, having the patient move his eye in the direction of the gonioscopic mirror often improves visibility.

The Glaucoma Laser Trial (GLT) was designed to minimize the complications of treatment without compromising the long-term pressure-lowering effect. Weinreb et al and other workers have reported that 180-degree treatment of the trabecular meshwork significantly reduces the incidence of an acute pressure rise compared to 360 degrees.[14]

However, despite the GLT protocol requiring placement of laser burns at the anterior border of the pigmented trabecular meshwork and dividing the treatment into two sessions of 180 degrees each, intraocular pressure spikes and the development of PAS were not eliminated.[15] Twelve percent of patients had an IOP rise of more than 10 mm Hg at one or both sessions. These patients were not pretreated with apraclonidine hydrochloride or other nonchronic medical therapy in an attempt to reduce the occurrence of pressure spikes.

I now routinely pretreat patients with significant cupping and visual field loss with apraclonidine hydrochloride, to prevent a significant pressure spike that could adversely affect visual function. Apraclonidine hydrochloride is an alpha-2 agonist that appears to work by decreasing aqueous production. Its effect is additive to beta blockers. Robin et al compared apraclonidine hydrochloride to placebo in 73 eyes receiving 360-degree ALT.[16] None of the eyes receiving apraclonidine hydrochloride had a pressure elevation greater than 10 mm Hg, while 18% of the placebo-treated eyes did. I reinstill the miotic if it has not been used within 2 hours of treatment and routinely monitor the IOP for at least 2 hours after ALT. However, if it is not feasible to monitor patients' IOP postoperatively, it seems prudent to routinely pretreat all patients with apraclonidine hydrochloride. If there is a significant IOP spike, I use an oral osmotic or a carbonic anhydrase inhibitor if not contraindicated for short-term use and if the patient is not already on it. The GLT study found that moderate or heavy pigment seems to be the strongest risk factor for a pressure rise after ALT (P = 0.001). Small-peaked PAS were found in 46% of eyes, and 33% of all eyes with ALT had PAS to the trabecular meshwork. Other possible complications are listed in the box on p. 303.

Dividing the treatment and applying the laser energy to the anterior border of the pigmented trabecular meshwork has almost eliminated the problem of a pressure elevation sustained beyond 24 hours. In my last 500 half-angle argon-laser trabeculoplasty treatments, only one patient has required semiemergent filtering surgery. This may also result from my evolving selection criteria; patients with juvenile glaucoma, uveitis, very high IOPs, or angle-recession are not offered argon-laser trabeculoplasty.

There are some concerns that argon-laser trabeculoplasty could adversely affect the success of future filtering surgery. Richter et al found an increased incidence of encapsulated filtering blebs in eyes with previous ALT.[17] The Advanced Glaucoma Intervention Study has undertaken an ancillary study on encapsulated filtering blebs and will be addressing this possible association in future reports. This is another reason to limit argon-laser trabeculoplasty to those eyes with a good chance for a long-term successful outcome.

Louis Schwartz et al reported on three groups of patients who had 100 burns placed on different parts of the meshwork and two grouups who had 50 burns placed on 180 degrees of the meshwork.[18] When they compared 50 burns spaced over 180 degrees in one eye versus 100 burns for 360 degrees in the other eye of the same group, they found little difference in the response between the two eyes. However, the average followup period was only four months, and differences may appear with longer followup.

## RETREATMENT

Long-term followup has shown a decreasing pressure-lowering effect with time. Since filtering surgery is often the next treatment, the natural question is whether

---

### Complications During and After Argon-Laser Trabeculoplasty

Bleeding
Corneal epithelial opacities
Fainting
Incorrect part of angle treated
Pressure elevation
Iritis
Peripheral anterior synechiae formation

---

repeat ALT will again improve outflow and provide a pressure-lowering effect for a reasonable time. My definition of retreatment involves eyes that have already had 360-degree treatment with a minimum 80 to 90 applications. At the 1982 meeting of the academy, I presented our 4-year experience with ALT, and reported six patients who were retreated after an initial 360-degree treatment.[7] None of these patients achieved a long-term success, and I stopped performing repeat treatment for this reason. Richter et al achieved only 14% incidence of success 21 months postoperative utilizing 180-degree retreatment.[19] Brown, Thomas, and Simmons reported that 12% of the patients were made worse after repeat 360-degree ALT and that only 38% of patients were successful at five months post-operatively.[20] Starita et al reported 17 eyes that had retreatment.[21] They found that 53% of their cases had a reduction but 12% had an increase in intraocular pressure of greater than or equal to 3 mm Hg at an average followup of only 12 weeks. With longer followup, a further decrease in success rate was found. If the long-term success rate equals the short-term complication rate, the therapeutic index does not favor the retreatment in most cases.

The only patients in whom I will perform retreatment are elderly patients with exfoliation syndrome or patients with primary open-angle glaucoma who had an excellent initial response but are poor surgical risks. My goal is to gain 6 to 18 months of additional pressure lowering. The major concern with repeat treatment is that it may cause additional scarring of the meshwork, with a sustained pressure elevation that may require emergency filtering surgery. However, all patients who are being retreated would otherwise require a trabeculectomy, albeit on a less emergent basis.

During this last decade, much work has to be done to evaluate the mechanism of action of ALT. Early reports found an increase in outflow using tonographic measurements. We reported the mean outflow facility in the treated eye was initially 0.10, and at two months post-treatment increased to 0.23, while the outflow facility in the untreated eye was unchanged. Wise proposed that the improvement in intraocular pressure may be due to "increased tension in the trabecular meshwork," with scar tissue contraction at the burn site pulling open the intertrabecular spaces.[22]

Van Buskirk stated the improvement in intraocular pressure control after ALT seems nonspecific for laser characteristics, including wave form, burn location, clock hours treated, and even to some degree laser power.[23] Photocoagulation of the trabecular meshwork focally destroys tissue but diffusely stimulates the mesh-work cells. Alterations in the trabecular meshwork function after laser may contribute to the outflow improvements. Van Buskirk feels that the cellular stimulation may activate a "molecular biological chain of events" within the trabecular extracellular meshwork that promotes improved aqueous outflow. Alexander and Grierson, who have demonstrated a gradual attrition of trabecular cells with age, suggest that this depopulation in the trabecular meshwork is accelerated in eyes with open-angle glaucoma.[24] Laser energy applied to these trabecular cells stimulates these cells to divide more frequently.

The effect of ALT on the trabecular meshwork is really still not fully understood. There may be both a mechanical effect and a biological alteration of the trabeculum. ALT may focally destroy but diffusely stimulate the trabecular tissue.

## THE FUTURE

The development of automated perimetry makes it possible to discover field defects at an earlier stage and to follow glaucoma patients more accurately. Also an improved understanding of glaucomatous damage to the optic nerve and nerve fiber layer and an increased utilization of optic nerve photographs and drawings now enable us to detect progressive damage to the optic nerve head earlier. Patients with glaucoma are being provided with improved care, even though this means that they are undergoing more surgical interventions because we are better able to document progressive damage. These developments, along with the relatively safe alternative to filtering surgery, argon-laser trabeculoplasty, have brought a renewed interest in glaucoma patients.

There have been no long-term evaluations comparing the two principal surgical interventions in advanced glaucoma. We know that argon-laser trabeculoplasty provides short-term success and is less invasive. However, the intraocular pressure-lowering effect may be of limited duration, compliance with medications is still required, and there may be pressure spikes that cause further glaucoma damage. Argon-laser trabeculoplasty may not obviate filtering surgery; it may merely delay it for several years. Recently in my practice and in residency training programs there has been a significant increase in filtering surgery as an increasing number of laser failures have made it necessary. Therefore, it seems important to compare these two surgical interventions.

The Advanced Glaucoma Intervention Study has been funded by The National Eye Institute in order to compare these two modalities. In this multicenter study, patients uncontrolled on maximal medical therapy will be randomized to argon-laser trabeculoplasty or filtering surgery. Automated perimetry will be used to follow patients and to provide information about long-term effects on visual function after medical therapy failure. The study is designed to provide the ophthalmic community with long-term followup information about the procedure that is more efficacious, allowing us to provide our patients optimal surgical management.

Another NIH collaborative study is the Glaucoma Laser Trial. This study is directed at the important question of whether argon-laser trabeculoplasty should be the initial treatment for patients with newly diagnosed primary open-angle glaucoma. This study compares initial ALT to standard medical therapy in previously untreated patients.[25] Patients have one eye randomly assigned to ALT and the other eye assigned to timolol maleate 0.5%. Medications were increased in a stepwise fashion in both the laser-first (LF) and medication-first (MF) eyes according to a set protocol. With two years of followup, the LF eyes had a 1 to 2 mm Hg lower mean IOP than the MF eyes. Fewer LF eyes required 2 or more medications (P < 0.001). Forty-four percent of LF eyes were controlled by ALT alone while 30% of MF eyes were controlled by timolol maleate alone, (P < 0.001), and 89% of LF eyes were controlled within the stepped medication regimen while only 66% of the MF eyes were controlled within the stepped regimen (P < 0.001). There was no significant difference in visual acuity or visual fields between the two groups over the 2-year followup.

On the basis of these results, the authors concluded that "the results of GLT are encouraging regarding the usefulness of ALT as an initial treatment for POAG (p 1412)."[25] Initial ALT seems to provide good pressure control, and it has the advantage of reducing the possibility of the side effects associated with the use of topical medications. The GLT study showed that ALT appears to be safe and effective for newly diagnosed glaucomas with a 2-year followup.

However, it is premature at this time to conclude that argon laser trabeculoplasty should be the initial treatment for all newly diagnosed primary open-angle glaucoma patients who do not have advanced disease, since this study did not address patients with advanced glaucoma. Followup of the GLT patient is continuing, and I think it prudent to wait for reports assessing a longer-term followup to help clarify any differences between the treatment groups. Primary open-angle glaucoma is a chronic disease, and a much longer followup is needed to determine the true benefit of initial ALT.

I think this report will nevertheless influence ophthalmologists to consider ALT earlier then they might have previously. In addition to its safety and efficacy, it is fascinating to patients, who are very accepting of having it performed. It is to be hoped that easy patient acceptance and the financial remuneration associated with the performance of argon-laser trabeculoplasty will not cloud the treating ophthalmologists' judgment regarding the changing role of this surgical technique in early glaucoma management.

During this last decade, argon-laser trabeculoplasty has achieved a preeminent position in the surgical management of the glaucoma patient with uncontrolled open-angle glaucoma. The followup of patients in the AGIS and GLT studies will help to determine its role in the next decade. It is also probable that other new techniques using laser energy to make a sclerostomy will be further refined and developed. The only certain thing is that there will be new and exciting developments to help our patients and to challenge our thinking. For this we are all grateful.

## Acknowledgments

I would like to thank Dr. Lucian Del Priore for reviewing the manuscript and Pat Kammann for her manuscript preparation.

## References


1. Krasnov MM. Laseropuncture of anterior chamber angle in glaucoma. Am J Ophthalmol 1973; 75:674-678.
2. Worthen DM, Wickham MG. Argon laser trabeculoplasty. Trans Am Acad Ophthalmol Otolaryngol 1974; 78:371-375.
3. Gaasterland D, Kupfer C. Experimental glaucoma in the Rhesus monkey. Invest Ophthalmol Vis Sci 1974; 14:455-457.
4. Schwartz AL, Whitten ME, Bleiman B, Martin D. Argon laser trabecular surgery in uncontrolled phakic open angle glaucoma. Ophthalmol 1981; 88:203-212.
5. Wise JB. Long-term control of adult open angle glaucoma by argon laser treatment. Ophthalmol 1981; 88:197-202.
6. Wilensky JT, Jampol LM. Laser therapy for open angle glaucoma. Ophthalmol 1981; 88:213-217.
7. Schwartz AL, Kopelman J. Four-year experience with argon laser trabecular surgery in uncontrolled open-angle glaucoma. Ophthalmol 1983; 90:771-780.
8. Schwartz AL, Love DL, Schwartz MA. Long-term follow-up of argon laser trabeculoplasty for uncontrolled open angle glaucoma. Arch Ophthalmol 1985; 103:1482-1484.
9. Shingleton BJ, Richter CU, Bellows AR, Hutchinson BT, Glynn RJ. Long-term efficacy of argon laser trabeculoplasty. Ophthalmol 1987; 94:1513-1518.
10. Wise JB. Ten year results of laser trabeculoplasty: does the laser avoid glaucoma surgery or merely defer it? Eye 1987; 1:45-50.
11. Simmons RJ, Kimbrough RL, Belcher CD, Dulit RA. Laser gonioplasty for special problems in angle closure glaucoma. In Trans New Orleans Acad Ophthalmol, St Louis, 1981, CV Mosby, pp 220-235.
12. Thomas JV, Simmons RJ, Belcher CD. Complications of argon laser trabeculoplasty. Glaucoma 1982; 4:50-52.
13. Traverso CE, Greenidge KC, Spaeth GL. Formation of peripheral anterior synechiae following argon laser trabeculoplasty. Arch Ophthalmol 1984; 102:861-863.
14. Weinreb RN, Ruderman J, Juster R, Zweig K. Immediate intraocular pressure response to argon laser trabeculoplasty. Am J Ophthalmol 1983; 95:279-286.
15. Glaucoma Laser Trial Research Group. The glaucoma laser trial. I. Acute effects of argon laser trabeculoplasty on intraocular pressure. Arch Ophthalmol 1989; 107:1135-1142.
16. Robin AL, Pollack IP, House B, Enger C. Effects of ALO 2145 on intraocular pressure following argon laser trabeculoplasty. Arch Ophthalmol 1987; 105:646-650.
17. Richter CU, Shingleton BJ, Bellows AR, Hutchinson BT, O'Connor T, Brill I. The development of encapsulated filtering blebs. Ophthalmol 1988; 95:1163-1168.
18. Schwartz LW, Spaeth GL, Traverso C, Greenidge KC. Variation of techniques on the results of argon laser trabeculoplasty. Ophthalmol 1983; 90:781-784.
19. Richter CU, Shingleton BJ, Bellows AR, Hutchinson BT, Jacobson LP. Retreatment with argon laser trabeculoplasty. Ophthalmol 1987; 94:1085-1089.
20. Brown SVL, Thomas JV, Simmons RJ. Laser trabeculoplasty re-treatment. Am J Ophthalmol 1985; 99:8-10.
21. Starita RJ, Fellman RL, Spaeth GL, Poryzees E. The effect of repeating full-circumference argon laser trabeculoplasty. Ophthalmic Surg 1984; 15:41-43.
22. Wise JB, Witter SL. Argon laser therapy for open-angle glaucoma—a pilot study. Arch Ophthalmol 1979; 97:319-322.
23. Van Buskirk EM. Pathophysiology of laser trabeculoplasty. Surv Ophthalmol 1989; 33(4):264-72.
24. Alexander RA, Grierson I. Morphological effects of argon laser trabeculoplasty upon the glaucomatous human meshwork. Eye 1989; 3:719-726.
25. The Glaucoma Laser Trial Research Group. The glaucoma laser trial (GLT). II. Results of argon laser trabeculoplasty verus topical medicines. Ophthalmol 1990; 97(11):1403-1413.

# 25 Laser Iridotomies: Then and Now

Irvin P. Pollack, MD

Irvin P. Pollack, MD

......................................................................................................

## THEN

Although lasers have been employed in medical research for more than 35 years, use of laser energy to treat glaucoma did not come into widespread practice until the 1980s. A variety of lasers have had a major impact on the way we treat the disease, and the use of laser energy continues to evolve as a significant method for treatment of many forms of glaucoma.

Before 1973, angle-closure glaucoma was routinely treated with a surgical iridectomy.* A small piece of peripheral iris was excised through a limbal-corneal incision or through a subconjunctival scleral incision just posterior to the limbus, and the patient was routinely hospitalized for 2 to 4 days. Outpatient laser iridotomy* was a revolutionary concept and gained acceptance slowly.[1-3]

Research and development have produced new lasers with different wavelengths and new techniques for delivering the laser energy, as well as new ways to create the iridotomy itself. We have come to recognize and respect the possible complications, and we take steps to avoid them wherever possible. Techniques to produce the desired lesion have evolved to the point where they allow us to make a satisfactory iridotomy in less time and with less expenditure of energy than previously.

## Synopsis of Original Work

Following the adaptation of the continuous-wave (c-w) argon laser to the slit lamp,[4] the argon laser soon became available in most centers of ophthalmic research, mainly for treatment of retinal disease.[4-6] Having a wavelength of 455-515 nm, the blue-green beam was transmitted by the optical system of the eye with relatively low absorption, while the quality of its burn was dependent on the presence of pigment and melanin (Figure 25-1). Its focusing quality made it wellsuited not only for the treatment of retinal vascular disease and retinal detachment but also for creation of iridotomies.

---

*By convention, laser photocoagulation of an iris hole is referred to as laser iridotomy while excision of an iris opening is a surgical iridectomy. (Laser Peripheral Iridotomy for Pupillary-Block Glaucoma. In Information about Eye Care, AAO Bulletin, June 25, 1988.)

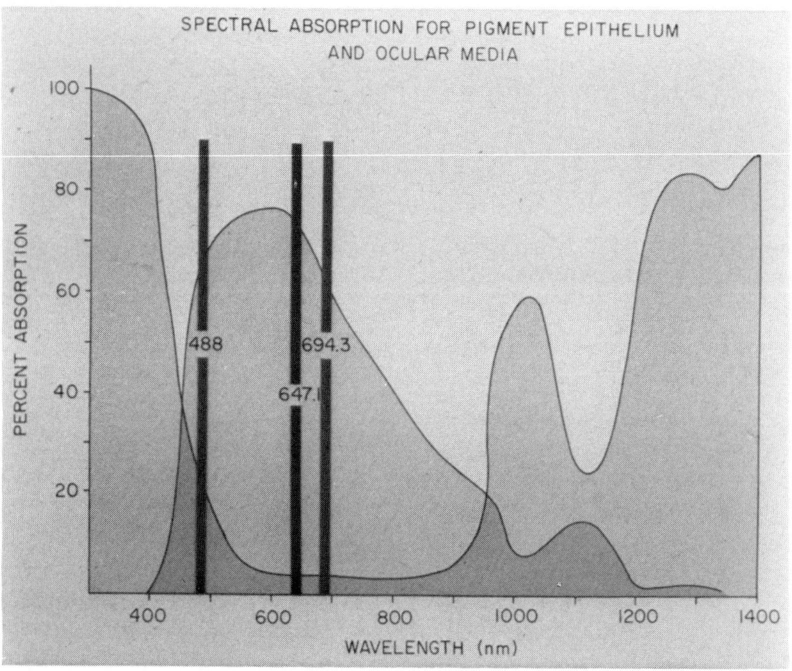



**FIGURE 25-1**    Laser energy is selectively absorbed by different tissues depending on wavelength. Melanin absorbs energy between 400 and 800 nm; therefore, argon blue-green (488 nm), krypton (647 nm), and ruby (694 nm) lasers are effective coagulators of the iris pigment epithelium. These same wavelengths are little absorbed by the ocular media. *(Adapted from Geeraets WJ, Williams RS, Chan G, et al. The relative absorption of thermal energy in retina and choroid. Invest Ophthalmol 1962; 1:340-347.)*

Using the continuous-wave (c-w) argon laser, iridotomies were successfully performed in monkeys,[7] Dutch-belted rabbits,[8] and in humans.[9-11] Spot sizes of 50 microns and powers of up to 1.5 watts for 0.2 to 0.5 seconds were used to perforate the iris after a series of burns at the same site.[12] Retreatment was occasionally required either because the iridotomy could not be completed during the first treatment session or because of subsequent closure.

## Laser Iridotomies

A major disadvantage of (c-w) argon lasers was that the long pulse (0.2-0.5 seconds) often produced a thermal insult to the overlying cornea and underlying lens. With shorter pulses, there occurred a corresponding reduction in heat loss from the target site to the other tissues. This resulted in greater focal rise in temperature and vaporization of the target tissue.[13] Although the pulsed ruby laser utilized these advantages and was very effective in vaporizing a hole in the brown iris, its weaker effect in the blue iris left something to be desired.[3] For this reason, there developed increased interest in a pulsed argon laser that was introduced as a tool not only to treat retinal disease but also to produce iridotomies with less thermal spread.

Early experience with the pulsed argon laser revealed that one could not produce a satisfactory iris burn with frequencies below 400 pulses per second when using the maximum available power of 3 watts.[12] With these high pulse repetition rates, the laser's effect on the iris, its associated side effects, and the ease with which the iridotomy could be produced were similar to those observed with a c-w argon laser.[12]

## DEVELOPMENT OF NEW IDEAS
### Techniques with the Argon Laser

In nearly every case, an iridotomy can easily be performed with powers of 1000 mW or less, using 0.2-second, 50-micron pulses.[14] Furthermore, with experience, a carefully made iridotomy can usually be completed with 1 to 50 burns (Figure 25-2). In some cases, as much as 1500 mW may be required, but longer pulses and more than 100 burns are likely to produce undesirable complications (see below).

A thick dark brown "velvety" iris or a light pigmented blue iris may be more difficult to penetrate with the argon laser, and modifications to the conventional technique have been described. The nonpigmented stroma of the blue iris is relatively transparent to argon laser light energy and poorly penetrated. On the other hand, the dark brown iris usually has a thick stroma, the anterior layers of which tend to shrink and char following argon laser application, and this seems to block any further laser effect. Several investigators have recommended the use of long-duration burns (0.5 to 1.0 second) combined with high power[15] or low power[16] to penetrate such difficult irides. The use of high power, particularly in combination with long pulses, is likely to produce many complications including corneal burns and large areas of iris atrophy (see the discussion of long-term considerations). Long pulses are likely to produce large burns on the iris because the Bell's phenomenon occurs between 0.2 and 0.5 seconds after the laser flash.

Other investigators have suggested the use of short-duration burns to "chip" the iris and avoid heat shrinkage.[16-19] This technique requires up to 250 applications of 1000-2000 mW using 50-micron spots for 0.01-0.05 seconds. Wise modified the short-duration technique by burning a 500-micron-long linear iridotomy parallel to the limbus across the radial fibers.[20]

---

### YAG Laser Iridotomy

The argon laser iridotomy is an effective and safe procedure,[21] but it is frequently accompanied by thermal burns to the anterior segment producing corneal endothelial opacities. Sometimes there is tissue destruction of the iris and the production of focal opacities of the lens behind the iridotomy. It is difficult to create an argon laser iridotomy in either lightly or heavily pigmented irides, in patients with nystagmus or head tremors, and in elderly patients who cannot maintain a steady head position and fixation.[22-24]

Earlier work with the Q-switched ruby laser revealed that pulsed lasers, from which energy was released as a large short pulse of light lasting only 10-20 nanoseconds, could punch a hole in even a thick iris by photodisruption rather than photocoagulation.[25-27] However, the neodymium (Nd):YAG laser has the distinct advantage over the Q-switch ruby laser in that it is smaller in size, less expensive, more reliable, and easier to use.

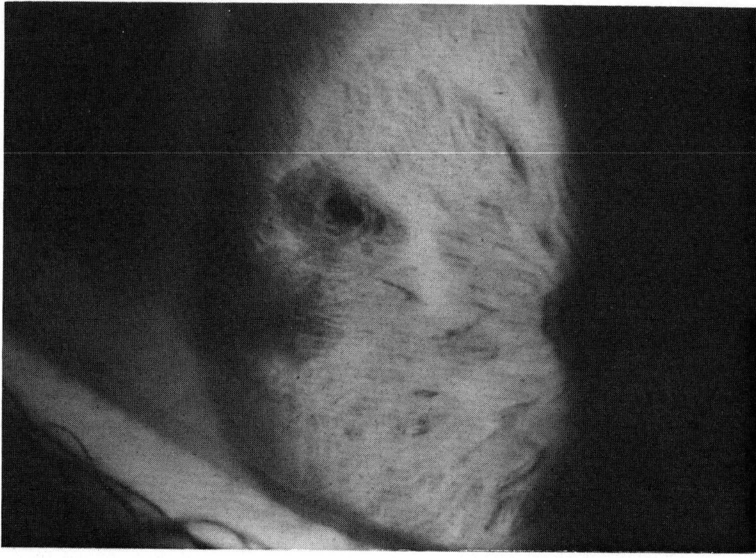

**FIGURE 25-2**   An argon laser iridotomy can usually be completed with less than 50 burns using 1,000 mw for 0.2 second with a 50-micron spot.

The Nd:YAG laser, like the Q-switched ruby laser, can reliably produce an iridotomy with fewer pulses and less energy.[24] In some cases, it is effective when argon laser iridotomy fails.[23] On the other hand, bleeding from the iridotomy site is a common complication and a major concern (Figure 25-3). Iris bleeding is more likely to occur in an inflamed eye; and many surgeons still prefer the argon laser iridotomy where bleeding almost never occurs, reserving Nd:YAG iridotomy for argon laser failures. One can also pretreat the site with the argon laser before completing the iridotomy with the YAG laser.

The Nd:YAG iridotomy usually can be completed with less than 5 double pulses (pulse train of 2) and 3-10 mJ.[24] The amount of total energy delivered is greater for brown irides than for blue. The long-term followup studies indicate that Nd:YAG iridotomy is as safe as argon iridotomy.[28]

## Effect of Various Wavelengths

The blue-green argon laser (455-515 nm) and the near infrared Nd:YAG laser (1064 nm) are the most commonly used wavelengths for creating an iridotomy. However, other lasers employing different wavelengths have been investigated.

The krypton laser (647 nm) has been successfully employed in the treatment of maculopathies. Our early experience with this (unpublished data) suggests that laser iridotomies can be produced using parameters similar to those employed with the c-w argon laser, but the maximum available power of approximately 800 mW is less than ideal in many cases. On the other hand, Yassur and coworkers achieved 100% success using exposure times of 0.01-0.04 second and 5 micron spots.[29] A major advantage of the krypton laser is that its wavelength is poorly absorbed by the cornea and lens.

An ideal laser might certainly be one that allowed any desirable wavelength to be dialed into use. Such a laser would produce a pulsed wavelength that could

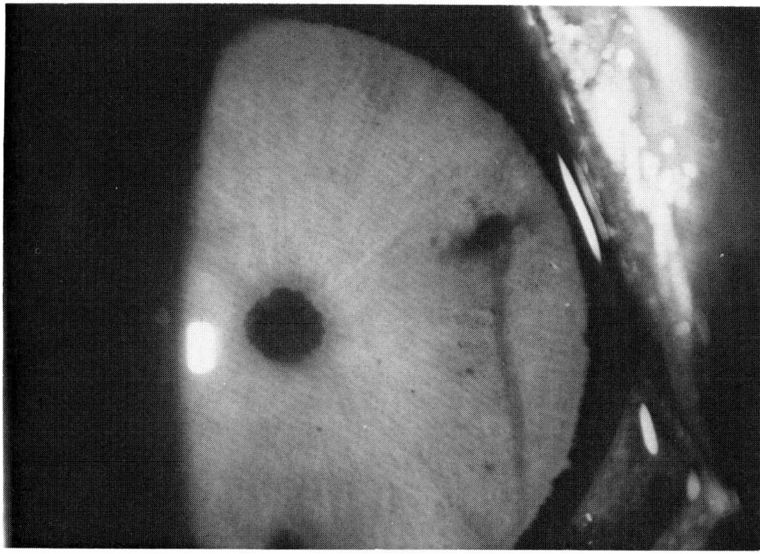

**FIGURE 25-3**    Bleeding that may occur from the iridotomy site is usually a minor complication although a major concern. *(Dragon DM, Robin AL, Pollack IP, et al. Neodymium: YAG laser iridotomy in the cynomolgus monkey. Invest Ophthalmol 1985; 26:789-796.)*

be completely transmitted by the cornea and completely picked up by the iris to produce an iridotomy with a single burst.[13] Wishart and Hitchings produced iridotomies with a pulsed dye laser using the organic dye, rhodamine 6G, and having a wavelength of 600 nm emitted in 3 microsecond pulses. A single burst of 41-65 mJ resulted in a patent iridotomy in 79% of cases. Although the iridotomies were larger than YAG iridotomies, there was a lower success rate, more bleeding, pigment dispersion and lens damage.[30]

The semiconductor diode laser (810 nm) may be another alternative. It has been shown to have a success and complication rate similar to that of the argon laser when used to produce iridotomies in rabbit eyes.[31]

## Long-Term Considerations

### Visual Acuity

In view of the fact that iridotomies made with the argon or Nd:YAG laser may cause localized damage to the underlying lens, it is only natural that we be concerned about gradual decrease in visual acuity due to cataract formation. However, this has not been easy to assess. Cataract formation with visual acuity loss is not at all unusual in an eye that has had an acute attack of glaucoma. Therefore, any assessment of the effect of laser surgery on visual acuity should include only normal eyes on which a laser iridotomy was performed prophylactically. Such a prospective, controlled, age-matched series is lacking. One five-year retrospective study showed evidence of visual acuity loss that compared closely to that of a normal office population over 45 years of age.[32]

One can find localized lens opacities following Nd:YAG laser iridotomy, but these too do not appear to lead to an increased rate of visual loss from clinically significant cataract formation.[33]

### Glaucoma

Postoperative pressure elevation within the first 3 hours after laser iridotomy is a potentially major problem because a rise in IOP greater than 10 mm Hg is not unusual. The current standard treatment of one drop of apraclonidine 1% one hour before and immediately after treatment will nearly always prevent this pressure rise and in many cases produce a fall in IOP (Figure 25-4).[34]

Postoperative IOP control has not been found to be significantly different in eyes treated with laser iridotomy and those treated with surgical iridectomy. More important, no eyes with a normal preoperative IOP had an elevated postoperative IOP five years after the treatment.[32] This has been corroborated by other clinical studies showing no tendency for late postoperative rises in IOP.[35-36]

One might be more concerned about the possibility of postoperative long-term rise in IOP following Nd:YAG laser iridotomy because of the high frequency of bleeding. Nevertheless, eyes with transient bleeding did not exhibit a higher incidence of IOP spikes, and Nd:YAG-treated eyes (with or without bleeding) did not require more medications or more surgical procedures for IOP control.[33]

A rather common finding, even 10 years after argon laser iridotomy, is the presence of pigment in the inferior trabecular meshwork. Studies of monkey eyes revealed no alteration in the facility of aqueous outflow 6 months after laser iridotomy and no ultrastructural alterations in the trabecular meshwork 12 months after treatment.[37]

### The Iridotomy

Although nearly all the iridotomies remain patent, about 30% of argon laser iridotomies show some tendency toward closure with regeneration of pigment epithelium across the opening. The same occasionally occurs after Nd:YAG iridotomy. If the iridotomy remains patent for six weeks, it generally remains permanently patent unless the eye suffers from recurrent uveitis or other inflammatory insult.

Iris necrosis is not uncommon following laser iridotomy, and it is much more common following argon laser iridotomy using long pulses. Pulses of 0.5 second are frequently associated with extensive iris necrosis around the iridotomy. The result is eventual enlargement of the iridotomy to form rather large and obvious openings (Figure 25-5).

### Posterior synechiae

Posterior synechiae frequently follow laser iridotomy and are often encountered in cases where miotics are employed for pressure control of chronic angle closure. These can be minimized by dilating the pupil soon after laser iridotomy has been performed, and repeating the dilation at periodic intervals during long-term miotic use.

## NOW

Both the argon and Nd:YAG lasers are widely available. Each is commonly used to make iridotomies for treating angle-closure glaucoma. In many cases, the laser of choice will depend on its availability and the level of comfort enjoyed by the surgeon with that laser.

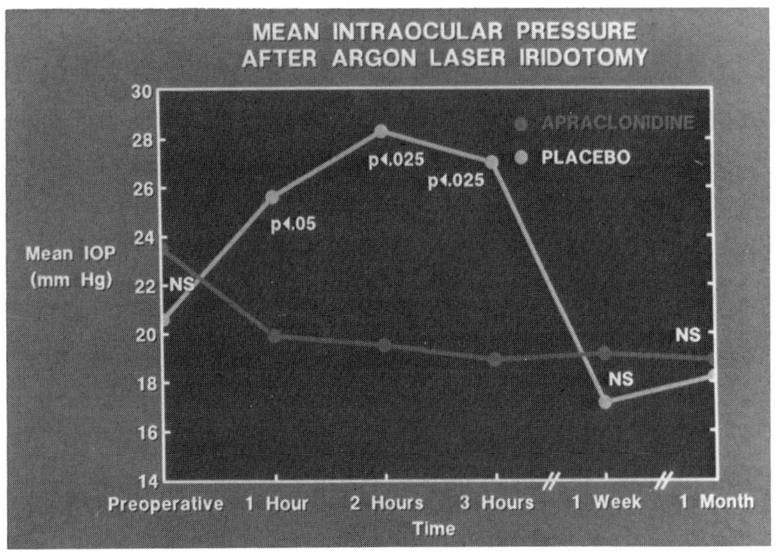


**FIGURE 25-4**    Line graph comparing mean IOP of apraclonidine- (dark line) and placebo- (light line) treated eyes following laser iridotomy. During the first 3 postoperative hours, eyes treated with apraclonidine had lower mean IOPs than eyes treated with placebo. There is no significant difference in the mean IOPs one week and one month after laser treatment. *(From Robin AL, Pollack IP, Defaller JM. Effects of topical ALO 2145 [p-aminoclonidione hydrochloride] in the acute intraocular pressure rise after argon laser iridotomy. Arch Ophthalmol 1987; 105:1208-1211.)*

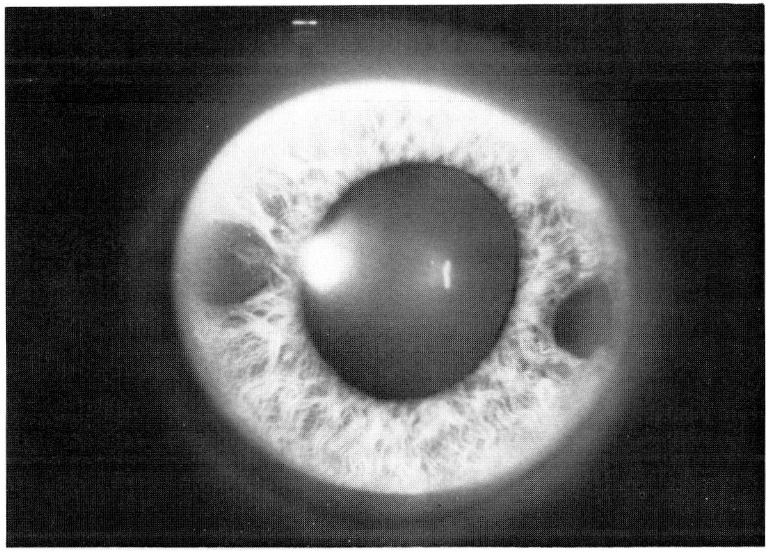

**FIGURE 25-5**    Use of an excessive number of burns with high powers and long pulses of 0.5 second are likely to cause stromal necrosis of the iris and progressive enlargement of the iridotomy over a period of years. *(From Pollack IP. Current concepts in laser iridotomy. Inter Ophthalmol Clinics 1984; 24:153-180.)*

Our experience has clearly shown that laser iridotomy is a relatively safe procedure, free of any major short-term or long-term side effects. Nevertheless, important facts we have gleaned over the years should be recognized.

When using the argon laser, one should treat the peripheral iris where there is less tendency to cause deflection of the pupil. Because of the anterior curvature of the lens, one is also less likely to produce posterior synechiae or focal cataracts in a peripherally placed iridotomy. At the same time, one should not remain within the arcus, because this may scatter the laser light. One should aim for iris crypts or thinner areas if they are in the periphery. However, if after 4 or 5 burns the iris reacts poorly to the laser light, then one should move to another spot. The iridotomy should be made superiorly where it is more likely to be covered by the upper eyelid. The Abraham contact lens is very helpful because it promotes ocular stability and increases the energy density and magnification to make the procedure easier. Extreme care should be made to aim away from the posterior pole. Nearly all argon iridotomies can be completed with fewer than 50 burns.

The Nd:YAG laser, which can produce an iridotomy faster, with less energy, and with fewer side effects than the argon laser, has become our first choice in routine cases. One nevertheless encounters eyes on which iridotomies cannot be performed with the Nd:YAG laser, and if 2 or 3 sites cannot be penetrated, one should switch to the argon laser without hesitation. There are definitely eyes that respond better to the argon less than to the Nd:YAG laser.

The argon laser may find the lightly pigmented blue iris difficult to penetrate while the Nd:YAG laser may make an effective iridotomy with one or two burns. Similarly the thick velvety dark brown iris that responds to intensive argon laser energy with little more than a char may be easily punctured with the Nd:YAG laser.

On the other hand, the argon laser should be used whenever the iris touches or comes close to the cornea. Then light laser burns of 200-400 mW cause the dilator muscle to contract and draw the iris away from the overlying cornea making it possible to avoid corneal damage with subsequent treatment. We prefer the argon laser to treat the inflamed eye because Nd:YAG iridotomy is more likely to produce not only a hyphema but a tremendous outpouring of protein into the aqueous.

The ease with which an iridotomy can be made with any laser is partly dependent on iris color and thickness, corneal tolerance and deturgessence, anterior chamber depth, patient cooperation, and instrument quality. However, the rate of success also depends in large measure on the surgeon's skill and experience. This human factor of acquired skill and experience should not be underestimated.

## References

1. Zweng HC, Flocks M, Kapany NS, et al. Experimental laser photocoagulation. Am J Ophthalmol 1964; 58:353-362.
2. Snyder WB. Laser coagulation of the anterior segment. I. Experimental laser iridotomy. Arch Ophthalmol 1967; 77:93-98.
3. Beckman H, Barraco R, Sugar HS, et al. Laser iridotomies. Am J Ophthalmol 1971; 72:393-402.
4. Zweng HC. Lasers in ophthalmology. In Wolbarscht ML, ed, Laser application in medicine and biology, New York, 1971, Plenum Press, pp 239-254.

5. L'Esperance FA Jr. An ophthalmic argon laser photocoagulation system: design, construction and laboratory investigations. Trans Am Ophthalmol Soc 1968; 66:827-904.

6. Patz A, Maumenee AE, Ryan SJ. Argon laser photocoagulation: advantages and limitations. Trans Am Acad Ophthalmol Otolaryngol 1971; 75:569-579.

7. Zweng HC, Paris GL, Vassiliadis A, et al. Laser photocoagulation of the iris. Arch Ophthalmol 1970; 84:193-199.

8. Khuri CH. Argon laser iridotomies. Am J Ophthalmol 1973; 76:490-493.

9. Hager H: Besondere mikrochirurgische Eingriffe. 2. Teil erste Erfahrungen mit dem Argon-Laser-Geraet 800. Klin Monatsbl Angenheilkd 1973; 162:437-450.

10. Abraham RK, Miller GL. Outpatient argon laser iridectomy for angle closure glaucoma: a two-year study. Trans Am Acad Ophthalmol Otolaryngol 1975; 79:529-538.

11. Pollack IP, Patz A: Argon laser iridotomy: an experimental and clinical study. Ophthalmic Surg 1976; 7:22-30.

12. Pollack IP. Use of argon laser energy to produce iridotomies. Trans Am Ophthalmol Soc 1979; 77:674-706.

13. Wheeler CB. Laser iridectomy. Phys Med Biol 1977; 22:1115-1135.

14. Pollack IP. Use of argon laser energy to produce iridotomies. Ophthalmic Surg 1980; 11:506-515.

15. Hoskins HD, Migliazzo CV. Laser iridectomy—a technique for blue irises. Ophthalmic Surg 1984; 15:488.

16. Ritch R, Palmberg P. Argon laser iridectomy in densely pigmented irides. Am J Ophthalmol 1982; 93:800.

17. Litwin RL. Argon laser iridotomy. technique in black people. Ophthalmol 1979, 86:137 (abstract).

18. Yassur Y, Melamed S, Cohen S, Ben-Sira I: Laser iridotomy in closed-angle glaucoma. Arch Ophthalmol 1979; 97:1920-1921.

19. Mandelkorn RM, Mendelsohn AD, Olander KW, Zimmerman TJ. Short exposure times in argon laser iridotomy. Ophthalmic Surg 1981; 12:805-809.

20. Wise JB. Iris sphincterotomy, iridotomy, and synechiotomy by linear incision with the argon laser. Ophthalmol 1985; 92:641.

21. Robin AL, Pollack IP. Argon laser peripheral iridotomies in the treatment of primary angle-closure glaucoma: long-term follow-up. Arch Ophthalmol 1982; 100:919-923.

22. Klapper EM. Q-switched neodymium:YAG laser iridotomy in closed-angle glaucoma. Ophthalmol 1984; 91:1017-1021.

23. Robin AL, Pollack IP. Q-switched neodymium:YAG laser iridotomy in patients in whom the argon laser fails. Arch Ophthalmol 1986; 104:531-535.

24. Robin AL, Pollack IP. A comparison of neodymium:YAG and argon laser iridotomies. Ophthalmol 1984; 91:1011-1016.

25. Krasnov MM. Q-switched ("cool") lasers in ophthalmology. Int Ophthalmol Clin 1976; 16:29-44.

26. Bonney CH, Gaasterland DE. Low-energy Q-switched ruby laser iridotomies in Maccaca mulatta. Invest Ophthalmol Vis Sci 1979; 18:278-287.

27. Pollack IP, Robin AL. Iridotomies in cynomolgus monkeys using a Q-switched ruby laser. Trans Am Ophthalmol Soc 1980; 78:88-106.

28. Del Priore LV, Robin AL, Pollack IP. Neodymium:YAG and argon laser iridotomy: long-term follow-up in a prospective, randomized clinical trial. Ophthalmol 1988; 95:1207-1211.

29. Yassur Y, David R, Rosenblat I, Marmour U. Iridotomy with grid krypton laser. Brit J Ophthalmol 1986; 70:295-297.

30. Wishart PK, Hitchings RA. Neodymium YAG and dye laser iridotomy—a comparative study. Trans Ophthal Soc UK 1986; 105:521-540.

31. Jacobson JJ, Schuman JS, Koumy HE, Puliafito CA. Diode laser peripheral iridectomy. Int Ophthalmol Clin 1990; 30:120.

32. Robin AL, Pollack IP. Argon laser peripheral iridotomies in the treatment of primary angle-closure glaucoma: long-term follow-up. Arch Ophthalmol 1982; 100:919-923.

33. Del Priore LV, Robin AL, Pollack IP. Neodymium :YAG and argon laser iridotomy: long-term follow-up in a prospective randomized clinical trial. Ophthalmol 1988; 95:1207-1211.

34. Robin AL, Pollack IP, DeFaller JM. Effects of topical ALO 2145 (p-aminoclonidine hydrochloride) on the acute intraocular pressure rise after argon laser iridotomy. Arch Ophthalmol 1987; 105:1208-1211.

35. Quigley HA. Long-term follow-up of laser iridotomy. Ophthalmol 1981; 88:218-224.

36. Abraham RK, Miller GL. Outpatient argon laser iridectomies for angle-closure glaucoma. A 3½ year study. Adv Ophthalmol 1977; 34:186-191.

37. Robin AL, Pollack IP, Quigley HA, D'Anna S, Addicks EM. Histologic studies of angle structures after laser iridotomy in primates. Arch Ophthalmol 1982; 100:1665-1670.

# 26 Retinopathy of Prematurity

**Arnall Patz, MD**

The retinopathy of prematurity (ROP), first correlated with prematurity by Terry in the early 1940s, within a decade became the largest cause of blindness in children in the United States and a major cause of blindness throughout the developed world. Terry originally designated the condition retrolental fibroplasia, based on his impression that the pathogenesis involved a proliferation of the embryonic hyaloid system that incorporated the retina.[43] As the basic process was clarified, the term *retinopathy of prematurity* has been generally adopted.

A large number of publications on ROP including several excellent monographs,[8,12,26,38] have appeared in the past decade. They include articles on current concepts of the pathogenesis of ROP, with attention given to the possible role of the spindle cells (Kretzer), to angiogenic substances and their inhibitors (Glaser), and to the physiology of developing retinal vessels and their response to oxygen (Flower), with the suggestion that the oxygen-induced marked vasoconstriction in the immature retina may be a defensive mechanism to protect it from elevated oxygen tensions.

The sophisticated management of the current CRYO-ROP study, compared to the multicenter study chaired by the late V. E. Kinsey[19] in the 1950s, reflects the progress made in controlled clinical trials. Indeed, Kinsey's cooperative study is one of the very early major multicenter clinical trials in American medicine. This early study documented the role of the *duration* of excess oxygen exposure as the major cause of ROP. There were no plans, nor experience to pursue the many leads and questions raised by the study results. It is also regrettable that at the time of the incrimination of excess incubator oxygen arterial blood gas measurement capability was not available, so that an unnecessarily large number of premature infants died or sustained brain damage as a result of rigid curtailment of oxygen that dramatically reduced the blindness from ROP. Flynn et al documented for the first time that not only the duration of exposure to oxygen but also the blood *level* of oxygen is a contributing factor to the development of ROP.[11]

During the epidemic of ROP in 1950s, the survival rate of premature infants with birth weights under 1,000 g was less than 10%. With the advent of the specialty of neonatology and the general availability of mechanical ventilation and other new technologies, the survival of low-birth-weight infants has increased significantly.

The most comprehensive review of survival was reported by Phelps et al from the CRYO/ROP study.[33] They noted during 1986 and 1987 that the 28-day survival for infants with birth weights of 500 g through 599 g was 30% while for

<table>
<tr><td colspan="3" align="center">Premature Infant Survival Rate</td></tr>
<tr><td>Year</td><td>Birth weight</td><td>Survival rate</td></tr>
<tr><td>1950</td><td><1,000 g</td><td>8%</td></tr>
<tr><td>1986-1987</td><td>500-599 g</td><td>30%</td></tr>
<tr><td></td><td>1,200-1,250 g</td><td>91%</td></tr>
</table>

Adapted from Phelps DL, Brown DR, Tung B. 28-day Survival rates of 6676 neonates with birth weights of 1250 grams or less. Pediatrics 1991; 87:7-17.

---

**Mechanism of Oxygen Action on the Immature Retina**

Primary Effect
   Vasoconstriction
   Vascular closure
Secondary Effect
   Neovascularization

---

those with birth weights 1,200 g through 1,250 g the survival rate was 91%. Gestational age was also found to be a highly significant predictor for survival, as shown in the upper box above.

The increased survival of extremely small premature infants, those with the most immaturely vascularized retinas, has produced a new population of infants at the highest risk of developing ROP; and indeed a significant number of new cases are occurring annually. These new cases are occurring in spite of meticulous monitoring of blood oxygen levels. Therefore a renewed interest in the identification of other potential factors contributing to the etiology and the investigation of methods of prophylaxis is being actively pursued in conjunction with further improvement in therapy.

## MECHANISM OF OXYGEN EFFECT

Since there is a renewed interest in possible treatment with oxygen of the early retinal neovascularization in acute ROP, an explanation of the presumed mechanism of oxygen action is appropriate. Experimental animal studies in the 1950s demonstrated that the primary effect of oxygen on immature retinal vessels is advanced vasoconstriction and subsequent vascular closure.[2,30] After removal from oxygen, neovascularization resulted. The degree of vascular closure and the subsequent degree of retinal neovascularization were directly proportional to the duration and concentration of oxygen and inversely proportional to the degree of maturity of the retinal vessels, as shown in the lower box above.

The animal models demonstrated that only the incompletely vascularized retina was susceptible to oxygen. These findings were consistent with the clinical observations that the premature infant with a more immature retina has a greater susceptibility to ROP. The infant with a fully vascularized retina has no risk of

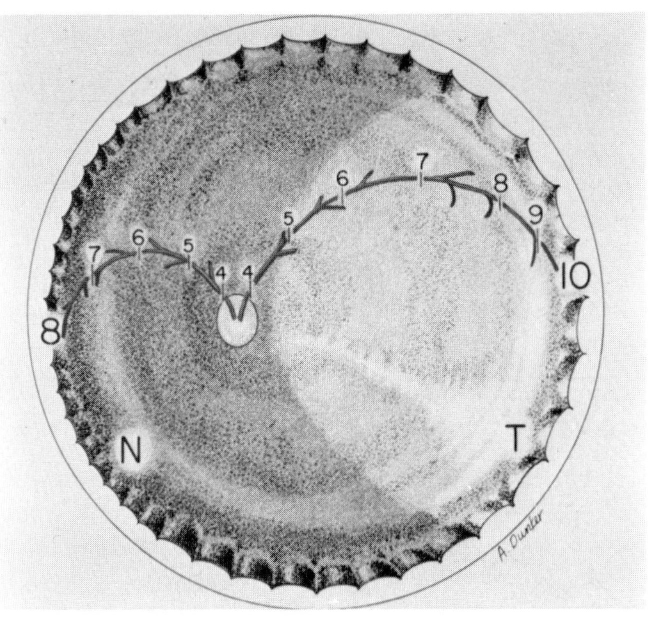


**FIGURE 26-1**    Schematic diagram of retinal vessel development in man. At 4 months gestation, vessels grow from the disc, reaching the ora serrata nasally at 8 months and temporally shortly after term. The vascularization of the newborn kitten corresponds to that of the human fetus at 6½ months gestation. *(From Patz A, Palmer EA: Retinopathy of prematurity. In Ryan SJ, ed, The retina, St Louis, 1989, Mosby–Year Book, p 510. Used with permission of author and publisher.)*

ROP. The predilection of the temporal retina for ROP, the last part of the retina to become vascularized, can also be explained on this basis (Figure 26-1).

An understanding of this mechanism suggests the rationale for the potential use of carefully monitored supplemental oxygen as a therapeutic agent in the early neovascular stages of ROP. This concept is discussed further in the section on STOP-ROP.

## International Classification of ROP

The international classification of ROP was reported in 1984. The retina is divided into three zones and the extent of disease by the meridians (hours of the clock) involved. The retinal changes are divided into four stages.[5]

The 3 zones are centered on the optic disc instead of the macula, as is the usual practice in standard retinal drawings (Figure 26-2). Zone I, the posterior pole, is a circle centered on the disc that subtends an arc of 60 degrees. It extends from the disc to twice the distance from the disc to the center of the macula, in all directions from the disc. Zone II extends from the peripheral border of Zone I to a circle tangential to the nasal ora serrata and temporally responds approximately to the anatomic equator. Zone III, which is the farthest from the disc, is the last to become vascularized and is most frequently involved with ROP.

### Extent of ROP

The extent of the ROP changes is specified by the hours of the clock involved.

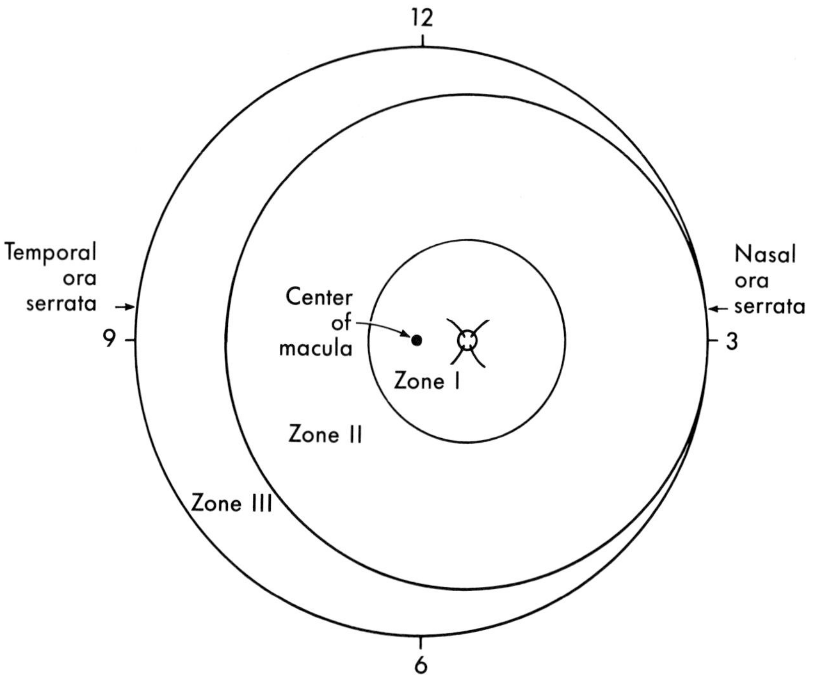


**FIGURE 26-2**   Schematic diagram showing the zones and clock hours of the retina that were adopted in the international classification of ROP to describe the location and extent of ROP. Note that Zone I is centered on the disc, in contrast to the usual retinal drawing in which the posterior zone is centered on the macula. *(Modified from Patz A, Palmer EA. Retinopathy of prematurity. In Ryan SJ, ed, The retina, St Louis, 1989, Mosby–Year Book, p 516. Used with permission of author and publisher.)*

## Staging of the disease

The abnormal vascular changes in the new international classification are divided into four stages.

**Stage 1: demarcation line.** Stage 1 is characterized by the presence of a demarcation line. This line represents a structure separating the anterior, avascular retina from the posterior, vascularized retina. It is essentially flat and white and lies within the plane of the retina. Abnormal branching or arcading of vessels leads up to the line.

**Stage 2: ridge.** In stage 2, the demarcation line of stage 1 has grown. It now has height and width, occupies a volume, and extends anterior to the plane of the retina. The ridge may change from white to pink, and vessels may leave the plane of the retina to enter it. Small tufts of new vessels may be seen posterior to the ridge structure. The absence of fibrovascular growth from the surface of the ridge separates this stage from stage 3.

**Stage 3: ridge with extraretinal fibrovascular proliferation.** Stage 3 is characterized by the presence of extraretinal, fibrovascular, proliferative tissue added to the ridge of stage 2. Proliferating tissue can be localized, continuous with the posterior aspect of the ridge, causing a ragged appearance of the ridge as proliferation increases into the vitreous perpendicular to the plane of the retina. Fibrovascular proliferation may be noted in either or both of these locations in stage 3. Vessels may leave the plane of the retina to enter the ridge.

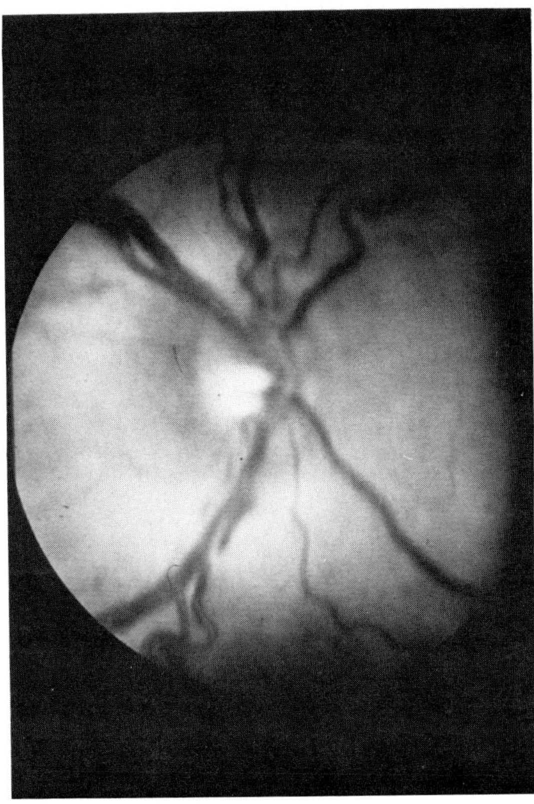

**FIGURE 26-3**　Plus disease with prominent dilatation and tortuosity of the retinal vessels in the posterior pole associated with stage 3 in the temporal periphery.

**Stage 4: retinal detachment.** Stage 4 is characterized by the presence of definite retinal detachment added to the above findings. It may be caused by an exudative effusion of fluid or traction or both.

"Plus" disease represents a more florid stage of ROP. Increasing dilatation and tortuosity of the peripheral retinal vessels, iris vascular engorgement, pupillary rigidity, and vitreous haze indicate progressive vascular incompetence. When the vascular changes are so marked that the posterior retinal veins are enlarged and the arterioles tortuous, to indicate "plus" disease a plus sign is added to the ROP stage number (Figure 26-3).

## Classification of retinal detachment

Retinal detachment (stage 4) findings of the 1984 classification are further described. The 1987 classification leaves unchanged the previous description of location and extent of disease published in 1984, but morphology, location, and extent of the retinal detachment are considered. Stage 4 has been expanded and a fifth stage of retinal detachment added.

## Regressed ROP

**Retinal findings.** Many patients with active ROP undergo partial regression. These residual changes have been divided in the classification into those affecting primarily the retinal periphery and those affecting the posterior fundus. In each location vascular abnormalities and the residual retinal changes are separately considered.

## ROP CLINICAL STUDIES
## Cryotherapy: CRYO-ROP Study

A multicenter, randomized trial of cryotherapy, the CRYO-ROP Study, chaired by Dr. Earl A. Palmer and supported by the National Eye Institute, documented earlier pilot studies of cryo treatment. This important collaborative study indeed represents the first confirmed effective therapy for ROP.[6]

The protocol for the multicenter trial included infants with birth weights less than 1,251 g. The first eye examination was performed when they were between 28 and 42 days of age, there were then biweekly examinations until the retinas were completely vascularized or until prethreshold ROP developed. After full vascularization of the retinas, examination was to be scheduled 3, 12, and 24 months after the original expected date of confinement (EDC).

Prethreshold disease was defined as any stage of ROP in Zone I, stage 2 with plus disease in Zone II, stage 3 without plus disease in Zone II, or stage 2 with plus disease in Zone I or II but less than five contiguous or less than eight cumulative clock hours of stage 3. When infants developed prethreshold disease, they were then followed at weekly intervals until regression of the prethreshold disease occurred or until progression to threshold ROP in one or both eyes was observed.

Threshold ROP was defined as five or more contiguous or eight or more cumulative clock hours of stage 3 ROP in Zone I or II with plus disease.

Once an infant patient reached threshold ROP, he or she became eligible for entry into the Randomized Study Group in the CRYO-ROP study. The amount of stage-3 disease that defined threshold ROP was selected in the planning phase of the study whenever it was the judgment of the investigators that a particular eye showed a 50% chance of either an adverse outcome or a good one without cryotherapy.

The treatment technique consisted of spots of transscleral cryotherapy directed at the entire avascular anterior cuff of premature retina, extending from the ora serrata posteriorly to the ridge of ROP (Figure 26-4). The freezes were contiguous but not overlapping. The eye to receive cryotherapy was randomly selected.

The results of the CRYO-ROP study were evaluated through a masked comparison of the incidence of objectively visible macular fold, retinal detachment, or retrolental mass in the eyes that received cryotherapy with those eyes not receiving it. Cryotherapy was found to reduce the frequency of photographically documented retinal detachment, retinal fold involving the macula, or abnormal retrolental tissue from 43% to 21.8%.

Documentation of the initial benefits of therapy represented Phase 1 of the study. Phase 2 of the CRYO-ROP study, which began in June 1989, was designed to determine the long-term effects of cryotherapy during the first 6 years of life.

New information was provided on the natural history of ROP in the study. For example, the earliest recording of threshold ROP was at approximately 6½ weeks; and for the overall study the average time was 11⅓ weeks. The general

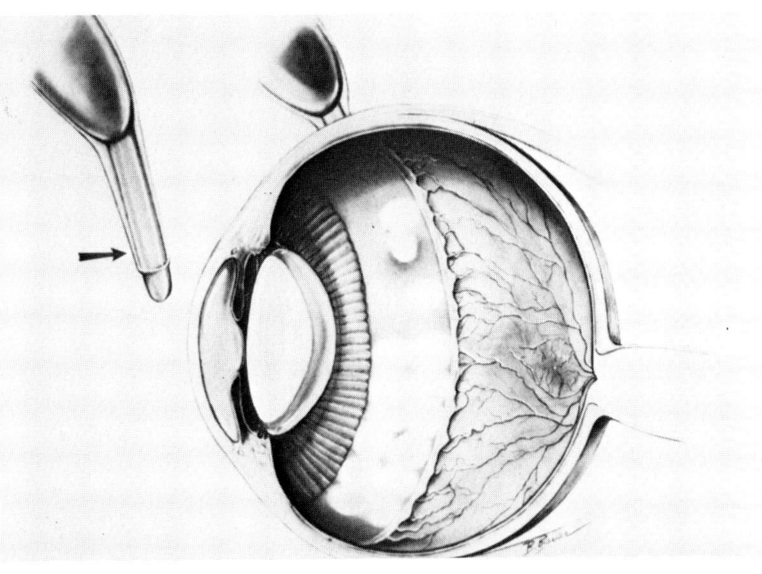

**FIGURE 26-4**    Schematic diagram of cryotherapy in stage 3 "plus" ROP. The freeze applications extend posteriorly to the ridge but do not spread through the ridge. Treatment inferiorly is complete and is in progress superiorly. Schematic of protective sleeve around the tip of the cryoprobe (arrow). *(From Patz A, Palmer EA. Retinopathy of prematurity. In Ryan SJ, ed, The retina, St Louis, 1989, Mosby–Year Book, p 526. Used with permission of authors and publisher).*

recommendation was that the initial eye examination be performed during the sixth week of life.

With definite evidence of regression of ROP in Zone III (loss of previously present plus disease, growth of retinal vessels into previously avascular retina, or fibrotic involution of extraretinal vascular proliferation on successive weekly examinations), examination was recommended at longer intervals with the patient evaluated at approximately 4- to 6-week intervals until the retinas are fully vascularized.

Because of the possible development of strabismus following cryotherapy, it was recommended that the patient should optimally be referred to a pediatric ophthalmologist, or to one experienced in visual development, for evaluation at six to nine months. The parents should be alerted to be aware of any obvious deviation of the eyes that would prompt earlier examination.

I have asked Dr. Palmer to provide a personal recommendation for his current management of patients with *bilateral* ROP. He has advised the following:

> In my personal opinion, cryotherapy is indicated for both eyes as soon as possible, whenever both eyes show threshold ROP that is located in *Zone 1*. If both eyes show threshold ROP in *Zone 2*, cryotherapy is recommended to the worse eye as soon as possible.
>
> Treatment of the second eye is always debatable, based upon current scientific knowledge; however, cryotherapy to the second eye seems justifiable whenever any of the following conditions exist:
>
> a) The threshold ROP is located posterior to the vortex vein ampullae.
> b) The threshold ROP has advanced relatively rapidly, as based upon clinical experience.

c) The majority of the stage 3 ROP in the threshold eye is classified in the "severe" category that is depicted in the International Classification of ROP, and according to the clinician's judgment.

d) The patient's parents understand that a spontaneously good outcome without treatment is slightly more likely than a bad outcome without treatment, that a bad outcome is still possible following cryotherapy, and that the long term risks of cryotherapy are not fully known—but nevertheless wish to accept these risks.

For cases in which only one eye has reached threshold ROP, and the other has not reached this stage, I would *not* always absolutely perform cryotherapy to every threshold eye. I would use the same criteria for recommending cryotherapy for the second eye, just listed, and would always recommend cryotherapy if it were a Zone 1 case. Whenever none of those special second-eye criteria are met, I would consider waiting, closely following both eyes with examinations at maximum intervals of three days, to assess:

a) rate of progression of ROP in both eyes,
b) likelihood that the second eye would reach threshold, and
c) the presence or absence of progression or regression in the threshold eye.

Then I would tailor the decision about this one threshold eye to the individual circumstances.

## LASER PHOTOCOAGULATION THERAPY

Xenon arc was first used as a photocoagulation treatment modality by Nagata and other Japanese investigators.[27] Difficulties in using the Xenon arc photocoagulator with its direct ophthalmoscope delivery system presented problems in treatment of the retinal periphery in these smaller infants' eyes, so that cryotherapy gradually supplanted Xenon arc photocoagulation in most institutions.

In 1972, Payne and Patz reported one of the first cases of ROP to be treated by the argon laser.[32] Utilizing a blue-green argon laser constructed at Johns Hopkins with a monocular *indirect* ophthalmoscope delivery unit, the active proliferative stage of ROP was treated in one eye of a patient with rapidly progressive proliferative ROP. The retinopathy would be considered grade 3 + of the current international classification. Significant vitreous hemorrhage was present; and at the time of laser therapy it was necessary to rotate the infant's head to allow shifting of the blood posteriorly. This maneuver enabled visualization of the neovascular tufts in the temporal periphery. The neovascularization was treated directly, and treatment extended anterior to the new vessels. Within two months, the vitreous was completely clear; and all the neovascularization had resolved. Followup over the next several years revealed no residual except mild tortuosity of the arterioles in the posterior pole. The patient developed 20/20 vision (Figure 26-5).

The recent availability of commercially manufactured binocular indirect laser photocoagulation delivery units has stimulated renewed interest in argon laser photocoagulation for active ROP. Landers et al used the recently available commercial laser indirect ophthalmoscope for treatment of acute proliferative ROP.[21] Utilizing the blue-green laser, photocoagulation treatment was delivered

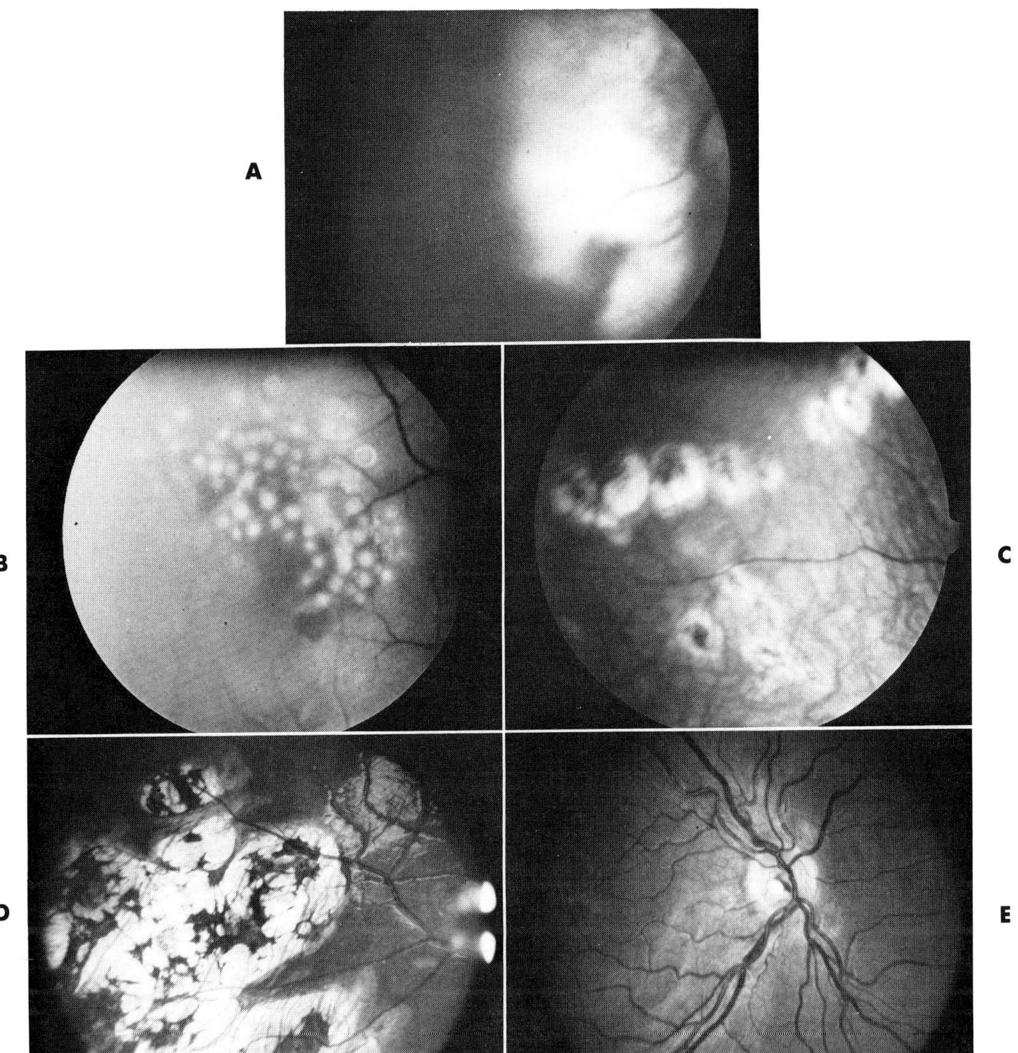

**FIGURE 26-5**   **A,** Vitreous hemorrhage obscures posterior pole and temporal periphery in premature infant with stage 3 "plus" ROP. Fundus photograph taken with camera aimed between disc and macula just prior to treatment. **B,** After tilting head, the hemorrhage shifted and the temporal periphery is visualized. Multiple laser burns were placed on the neovascular ridge and extended anteriorly. **C,** Most posterior laser scars 2 months after treatment. *(**A, B, C,** from Payne JW, Patz A. Treatment of acute proliferative retrolental fibroplasia. Am Acad Ophthalmol Otolaryngol 1972; 76:1234-1246. Used with permission of authors and publisher.)* **D,** At age 10, laser scars are noted in the temporal periphery. **E,** Optic disc photo at age 10 shows only residual of ROP is mild increased tortuosity of the retinal arterioles. Visual acuity measured 20/20. *(**D, E,** courtesy Dr. John W. Payne, Baltimore.)*

to the avascular retina anterior to the ridge of extraretinal fibrovascular proliferation. Treatment resulted in a regression of the active proliferative changes. The authors point out the relative ease of applying scleral depression with a small lens loop.

McNamara et al reported on a prospective randomized trial to compare the efficacy of argon green laser photocoagulation with transscleral cryotherapy.[25] The early results with a followup of at least three months revealed 15 of the 16 eyes randomized to laser treatment (versus 9 of 12 eyes receiving cryotherapy) showed regression of active proliferative ROP. These investigators reported that "laser photocoagulation seems to be at least as effective as cryotherapy in achieving a favorable outcome" and are continuing the controlled study.

## Oxygen As a Therapeutic Agent: STOP-ROP

Dr. Dale L. Phelps (personal communication) has reintroduced the concept of treating ROP at the prethreshold level with added oxygen. The study is designated "STOP-ROP." Small increases in supplemental oxygen—raising the arterial saturation from levels of 89% to 94%, which are currently advocated, to levels of 98% to 99%—are planned on a randomized basis for infants with "pre-threshold" disease. Careful monitoring of the infants in this prospective study will be accomplished by the use of pulse oximetry. The sound basis for testing the hypothesis that slight increases in blood oxygen levels might prove beneficial in the acute proliferative stage of ROP are summarized.

In more recent laboratory studies where retinal capillary endothelial cells were grown in cell culture, the rate of proliferation of the endothelial cells was found to be significantly increased when the oxygen tension was reduced from room air level of 21% to 14%. On the other hand, when the oxygen concentration was increased above room air level, the endothelial cell proliferation decreased. It stopped completely when the oxygen concentration measured 80%.[37]

Phelps[34] repeated some of the earlier studies by Ashton on kittens[2] and observed that on removal of animals, after initial exposure to high oxygen, to incubator concentrations of 13% the amount of secondary neovascularization was increased. When the animals, after exposure to high oxygen, were transferred to 28% oxygen concentrations instead of room air, there was a slight decrease in the neovascularization observed.

It is of interest that Szewczyk[40] reported in the early 1950s that placing premature infants back into higher incubator oxygen concentrations appeared to have a beneficial effect on active ROP. These observations, which may have been correct, were uncontrolled. They were not given serious consideration at the time for several reasons. First, the known spontaneous remission of active ROP in selected cases might have influenced these observations. Second, the role of excess oxygen as the major cause of ROP was being documented in prospective controlled clinical studies. The experimental production of retinal neovascularization, somewhat resembling the early proliferative stages of ROP, following oxygen treatment supported the clinical studies. Bedrossian et al reported on treatment of several infants with progressive severe ROP by returning them to oxygen.[3] They also noted in a small controlled study that gradually weaning infants by reducing the incubator oxygen concentration reduced the incidence of ROP among these infants compared with infants suddenly removed from oxygen. Seven infants with progressive ROP, after being placed back in 50% to 60% incubator oxygen, had regression of the ROP.

The general practice of rigid restriction of supplemental oxygen became so widespread that there was no suitable climate to test the possible benefits of oxygen to treat active ROP. Finally, blood gas monitoring capability was not available, so that there would have been a significant risk to an infant to provide added incubator oxygen without the ability to know the blood oxygen levels achieved.

One other consideration in the oxygen mechanism is fundamental to the consideration of administering small and carefully measured supplemental oxygen to an infant with active proliferative ROP. As discussed in describing the mechanism of oxygen action, only animals with an *immature* retinal vasculature demonstrate oxygen-induced vasoconstriction and vascular closure followed by neovascularization after removal from high oxygen to room air. Once the retina was fully vascularized, no permanent vascular closure occurred and secondary neovascularization never developed.

The small doses of added oxygen recommended by Phelps should have essentially no risk in causing further vascular closure. The potential benefit to the patient of controlling the neovascularization should far outweigh any theoretical risk of causing further vascular closure. Indeed the animal studies suggest that these small doses of closely monitored added oxygen would be incapable of producing vascular closure and new neovascularization.

At my request, Dr. Phelps has supplied this overview and background to the STOP-ROP planned study:

> Supplemental Therapeutic Oxygen for Prethreshold ROP (STOP-ROP) is a treatment that was used by Szewczyk in the 1950's, but one that was not tested in controlled trials (except one small trial that was prematurely stopped) and has never been accepted. Theoretically, it is attractive because our best current understanding of ROP is that avascular and hypoxic retina is the source of an angiogenic factor that drives the retinopathy. The success of cryotherapy in controlling ROP is indirect support of this theory because it destroys that avascular retina. Additional support comes from an animal model of ROP that is worse when systemic hypoxia is added to the model and improves when mild hyperoxia is put into the equation. The animal and bench research on hypoxia and angiogenesis have provided the reassurance needed for clinicians to face the difficulty of giving extra oxygen to infants who have a disease that is strongly connected to excess oxygen. In addition, the development of pulse oximetry over the past few years has made this trial technically feasible, whereas previously it has not been practical to continuously monitor the blood oxygen levels of convalescent premature infants who no longer have arterial lines in place.
>
> Therefore, the multicenter STOP-ROP trial will test whether increasing an infant's oxygenation saturation in a controlled manner will be able to prevent Prethreshold ROP from progressing to Threshold ROP requiring cryotherapy.

## THE EFFECT OF LIGHT ON ROP

Hepner et al in 1949 tested the concept of "light" as an etiological agent by patching both eyes of 5 premature infants from shortly after birth until the infants had reached 8 weeks of age.[16] Four of the five developed significant ROP.

Locke and Reese further tested the "light" hypothesis.[22] One eye of 22 premature infants was occluded, and the fellow eye served as a control. No difference in ROP was noted.

Both these early studies were conducted prior to the incrimination of oxygen. The high oxygen routinely administered could have masked any theoretical protective effect of light restriction on the development of ROP. Once excess oxygen was identified, the interest in light as a risk factor waned.

Two decades later, Glass et al reexamined the light hypothesis.[14] They compared the incidence of ROP in 74 infants exposed to standard nursery lighting with a group of 154 infants exposed to significantly reduced light levels. A neutral-density filter was placed over each incubator to reduce the intensity of the light at each infant's face by approximately 50%. The investigators noted a lower incidence of ROP in infants exposed to reduced light levels when compared with historical controls exposed to high levels of ambient nursery lighting.

Ackerman and coworkers examined 161 infants. Each isolette was partially covered with a blanket to shield the baby's eyes. They compared their findings with the ocular findings for 129 premature infants who had no shielding.[1] They found no difference in the severity or incidence of ROP in the two groups of infants. As in the Glass study, only historical controls were utilized.

There are several experimental studies demonstrating the retinotoxic effect of light exposure. Sisson et al observed that light-induced retinal damage is increased when oxygen concentrations are increased.[39] O'Steen reported that retinal damage was greater in younger animals.[28] Small elevations in body temperatures have been reported to increase light damage.[9] Gottsch et al proposed that the initial mechanism of injury in ROP occurs by photosensitization from blood-borne photosensitizers which damage developing vascular endothelium.[15] It remains to be proven that light exposure has an effect on the pathogenesis of ROP, but there is an important need to test the concept of "light" exposure in a prospective, controlled, clinical investigation.

Dr. Rand Spencer (personal communication) is in the process of organizing a multicenter collaborative clinical trial to test the "LIGHT-ROP" hypothesis. The plan for this study will involve the random assignment of infants with birth weights of 1,000 grams or less to wearing goggles that reduce light by 2 log units from the first day of life through 31 weeks gestational age. The control group will have standard nursery lighting. Ophthalmological examination will be done every two weeks until the retinal vasculature is mature or until the infant reaches prethreshold ROP, when they would be eligible to enter the "STOP-ROP" study. For infants not included in a "STOP-ROP" study, if progression occurs to threshold ROP, cryotherapy would be instituted.

## VITAMIN E IN PROPHYLAXIS OF ROP

Owens and Owens investigated the role of vitamin E supplements on ROP in the late 1940s, before the incrimination of oxygen and without consideration of its antioxidant effects.[29] Two decades later, the "antioxidant" property of vitamin E and its possible prophylactic role in ROP were examined. Controlled clinical trials testing the role of large doses of vitamin E in the prevention of ROP were reported by several investigators. These are summarized in Institute of Medicine report.[17]

The Institute of Medicine report published in 1986, provides the following conclusion and recommendation of a special committee assigned to review the vitamin E results:

> Vitamin E as prophylaxis for retinopathy of prematurity was subject to a detailed analysis. This committee found no conclusive evidence either of benefit or harm from vitamin E administration. Risks from vitamin E appear to be minimal for premature infants provided that doses are kept moderate to achieve a blood level no higher than 3 mg/dl.[17]

Patz and Palmer commented in 1989 that "there is ample evidence that vitamin E deficiency should be avoided in the premature infant."[31]

## Surfactant and ROP

Repka et al have reported from a retrospective study with historical controls that prophylactic administration of surfactant extract had an apparent beneficial effect in reducing the frequency and severity of ROP.[36] These investigators observed that 3 of 87 patients on surfactant therapy developed threshold (stage 3 plus) ROP when compared with 8 of 80 patients not on therapy. The incidence of *any* stage of ROP occurring was reduced from 85% (68/80) in the control group to 63% (55/87) in the surfactant-treated infants (P < 0.003).

Repka et al also point out that it would have been desirable to conduct a prospective randomized controlled study. However, the apparent benefits of surfactant in preventing the complications of the respiratory distress syndrome raise questions on randomly assigning infants to a no-surfactant treatment. The historical controls used by Repka consisted of infants in the period immediately preceding the routine use of surfactant in the nursery. We await the continued followup of this investigation, which suggests that this form of therapy may have a significant impact in reducing the incidence and severity of ROP.

## MANAGEMENT OF REGRESSED ROP

Children with a history of mild cicatricial or regressed ROP have an increased incidence of peripheral retinal breaks, which frequently occur even when there is no residual abnormality posteriorly. Tasman pointed out the risk of retinal detachment occurring late in life in these cases.[41] The patient and responsible members of the patient's family should be advised of the potential for retinal detachment in future years and alerted to both the symptoms and signs of detachment and the need for periodic examinations.

Kushner cautioned that children with a history of even the most mild ROP with total regression have a significant incidence of high refractive errors, amblyopia, and strabismus.[20] I have observed several cases with mild active ROP in the nursery and no residual disease after remission. Several of these cases have developed a high degree of myopia, present before preschool years, in contrast to typical myopia which starts later. Indeed, it is recommended that the examining ophthalmologist question the family on the birth history whenever high myopia is detected in early childhood. If prematurity is established, the myopia could be the only finding of regressed ROP.

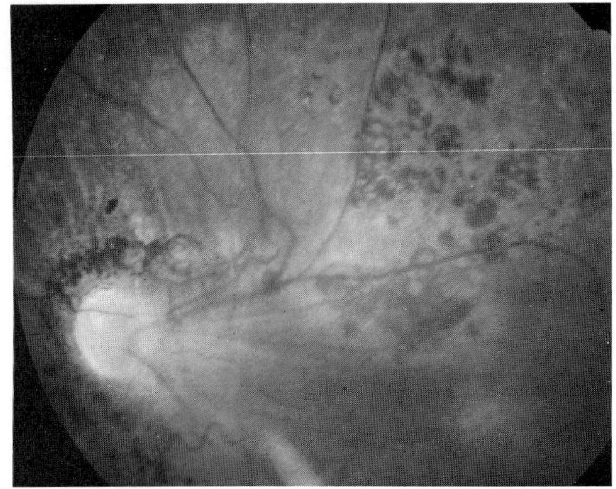
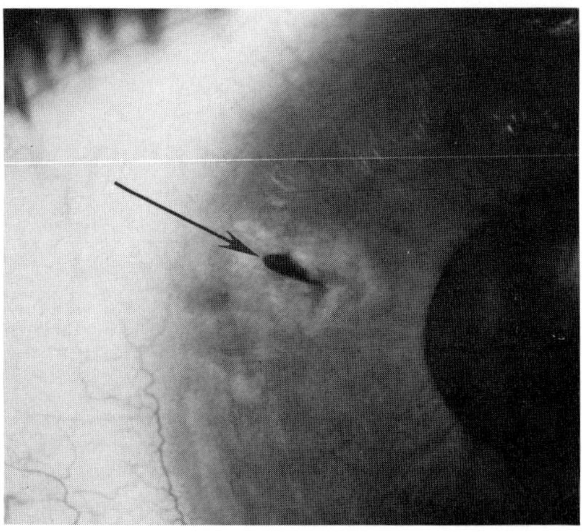



**FIGURE 26-6**     **A,** Fundus photograph of patient with regressed ROP. Note dragging of vessels across the disc and heterotopia of the macula. The patient developed acute narrow-angle glaucoma at the age of 20. **B,** Laser iridotomy (arrow) controlled the acute angle closure attack, and a prophylactic iridotomy was also performed in the fellow eye. *(From Patz A, Palmer EA: Retinopathy of prematurity. In Ryan SJ, ed, The retina, St Louis, 1989, Mosby–Year Book, p 520. Used with permission of authors and publishers.)*

## Angle-Closure Glaucoma in Regressed ROP

Eyes with regressed ROP are at increased risk of developing acute angle-closure glaucoma, with the risk extending to adulthood. I have observed several of these cases and have followed two patients with regressed ROP from childhood who between regular examinations, at age 20 and 30 respectively, developed angle-closure glaucoma. Laser iridotomy was used successfully in treatment of the eye with angle closure in each patient. Prophylactic iridotomy in the fellow eye, which showed extremely narrow angles, was performed uneventfully in both patients (Figure 26-6).

Since the complication of angle-closure glaucoma in regressed ROP has been recognized only relatively recently, many patients are neither aware of the risk nor receiving regular ophthalmologic care. Because this form of glaucoma may develop when the patient is older and since it is usually treatable by laser surgery, the ophthalmologist should be aware of this potential complication and of its management. Patients and their families should also be advised of this risk and alerted to the symptoms of acute angle-closure glaucoma.

## Retinal Detachment and Vitrectomy for ROP

There have been several detailed reports on the use of scleral buckling and vitrectomy for retinal detachments occurring in advanced ROP.[4,23,44,45] These procedures have resulted in "anatomically reattached" retinas in many instances. The 1991 report by Quinn et al[35] provides new information on visual development by testing "pattern vision" that is applicable to these cases.[24,42] Using this technique, they found poor visual outcomes in patients with a previous history of retinal detachment who had been anatomically reattached by surgery or spontaneously without surgery. Quinn et al used masked examiners and techniques to avoid auditory and other clues to the infant being tested. Kalina[18] in an accompanying editorial pointed out that the more favorable results in other surgical studies may have been influenced by these clues, as well as the motivation of the parents and the operating surgeons, all understandably hoping that the child would have useful vision. The fact that many very low birth weight infants may have neurological damage also makes assessing the true visual status difficult. The poor visual development in patients with retinal detachment reported by Quinn and coworkers gives further priority to the development of more effective therapy to prevent the advanced stages of ROP.

## References


1. Ackerman B, Sherworit E, Williams J. Reduced incidental light exposure: effect on the development of retinopathy of prematurity in low birth weight infants. Pediatrics 1989; 83:958-62.
2. Ashton N, Ward B, Serpell G. Effect of oxygen on developing retinal vessels with particular reference to the problem of retrolental fibroplasia. Br J Ophthalmol 1954; 38:397-432.
3. Bedrossian RH, Carmichael P, Ritter J. Retinopathy of prematurity (retrolental fibroplasia) and oxygen: clinical study: further observations on disease. Am J Ophthalmol 1956; 41:619.
4. Charles S: Vitrectomy with ciliary body entry for retrolental fibroplasia. In McPherson AR, Hittner HM, Kretzer FL, eds, Retinopathy of prematurity: current concepts and controversies. Toronto, 1986, BC Decker, pp 225-234.
5. Committee for the Classification of Retinopathy of Prematurity. An international classification of retinopathy of prematurity. Arch Ophthalmol 1984; 102:1130-1134.
6. Cryotherapy for Retinopathy of Prematurity Cooperative Group. Multicenter trial for retinopathy of prematurity: one year outcome. Arch Ophthalmol 1990; 108:1408-1413.
7. Dobson V, Quinn GE, Biglan AW. Acuity card assessment of visual function in the cryotherapy for retinopathy of prematurity trial. Invest Ophthalmol Vis Sci 1953; 31:1702-1708.
8. Eichenbaum JW, Mamelok A, Mittl RN. Treatment of retinopathy of prematurity, St Louis, 1990, Mosby–Year Book.
9. Fielder AR, Levene NI, Russell-Eggitt IM, Weale RA. Temperature—a factor in ocular development? Devel Med Clin Neurol 1986; 28:279-284.
10. Flower RW. Perinatal retina vascular physiology. In Silverman WA, Flynn JT, eds, Retinopathy of prematurity, Boston, 1985, Blackwell Scientific, pp 97-120.
11. Flynn JT, Bancalari E, Bawol R, Fever W, Roberts J, Gillings D, Sim E, Buckley E, Bachynski BN. Retinopathy of prematurity: a randomized, prospective trial of transcutaneous oxygen monitoring, Ophthalmol 1987; 94:630-638.
12. Flynn JT, Phelps DL. Retinopathy of prematurity: problem and challenge, New York, 1988, Wiley-Liss.
13. Foos, RY. Retinopathy of prematurity—pathologic correlation of clinical stages. Retina 1987; 7:260-276.
14. Glass P, Avery GB, Subramanian KNS, et al. Effects of bright light in the hospital nursery on the incidence of retinopathy of prematurity. N Engl J Med 1985; 313:401-404.
15. Gottsch JD, Pou S, Bynoe LA, Rosen GM. Hematogenous photosensitization: a mechanism for the development of age-related macular degeneration. Inv Ophthalmol 1990; 31:1674.
16. Hepner WR, Krause AC, Davis ME. Retrolental fibroplasia and light. Pediatrics 1949; 3:824-28.
17. Institute of Medicine. Report of a study: vitamin E and retinopathy of prematurity. Washington, DC, 1986 National Academy Press, pp 1-24.
18. Kalina RE. Normal and pathologic anatomy of the immature eye. Trans Pac Coast Oto-Ophthalmol Soc 1970; 51:185-193.
19. Kinsey VE. Retrolental fibroplasia: cooperative study of retrolental fibroplasia and the use of oxygen. Arch Ophthalmol 1956; 56:481-543.
20. Kushner BJ. Long-term follow-up of regressed retinopathy of prematurity. In. Flynn JT, Phelps DL, Retinopathy of prematurity: problem and challenge, New York, 1988, Wiley-Liss, pp 193-199.
21. Landers MB III, Semple HC, Rueben JB, and Serdahl, C. Argon laser photocoagulation for advanced retinopathy of prematurity. Am J Ophthalmol 1990; 110:429-31.
22. Locke JC, Reese AB. Retrolental fibroplasia. Arch Ophthalmol 1952; 48:44-47.
23. Machemer, R. Closed vitrectomy for severe retrolental fibroplasia in the infant. Ophthalmol 1983; 90:436-441.

24. Mayer DL, Trese MT. Visual function evaluation of patients with retinopathy of prematurity. In Noninvasive assessment of the visual system: summaries of papers presented at the noninvasive assessment of the visual system topical meeting, Feb. 5-8, Incline Village, Nevada, Washington, DC, 1990; Optical Society of America. pp 22-25.

25. McNamara JA, Tasman W, Brown GC, Federman, JL. Laser photocoagulation for stage 3 + retinopathy of prematurity. Ophthalmol 1991; 98:576-580.

26. McPherson AR, Hittner HM, Kretzer FL. Retinopathy of prematurity: current concepts and controversies. Toronto, 1986, BC Decker.

27. Nagata M, Isuruoka Y. Treatment of acute retrolental fibroplasia with xenon arc photocoagulation. Japan J Ophthalmol 1972; 16:181-243.

28. O'Steen WK. Retinal and optic nerve serotonin and retinal degeneration as influenced by photoperiod. Exp Neurol 1970; 27:194-205.

29. Owens WC, Owens EU. Retrolental fibroplasia in premature infants. Am J Ophthalmol 1949; 32:1-29.

30. Patz A, Eastham A, Higginbotham DH, Kleh T. Oxygen studies in retrolental fibroplasia: the production of the microscopic changes of retrolental fibroplasia in experimental animals. Am J Ophthalmol 1953; 36:1511-1522.

31. Patz A, Palmer EA. Retinopathy of prematurity. In Ryan SJ, ed, The retina, St Louis, 1989, Mosby–Year Book, pp. 509-530.

32. Payne JW, Patz A: Treatment of acute proliferative retrolental fibroplasia. Trans Am Acad Ophthalmol Otolaryngol 1972; 76:1234-1246.

33. Phelps DL, Brown DR, Tung B. 28-day survival rates of 6676 neonates with birth weights of 1250 grams or less. Pediatrics 1991; 87:7-17.

34. Phelps DL. Oxygen and developmental retinal capillary remodeling in the kitten. Invest Ophthalmol Vis Sci 1990; 31:2194-2197.

35. Quinn GE, Dobson V, Barr CC. Visual acuity in infants after vitrectomy for severe retinopathy of prematurity. Ophthalmol 1991, 98:5-13.

36. Repka MX, Hudak ML, Parsa CF, Tielsch JM. Calf-lung surfactant extract prophylaxis and retinopathy of prematurity. Ophthalmol 1992, (in press).

37. Rosen P, Boulton M, McLeod D. The effect of different oxygen concentrations on the proliferation of retinal microvascular endothelial cells and pericytes in vitro. Invest Ophthalmol 1989; 30(supp):316.

38. Silverman WA, Flynn JT. Retinopathy of prematurity: contemporary issues in fetal and neonatal medicine. Boston: 1985, Blackwell Scientific Publications.

39. Sisson TR, Glauser SC, Glauser EM, et al. Retinal changes produced by phototherapy. J Pediatr 1970; 77:221-227

40. Szewczyk TS. Retrolental fibroplasia: etiology and prophylaxis. Am J Ophthalmol 1952; 35:301-311.

41. Tasman W. Late complications of retrolental fibroplasia. Ophthalmol 1979; 86:1724-1740.

42. Teller DY, McDonnald MA, Preston K, et al. Assessment of visual acuity in infants and children: the acuity card procedure. Dev Med Child Neurol 1986; 28;779-789.

43. Terry TL. Fibroblastic overgrowth of persistent tunica vasculosa lentis in premature infants: II. report of cases-clinical aspects. Arch Ophthalmol 1943; 29:36-53.

44. Topilow HW, Ackerman AL, Wang FM. Successful treatment of advanced retinopathy of prematurity. Ophthalmic Surgery 1988; 19:781-785.

45. Trese MT. Surgical results of stage V retrolental fibroplasia and timing of surgical repair. Ophthalmol 1984; 91:461-466.

# 27 Acute Retinal Necrosis

**Michael J. Potter, MD**
**Julia A. Haller, MD**

Acute retinal necrosis (ARN) syndrome is a disorder characterized by viral retinitis, vaso-occlusion, vitritis, and retinal detachment that typically affects healthy patients. Since its description in 1971, numerous investigators have elucidated the clinical course and etiology of the disease. We will review and discuss the original case reports of ARN, subsequent clinical research, and management strategies.

In 1971 Urayama et al described six patients with a unilateral acute uveitis, retinal periarteritis, and retinal detachment.[1] The authors proposed the name "Kirisawa's uveitis" for this disease, naming it after their mentor. The first report in the English literature, by Willerson, Aaberg, and Reeser in 1977, described two patients with an acute bilateral retinal vaso-occlusive disease of unknown etiology.[2] The first patient was a 65-year-old man with a history of vesicular eruption and a cold sore on his upper lip. Two days later, he developed a hypopyon uveitis with prominent keratic precipitates in the left eye, and visual acuity dropped to 20/300. There were confluent yellow-white intraretinal opacities for 360 degrees and sheathed posterior retinal blood vessels. Visual acuity in the right eye was 20/30, with a single white intraretinal lesion. Complement fixation titers for herpes, cytomegalovirus, and fungi were negative. VDRL and RTA-ABS were non-reactive. A clinical diagnosis of Behçet's disease was made, and therapy with oral prednisone and chlorambucil was begun. Despite treatment, disease progressed in both eyes. A rhegmatogenous retinal detachment developed in the left eye with a retinal hole in an area of retinal atrophy and necrosis. Retinal reattachment with a scleral buckling procedure was initially successful, but a new posterior tear and redetachment developed subsequently. In the right eye, an epiretinal membrane caused a tractional retinal detachment that progressed to a combined traction-rhegmatogenous detachment over a two-week period. Chlorambucil had to be discontinued because of bone-marrow suppression. The patient went on to develop herpetic lesions on the skin.

The second patient described by Willerson et al was a 30-year-old white woman who had an acute decrease in vision in her left eye, followed one week later by similar symptoms in the right eye. Visual acuity was finger counting in both eyes. Visual fields were constricted bilaterally. There were mutton-fat keratic precipitates in the left eye. Retinal vasculitis and panuveitis were present. Diffuse areas of leakage and obstruction of retinal vessels were seen on fluorescein angiography. The right eye developed an apparently exudative retinal detachment. Final visual acuity was hand motions in the right eye and light perception in the left.

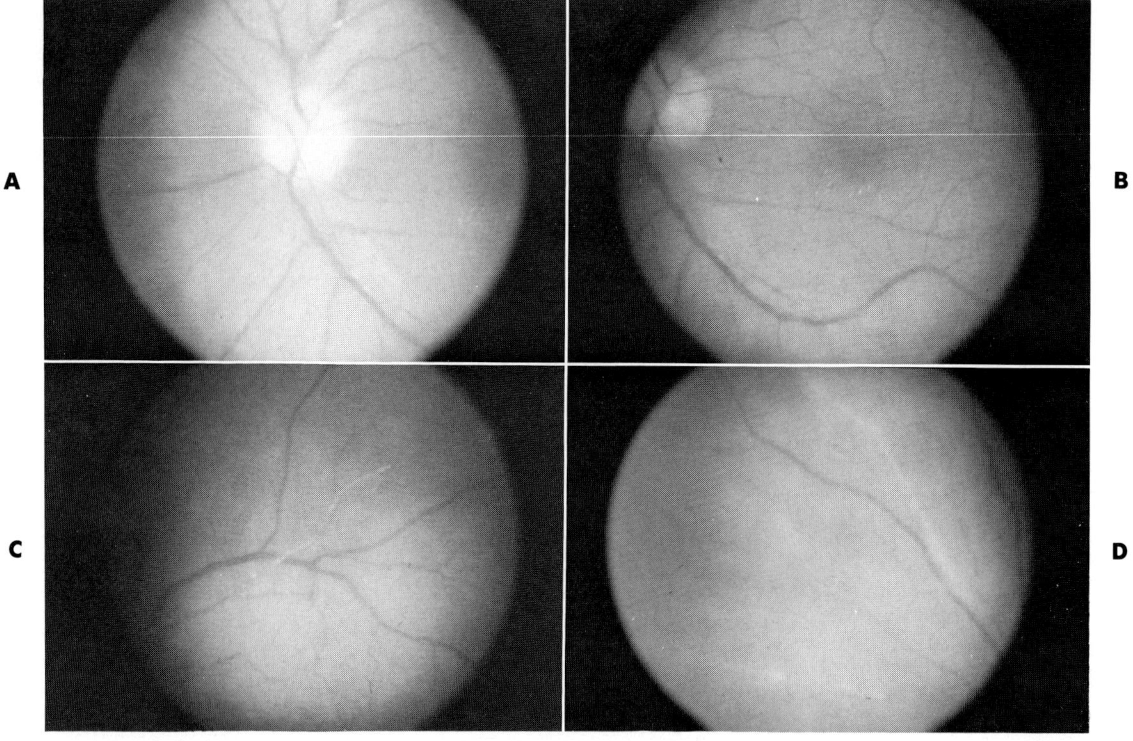

**FIGURE 27-1**    This 30-year-old white male had a 3-day history of floaters in the left eye. Vision was 20/30. **A,** Fundus examination revealed vaso-occlusion posteriorly. **B,** There was some thickening of the inferior macula with lipid deposition. **C, D,** Vaso-occlusion extended into the periphery.

In their report, Willerson and coworkers made note of the presence of herpetic vesicles in the first patient and of the similarity of this disorder to the clinical description of herpetic retinitis. There was no direct proof of an infectious etiology, however.

## FURTHER DESCRIPTIONS OF THE CLINICAL COURSE OF ARN

In 1978, Young and Bird reported four patients with bilateral acute retinal necrosis, to which they gave the acronym BARN syndrome.[3] The clinical course was similar to that seen by Willerson et al. There was also a resemblance to cytomegalovirus (CMV) retinitis at the height of the disease. Similarities included white patches of inflammatory retinitis that became confluent, vascular sheathing, and hemorrhage (Figures 27-1 through 27-3). The disease was different from CMV in that CMV retinitis progresses much more slowly and is almost always seen in immunocompromised patients. New lesions evolve in CMV retinitis as older patches of infection subside into areas of necrotic retina. BARN lesions, by contrast, all appear nearly simultaneously. BARN patients are by definition not immunocompromised. In 1982, Fisher et al reported 11 new cases and reviewed the previous 30 published cases.[4] That review demonstrated that 66% of cases were unilateral and that the term ARN was therefore more appropriate than BARN. Of all affected eyes in this

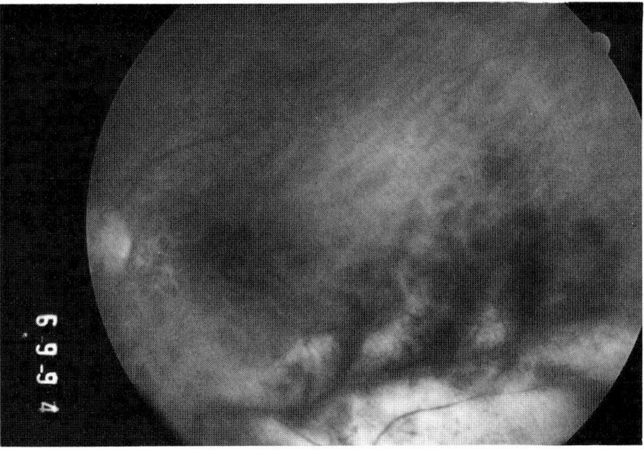

**FIGURE 27-2**    This 45-year-old patient had progression of disease after one week to involve the posterior pole. Confluent creamy lesions were present in the periphery and extended posteriorly along the inferotemporal arcade. There was a prominent component of hemorrhage in this case.

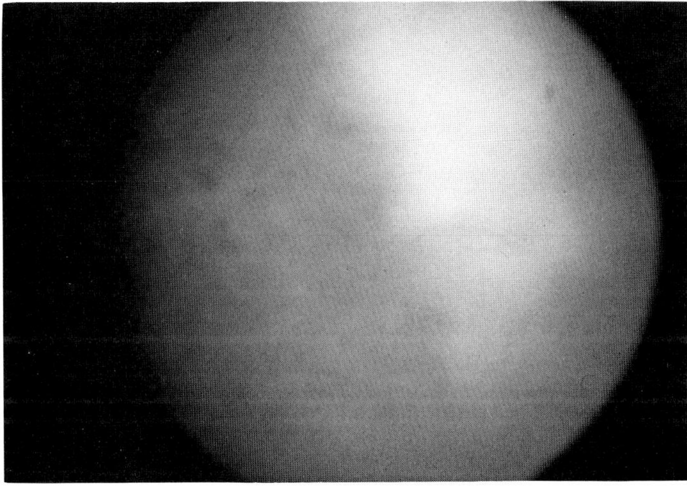

**FIGURE 27-3**    This 15-year-old female with a one-week history of floaters and decreased vision presented with acuity 20/40 and typical confluent peripheral lesions. The media were hazy.

series, 75% eventually developed retinal detachments, almost all of which occurred within three months of the onset of symptoms. In bilateral cases, retinitis in the second eye developed within six weeks. Corticosteroid treatment was generally ineffective in altering the outcome. Only 4 of 18 (22%) of eyes surgically treated for retinal detachment achieved anatomic success, and only two of these had a final visual acuity better than 20/400.

Subsequent reports have further characterized the clinical course of ARN.[5-18] Over 60% of patients are male. There is no age or racial predilection. Case reports record patients as old as 89 years, and reports of infantile herpes simplex retinopathy may be equivalent to cases of ARN.[11] The ARN syndrome typically begins with symptoms of blurred vision, floaters, and sometimes pain. Examination reveals episcleritis, keratic precipitates, anterior segment inflammation, and vitritis. Intraocular pressure may be elevated. Within days to weeks, multifocal patches of yellow-white necrotizing retinitis develop in the retinal periphery. These patches progress circumferentially, become confluent, and may move posteriorly. The macula is often spared. There is a typical serrated appearance to the border between involved and normal retina. A hemorrhagic occlusive vasculitis is present, and optic nerve swelling and hemorrhage are frequently seen. In approximately one third of cases, bilateral involvement develops, usually within 6 weeks of involvement of the first eye. With resolution of the disease, scarring, retinal tears, and epiretinal membrane growth may complicate the course. Detachment develops in up to 90% of patients, with retinal breaks occurring at the interface of involved and uninvolved retina.

## DIAGNOSTIC TESTING

Fluorescein angiography of eyes with ARN reveals extensive occlusion of the retinal vessels, capillary leakage, and focal choroidal nonperfusion.[4] The discs leak late. Visual fields are markedly constricted, which may reflect an accompanying optic nerve dysfunction as well as peripheral retinal disease.[23] Electrophysiologic testing has, in one patient, revealed a normal a wave but moderately reduced b wave.

Sergott et al described neuroimaging performed on two patients with an optic neuropathy associated with ARN.[23] The computed tomographic (CT) findings included diffusely enlarged optic nerve silhouettes in two eyes, while a third eye featured thickening of the nerve at its junction with the globe, with thinning posteriorly. One patient had an improvement in vision from light perception to 20/200 (final acuity 20/70) following optic nerve sheath decompression.

Farrell et al have recently reported a patient with herpes zoster ophthalmicus of the right eye followed two weeks later by ARN in the fellow eye.[30] MRI studies showed bilateral enhancement of the trigeminal roots, which resolved after intravenous acyclovir and oral prednisone therapy.

B-scan ultrasonography may be useful to determine whether retinal detachment is present when the media is quite hazy. A thickened choroid is sometimes seen.[23] An enlarged optic nerve shadow may also be present, but is better demonstrated on CT or MRI scans.

The majority of cases in the literature that report lumbar puncture findings describe normal cell counts, glucose, and protein levels. A cerebrospinal fluid (CSF) pleocytosis may occur in ARN syndrome, with an elevated number of monocytes or lymphocytes.

## ETIOLOGY

Early attempts to identify an infectious agent in ARN were unsuccessful. In 1982, Fisher et al reported culturing a herpes-class virus from the enucleated eye of a patient with ARN.[5] Electron microscopy confirmed the presence of herpes-type virus particles. Immunofluorescent staining was negative for herpes simplex types I and II. The patient had serologic evidence of previous infection by CMV, Epstein-Barr virus, HSV I, and varicella zoster virus, without evidence of rising titers to any of these infectious agents.

Ludwig et al described a case of ARN associated with an outbreak of culture-positive herpes simplex skin vesicles.[24] Rungger-Brandle et al reported a case of bilateral ARN in which electron micrographic studies showed herpes-family virus particles in involved retinal tissue.[15] The virus was cultured in human embryo fibroblast cells, and immunofluorescent antibody staining was positive for CMV. In addition, CMV titers increased from 1:16 to 1:256 within six months after onset of the eye disease. Histology was atypical of CMV infection, however, in that no cytomegaly was found. Yeo et al described two cases of ARN following herpes zoster dermatitis, one of which was associated with auricular herpes zoster with otalgia and facial nerve paralysis (Ramsay-Hunt syndrome).[16] Serologic testing was diagnostic of recent varicella-zoster (VZ) infection and not of CMV or HSV. Culbertson et al were able to culture varicella zoster virus from the enucleated eye of a patient with ARN in 1986.[17] They were able to confirm the presence of VZ DNA by restriction endonuclease analysis.

Three years later, Lewis et al cultured herpes simplex virus type I (HSV-I) from the vitreous of two patients with ARN.[25] In one patient, the disease was a new infection (inferred from serologic evidence); the other was apparently a reactivation with stable HSV I titers and a history of previous vesicular eruptions. Culbertson et al have recently reported four cases of ARN occurring 5 to 28 days after primary chicken pox. These cases were less severe than most, with no retinal detachment or decrease in visual acuity.[31]

Thus ARN appears to result from infection with at least two herpes-class viruses: varicella zoster and herpes simplex. CMV is a less well-established etiologic agent.

## HISTOPATHOLOGY

Corneal histopathology may reveal keratic precipitates with mixed populations of leukocytes. Inflammatory cells can also be seen in the trabecular meshwork and iris. A perivasculitis in the iris has been described. Vitrectomy specimens have demonstrated fibrocellular membranes containing lymphocytes and histiocytes. Multinucleated giant cells, epithelioid cells, and plasma cells have been seen.

Retinal sections demonstrate necrosis, especially peripherally, with occasional intact blood vessels (Figures 27-4 through 27-7). Inflammatory debris, erythrocytes, macrophages, and polymorphonuclear leukocytes are seen. Although the posterior pole is often relatively spared, it may contain necrotic foci. Some authors have taken the abrupt transitions from normal to necrotic retina to indicate that direct cell-to-cell transmission of virus is taking place, with involved areas surrounding a focus of infection.[5,18] Eosinophilic intranuclear inclusions may be observed in the ganglion cell layer, the inner nuclear layer, and the retinal pigment epithelium. Cytomegaly has occasionally been seen.

Choroidal thickening, which often accompanies ARN, is due to inflammatory cell infiltrates. Plasma cells and lymphocytes may similarly be present in the choriocapillaries, ciliary nerves, sclera, and episclera. Optic nerve inflammation, perivasculitis of vessels in the optic nerve head, and necrosis are frequently seen.

In a series of eyes treated with acyclovir, which included five eyes with visual function worse than 20/40 attributed to optic neuropathy, it was suggested that the optic nerve dysfunction may be secondary to vasculitis rather than a direct neurocytopathic effect of the viruses.[19] This was based on the previous histopath-

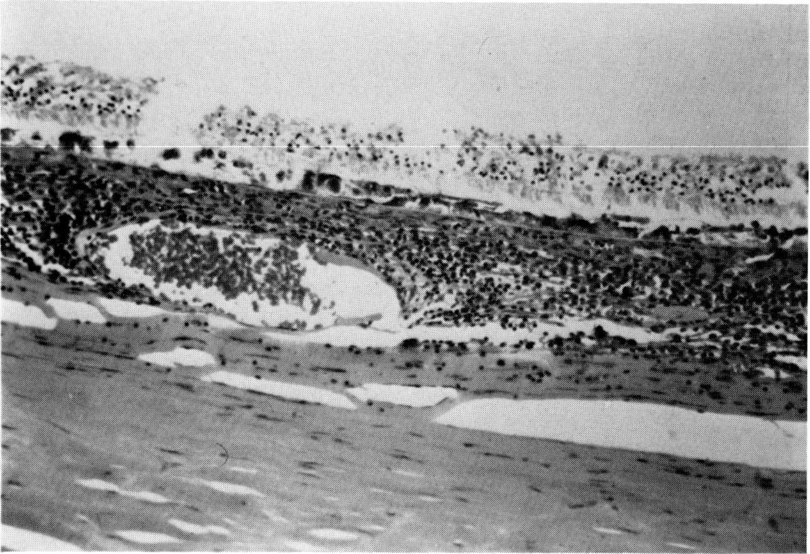

**FIGURE 27-4**     Histopathological sections reveal necrosis with loss of retinal structure and photoreceptor drop out. Marked inflammation is seen in the choroid and choriocapillaris. *(Courtesy of Dr. J. S. Pepose.)*

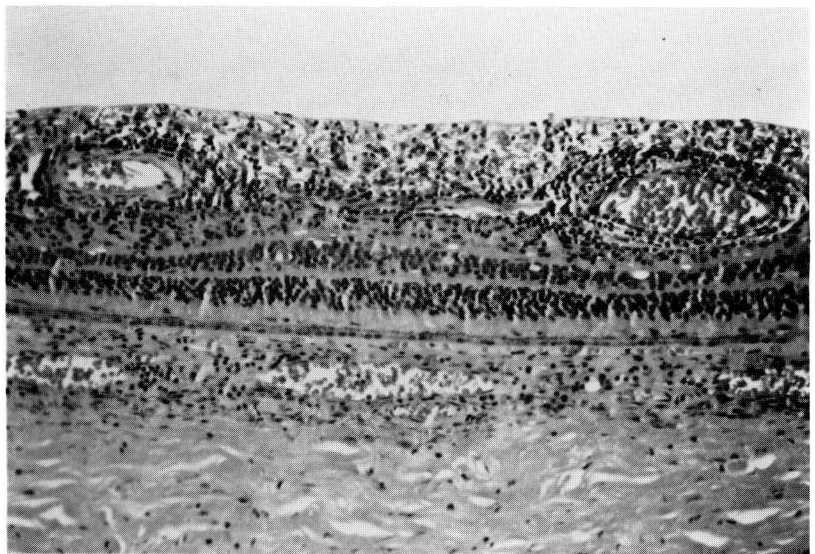

**FIGURE 27-5**     Marked retinal inflammation can be seen in this acutely infected eye, which has not yet undergone retinal necrosis in this area. A prominent component of perivasculitis with round cell infiltrate is seen. *(Courtesy of Dr. J. S. Pepose.)*

ologic findings of inflammatory cell infiltrates, vascular endothelial swelling, and arteriolar thromboses but no evidence of viral particles in the optic nerve or associated vessels. This presumed form of anterior ischemic optic neuropathy may explain the sudden visual loss sometimes seen in ARN patients.[4]

Electron microscopy demonstrates virus particles in all layers of the retina, as well as the pigment epithelium and vascular endothelium. A typical herpes-

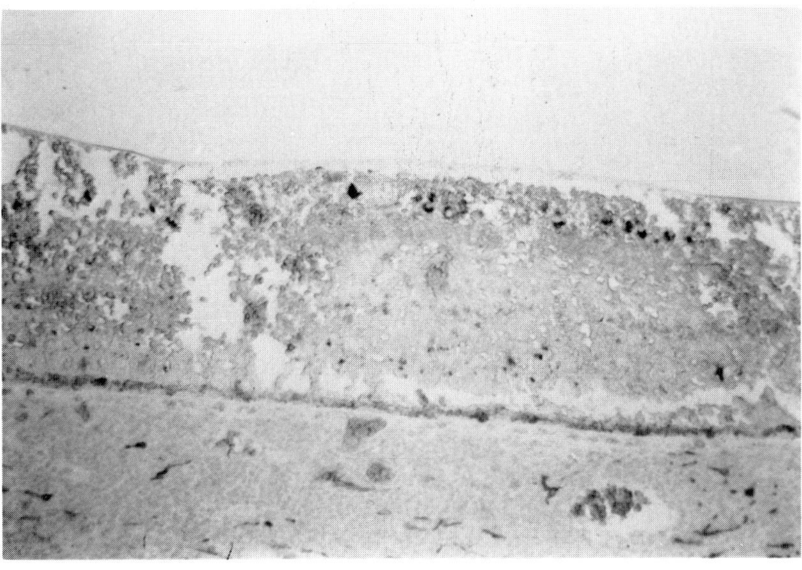

**FIGURE 27-6**  Dark staining of viral particles can be seen in the necrotic intraretinal layers. *(Courtesy of Dr. J. S. Pepose.)*

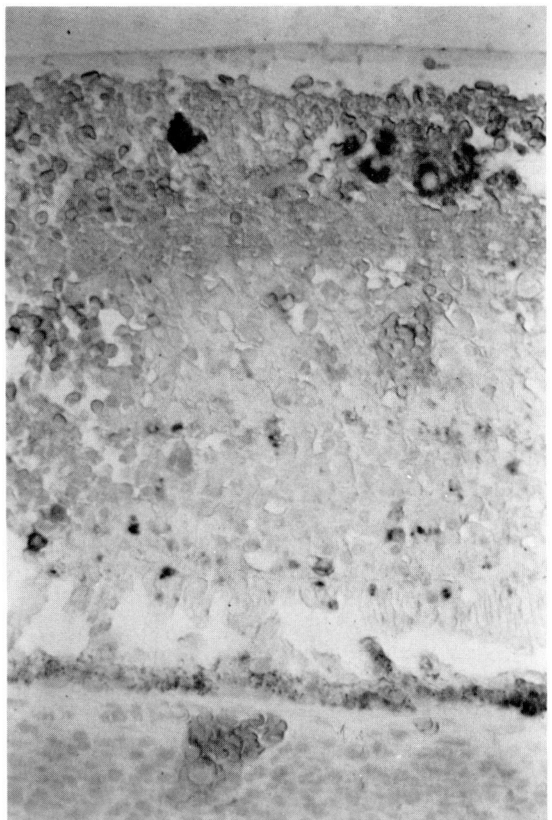

**FIGURE 27-7**  At higher power, viral protein picks up dark stain in infected cells in the inner layers of the retina. *(Courtesy of Dr. J. S. Pepose.)*

type hexagonal nucleocapsid, 80-100 nm in size, is seen, with enveloped virus particles, 180-120 nm in diameter.[5]

## MANAGEMENT

Appropriate management of ARN patients requires timely diagnosis and intervention with antiviral, anti-inflammatory, and surgical treatment. Blumenkranz and coworkers pioneered the use of acyclovir in patients with ARN, after early evidence suggested a herpes virus as the culpable agent.[19] Acyclovir is specific for this group of viruses. Herpes virus thymidine kinase phosphorylates acyclovir into acyclovir monophosphate. A series of host enzymes further modifies it to a nucleoside triphosphate, a potent selective inhibitor of viral DNA polymerase. Pepose et al tested the in vitro sensitivity of a VZ virus isolated from an ARN patient to acyclovir.[28] They found that the intravitreal levels achieved following intravenous acyclovir administration were over three times the $ED_{50}$ of the ARN-associated virus. Serum levels achieved after oral acyclovir dosing are often subtherapeutic. Thus the current treatment recommendation for intravenous acyclovir administration is 1500 mg/m²/day in 3 divided doses, usually for 10 days to 2 weeks. There are no reports of acyclovir toxicity in ARN patients. Known complications of high-dose systemic acyclovir administration include phlebitis, rash, transient elevation of serum creatinine, encephalopathy, and hypersensitivity. Gancyclovir (DHPG) is 10 to 100 times more effective against cytomegalovirus *in vitro* than acyclovir, but it is not the first-line drug used in ARN unless the disease is unresponsive to acyclovir or there is evidence of CMV infection.

In the first reported series of ARN patients treated with acyclovir, Blumenkranz and coworkers treated 13 eyes of 12 patients with the intravenous drug for an average of 10.9 days.[19] Progression of retinal lesions stopped by 48 hours in all cases, and regression began an average of 3.9 days after starting acyclovir. Intravitreal acyclovir has been used in vitrectomy infusion during prophylactic vitrectomy in two patients by Peyman et al with good results.[26]

Blumenkranz et al also reported the use of oral aspirin or coumadin to reduce the incidence of vaso-occlusive events. Ando and coworkers have noted platelet hyperaggregation in six of seven ARN patients.[29] Various investigators have tried antithrombotic therapy in an uncontrolled fashion without conclusively demonstrating a benefit. The risks entailed in treating patients with aspirin, 75% of whom will need semi-emergent surgery, may be significant. Although the effects of heparin and coumadin can be reversed, these drugs increase the risk of systemic hemorrhagic complications.

Anterior segment inflammation in ARN responds to topical treatment with corticosteroids and cycloplegic agents. Blumenkranz and coworkers have reported the use of oral prednisone at doses of 30 to 120 mg daily to improve the vitritis.[19] In that series, systemic steroids were begun 2 to 10 days after antiviral therapy was initiated. Steroids may theoretically worsen the infection if used without accompanying antiviral therapy. Patients with severe vitritis seem to have a worse outcome; whether final visual acuity or retinal detachment rates are altered by steroid treatment is unknown.

Prophylactic laser photocoagulation to prevent retinal detachment was re-

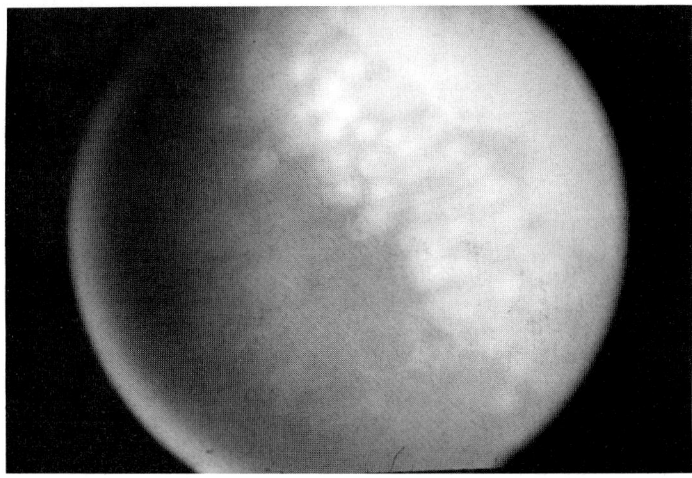

**FIGURE 27-8**    Argon photocoagulation has been placed in confluent rows posterior to the zones of retinitis to create a tight chorioretinal adhesion. It is at this interface between involved and uninvolved retina that retinal breaks develop in eyes with ARN.

ported by Yeo et al in 1986.[16] Confluent argon laser photocoagulation was applied posterior to the zone of peripheral retinal necrosis to create a band of chorioretinal adhesion (Figure 27-8), in addition to treatment with acyclovir and systemic steroids. The retina remained attached nine months after the episode of acute inflammation subsided. Han et al later described five patients treated prophylactically with argon or krypton laser. Treatment was applied confluently in two to three rows using a spot diameter of between 300 and 500 microns.[20] Power and duration were adjusted in order to obtain a white burn. The patients were also given acyclovir and steroids. All five retinas remained attached after fifteen months followup. Four of the five had confluent areas of retinitis limited to 150 degrees of the fundus.

Sternberg et al later reported results in 12 eyes of 10 patients treated with laser.[21] Retinal detachment occurred in two eyes (17%). Seven eyes with ARN were not treated with laser, most often because of dense ventritis, with a 67% detachment rate. The two eyes that detached after laser photocoagulation had a relatively good surgical and visual outcome. These authors hypothesized that strong chorioretinal adhesions may counteract the vitreoretinal traction at the edge of necrotic patches of retina. At these junctures, a posterior vitreous detachment is likely to develop as a corollary to severe inflammation with resultant retinal tears. Without a randomized, controlled trial, it is impossible to determine with certainty whether laser improves the outcome in ARN or cases with clear enough media to allow photocoagulation simply represent the more favorable end of the spectrum of disease in ARN. Nevertheless, photocoagulation is apparently safe, and it may have significant benefit.

Neovascularization of the optic disc may occasionally be seen in ARN, as well as other sequelae of retinal ischemia, including retinal neovascularization, neovascular glaucoma, cataract, and vitreous hemorrhage.[9] Han and coworkers reported complete regression of disc neovascularization in one patient within 16 days of panretinal photocoagulation.[22] Laser burns were placed in areas of non-

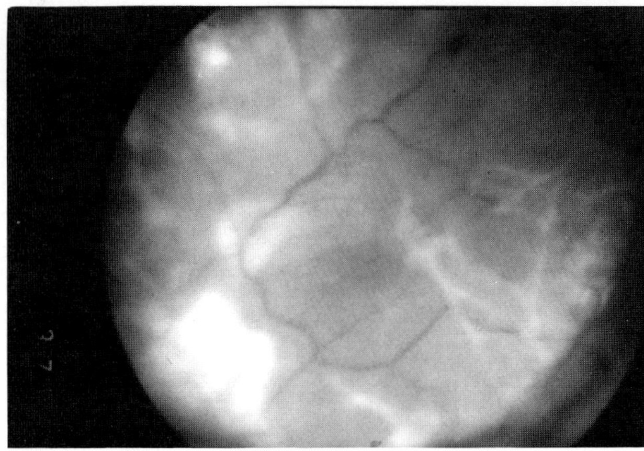

**FIGURE 27-9**    Despite successful retinal reattachment in this patient with ARN, final visual acuity is at the count-fingers level with macular distortion and epiretinal membrane formation.

necrotic and segmentally nonperfused retina as shown by fluorescein angiography. The krypton wavelength was felt to offer advantages for penetration of hazy media.

A number of surgical approaches to the treatment of ARN and associated retinal detachment have been described. In 1984, Clarkson et al reported the results of retinal detachment surgery in thirteen eyes.[14] Vitrectomy was performed in eight of the ten successful cases. Only one eye remained attached with a single scleral buckling procedure. Five of the nine eyes that remained attached with more than three-month followup had 20/200 vision or better. All six eyes that remained detached had proliferative vitreoretinopathy. Optic atrophy, possibly due to papillitis, and macular pucker were frequent complications causing poor vision (Figure 27-9).

Peyman et al treated two patients with no retinal detachment with vitrectomy, intravitreal infusion of acyclovir and prophylactic scleral procedures. Followup times were five and fourteen months. The retinas in both eyes remained attached, with visual acuities of 20/50 and 20/30.[26]

In an effort to clarify the most appropriate surgical approach, Blumenkranz and coworkers contrasted their series of eight patients treated with primary scleral buckling and cryotherapy, with or without vitrectomy, to eight eyes treated without primary scleral buckles, but with vitrectomy, and in most cases lensectomy, intravitreal gas, and endophotocoagulation.[27] All patients had been treated with acyclovir, oral prednisone, aspirin, and in some instances, heparin and coumadin. The groups were comparable in terms of preoperative characteristics. There was a 93.8% rate of final reattachment overall, with fewer operations (a mean of 1.5 per eye compared to 2.25 per eye) required in the nonbuckle group. Three of the buckled eyes and none of the others required silicone injection. Two eyes in each group had previously undergone prophylactic vitrectomy, two with scleral buckles and two without, prior to retinal detachment development. Excluding eyes treated prophylactically, two of six (33%) in the scleral buckle were reattached with a single operation, as compared to six out of six (100%) in the nonbuckle category. It is difficult to make firm recommendations based upon these relatively small numbers of patients, numbers reduced further if one eliminates the case in the buckle group treated with a scleral buckle alone. In addition, the eyes with primary scleral buckles received cryotherapy, which may have altered the prognosis by comparison with the vitrectomy-alone group, where laser was used instead. Nevertheless, this is the largest reported surgical series we have for evaluation, and it both serves to underline the value of vitrectomy in eyes with ARN and to suggest that in selected cases lensectomy may be useful while extensive scleral buckling may not always be necessary.

In this series, it is not surprising to find that eyes with scleral buckles and cryotherapy had a higher rate of choroidal detachment, fibrinoid reaction, and elevated intraocular pressure than eyes treated with vitrectomy alone. Also as expected, cataract development was more common in the vitrectomy and long-acting gas group.

There are too few patients treated with prophylactic surgery to draw conclusions about its efficacy. Peyman and coworkers reported successful outcomes in two patients treated with prophylactic vitrectomy and scleral buckling.[26] However in the series described by Blumenkranz et al, the only eyes in the nonbuckle group requiring reoperation were those prophylactically treated, and all four eyes (two in the buckle group and two in the nonbuckle group) so treated required reoperation.[27]

---

## References


1. Urayama A, Yamada N, Sasaki T, et al. Unilateral acute uveitis with retinal periarteritis and detachment. Japan J Clin Ophthalmol 1971; 25:607-619.
2. Willerson D Jr, Aaberg TM, Reeser FH. Necrotizing vaso-occlusive retinitis. Am J Ophthalmol 1977; 84:209-219.
3. Young NJ, Bird AC. Bilateral acute retinal necrosis. Br J Ophthalmol 1978; 62:581-590.
4. Fisher JP, Lewis ML, Blumenkranz M, Culbertson WW, Flynn H, Clarkson JG, Gass JDM, Norton EWD. The acute retinal necrosis syndrome part 1: clinical manifestations. Ophthalmol 1982; 89:1309-1316.
5. Culbertson WW, Blumenkranz MS, Haines H, Gass JDM, Mitchell KB, Norton EWD. The acute retinal necrosis syndrome part 2: histopathology and etiology. Ophthalmol 1982; 89:1317-1325.
6. Sagu U, Ozawa H, Sishi S, Nagahara K, Akeo K, Kimura C, Uemura Y. Acute retina necrosis (Kirisawa's uveitis). Japan J Ophthalmol 1983; 27:353-361.
7. Culbertson WW, Clarkson JG, Blumenkranz M, Lewis ML. Acute retinal necrosis. Am J Ophthalmol 1983; 96:5 638-685.
8. Price FW Jr, Schlaegel TF Jr. Bilateral acute retinal necrosis. Am J Ophthalmol 1967; 62:581-590.
9. Hayreh MMS, Kreiger AE, Straatsma BR et al. Acute retinal necrosis. Invest Ophthalmol Vis Sci 1980; 19(suppl):48.
10. Brando K, Kinoshitra A, Mimua Y. Six cases of so-called "Kirisawa type" uveitis. Japan J Clin Ophthalmol 1979; 33:115-1521.
11. Cogan DG, Kuwabara T, Young GF, Knox DL. Herpes simplex retinopathy in an infant. Arch Ophthalmol 1964; 72:641-645.
12. Cibis GW, Flynn JT Jr. Bilateral acute retinal necrosis. Am J Ophthalmol 1980; 89:419-424.
13. Sternberg P Jr, Knox DL, Finkelstein D, et al. Acute retinal necrosis syndrome. Retina 1982; 2:145-151.
14. Clarkson JG, Blumenkranz MS, Culbertson WW, Flynn HW Jr, Lewis ML. Retinal detachment following the acute retinal necrosis syndrome. Ophthalmol 1984; 91:1665-1668.
15. Rungger-Brandle E, Rous L, Luenberger PM. Bilateral acute retinal necrosis (BARN): identification of the presumed infectious agent. Ophthalmol 1984; 91:1648-1658.
16. Yeo JH, Pepose JS, Stewart JA, et al. Acute retinal necrosis syndrome following herpes zoster dermatitis. Ophthalmol 1986; 93:1418-1422.
17. Culbertson WW, Blumenkranz MS, Pepose JS, Stewart JA, Curtin VT. Varicella zoster virus is a cause of the acute retinal necrosis syndrome. Ophthalmol 1986; 93:559-569.
18. Olson RM, Holland GN, Goss SJ, Bowers WD, Meyers-Elliott RH. Routes of viral spread in the Von Szily model of herpes simplex virus retinopathy. Curr Eye Res 1987; 6:1 59-62.
19. Blumenkranz MS, Culbertson WW, Clarkson JG, Dix R: Treatment of the acute retinal necrosis syn-

drome with intravenous acyclovir. Ophthalmol 1986; 93:296-300.

20. Han DP, Lewis H, Williams GA, et al. Laser photocoagulation in the acute retinal necrosis syndrome with intravenous acyclovir. Ophthalmol 1986; 93:296-300.

21. Sternberg P Jr, Han DP, Yeo JH, Barr CC, Lewis H, Williams GA, Mieler WF. Photocoagulation to prevent retinal detachment in acute retinal necrosis. Ophthalmol 1988; 95:1389-1393.

22. Han DP, Abrams GW, Williams GA. Regression of disc neovascularization by photocoagulation in the acute retinal necrosis syndrome. Retina 1988; 8:244-246.

23. Sergott RC, Belmont JB, Savino PJ, et al. Optic nerve involvement in the acute retinal necrosis syndrome. Arch Ophthalmol 1985; 103:1160-1162.

24. Ludwig IH, Zegarra H, Zakov ZN. The acute retinal necrosis syndrome possible herpes simplex retinitis. Ophthalmol 1984; 91:1659-1664.

25. Lewis ML, Culbertson WW, Post MJ, Miller LD, Kokame GT, Dix R. Herpes simplex virus type 1: a cause of the acute retinal necrosis syndrome. Ophthalmol 1989; 96:875-878.

26. Peyman GA, Goldberg MF, Uninsky E, Tessler H, Pulido J, Hendrix R. Vitrectomy and intravitreal antiviral drug therapy in acute retinal necrosis syndrome. Arch Ophthalmol 1984; 102:1618-1621.

27. Blumenkranz M, Clarkson J, Culbertson WW, Flynn HW, Lewis ML, Young GM. Visual results and complications after retinal reattachment in the acute retinal necrosis syndrome: the influence of operative technique. Retina 1989; 9:170-174.

28. Pepose JS, Biron K. Antiviral sensitivities of the acute retinal necrosis syndrome virus. Current Eye Res 1987; 6:(1) 201-205.

29. Ando F, Kato M, Goto S, Kobayashi K, Ichikawa H, Kamiya T. Platelet function in bilateral acute retinal necrosis. Am J Ophthalmol 1983; 96:27-32.

30. Farrell TA, Wolf MD, Folk KJC, Pulido JS, Yuh WTC. Trigeminal nerve involvement by herpes zoster leading to keratouveitis and contralateral acute retinal necrosis. Ophthalmol 1990; 97(supp):152.

31. Culbertson WW, Brod RD, Flynn HW, Taylor BC, Brod BA, Lightman DA, Gordon G. Acute retinal necrosis (arn) following chicken pox. Ophthalmol 1990; 97(supp):110.

# CONTROVERSY IN CURRENT PRACTICE

# 28

# Rigid Gas Permeable versus Soft Contact Lenses

## *The Superiority of Soft Contact Lenses*

**Daniel J. Sigband, MD, FACS**

Theoretically speaking, rigid lenses have numerous advantages over soft contact lenses, but theory has to take a back seat to reality in terms of success and utilization, soft lens being preferred by more than 5 to 1 persons—both practitioners and patients.

Soft lenses are being used by approximately 85% of contact lens wearers in the United States. This is true despite the advances in rigid gas-permeable technology and the presumed physiological, visual, and durability factors possessed by the rigid products. Patient acceptance and success with soft lenses make this product the lens of overwhelming choice by both doctor and patient. Although both categories of products have disadvantages, soft lenses have recently made great strides forward. Introduction of new manufacturing methods has made possible disposable lenses and reliable soft toric lenses. These soft lens products, in my opinion, will make the most outstanding contributions in contact lens technology in the 1990s. The purpose of this discussion is to illustrate why rigid lenses have fallen short of expectations and, therefore, why soft lenses have been so successful and demand such a large share of the contact lens market.

A primary goal of manufacturers has been to overcome the major and overriding problem with rigid lenses, namely comfort. Despite the improvement in materials made by the introduction of oxygen-permeable polymers (RGPs) compared to nonoxygen materials (PMMA) and improvements in fitting techniques and designs (i.e., aspherics), rigid lenses are uncomfortable for most patients. Unfortunately, the initial foreign-body sensation, as well as continued discomfort during adaptation discourages both patients and practitioners alike. Because of the excellent comfort of soft lenses from the outset of wear, patients readily accept these lenses; and there is considerably less discontinuation of wear (drop out) among them than among rigid lens wearers.

An examination of the fundamental difference in design between rigid and soft lenses reveals why soft lenses are so much more comfortable. Rigid lenses must be made smaller than the corneal diameter. Because of this limitation in size and because of the hardness of the material, the presence of corneal and lid sensation for the patient constitutes the major and unavoidable comfort problem inherent with rigid lenses. More flexible rigid materials, improved edge designs, and aspheric lenses have been disappointing in terms of marked improvement in overall RGP lens comfort.

Because of the limitation on the size of rigid lenses, entrapment of foreign bodies under them continues to constitute one of their major disadvantages. Rigid lenses are thus avoided by many individuals engaged in activities where foreign-body entrapment poses a serious hazard to their jobs or leisure time pursuits. In addition to this problem, the size limitation of rigid lenses can cause lens displacement, excessive lens movement, or lens displacement commonly caused by rapid gaze or rubbing. Excessive lens movement and lens loss result in the problem of transient or total visual loss for the individual patient. Patients in critical professions, such as law enforcement, and those engaged in numerous sporting activities, find rigid lenses to be a major disadvantage for their occupations or advocations.

On the other hand, the large size of soft lenses, which bridge the corneal limbus by at least 1 mm, gives the patient comfort by eliminating corneal sensation. More important, proper fit of soft lenses prevents foreign body entrapment, excessive lens movement, lens displacement, and lens loss. This major advantage of soft lenses weighs heavily in lens choice for the active patient engaged in numerous vocational and recreational activities.

Another disadvantage of the relatively small size of rigid lenses is the impossibility of ocular iris enhancement that is possible with soft lenses which completely cover the iris from limbus to limbus. Tinted or opaque-colored soft lenses are popular alternatives for patients to enhance lens handling, provide glare reduction, and make cosmetic improvement. This advantage extends to those individuals who have congenital iris defects (aniridia, colomboma), traumatic or surgical iris defects (iridectomy), and disfigured or damaged eyes. Thousands of individuals have been helped by standard or custom-tinted colored soft lenses.

Another advantage of soft lenses has been their successful use as therapeutic devices following corneal trauma or corneal disease or as an adjunct to anterior-segment surgery.

The greater comfort of soft lenses ensures longer daily wear and the possibility of overnight wear. Whereas approved extended-wear, rigid, oxygen-permeable lenses have been a disappointing failure because of comfort problems, displacement possibility, and adherence problems, extended-wear soft lenses have been a resounding success, with 1 out of 4 soft-lens wearers choosing this modality. It is estimated that about 5 million Americans wear extended-wear soft lenses. Ease of adaptation and greater comfort have allowed these millions to enjoy the continuous good vision and convenience afforded by extended wear. The introduction of disposable lenses has further increased the convenience and safety of extended-wear lenses, with thousands of new patients choosing them. The ease of adaptation and comfort of soft lenses also permit occasional wear. If rigid lenses are not worn every day, readaptation is uncomfortable and time consuming, discouraging most patients interested in occasional wear. Thus, a patient interested in extended wear or flexible wear will certainly prefer soft lenses.

Arguments that rigid lenses provide crisper vision due to correction of astigmatism fail to consider numerous other problems of vision correction inherent in rigid lenses. If the astigmatism is purely corneal and 2 diopters or less in amount, visual correction with rigid lenses is usually excellent. However, flexure of the newer, improved, rigid, oxygen-permeable material, especially if corneal astigmatism is more than 2 diopters, creates visual problems for many patients.

Furthermore, many patients with "lenticular" or noncorneal astigmatism have had greater success with the newly designed, better-manufactured soft toric lenses than with rigid-front toric lenses. Because back toric or bitoric rigid lenses have numerous disadvantages, many practitioners choose soft torics for astigmatism problems. Among other visual problems commonly seen with rigid lenses are edge flair due to lens size; the common flair problem induced by planned lens displacement (upper lid attachment fit); or unplanned lens displacement, commonly seen in against-the-rule astigmates. Spectacle blur is another common problem, caused by the corneal molding induced by rigid lenses. Both problems of flair and spectacle blur are usually avoided in the soft lens wearer.

Another problem encountered among rigid-lens patients but not commonly seen in soft lens wearers is corneal desiccation. The cause of this problem can be traced to the relatively small size of the rigid lenses which interrupt the corneal tear film meniscus in that palpebral fissure region. This rigid-lens limitation leads to corneal dehydration, the common problem of 3-9 staining, vascularization, and finally pseudo-pterygium formation. Not only chronic discomfort but also the cosmetically unappealing palpebral 3-9 conjunctival injection are the results of this common problem, found primarily in rigid-lens wearers.

It was commonly argued in the past that rigid lenses were more durable and required less care than soft lenses. In the era of PMMA lenses, this was true; but the newer, rigid gas-permeable polymers are often as fragile as many of the better-manufactured soft lenses. Also, the newer gas-permeable polymers require as much care as soft lenses in terms of cleaning, soaking, and disinfection. Improved cold disinfection methods for soft lenses (such as Renu, Optifree) have simplified lens care and placed rigid and soft lens maintenance on par for simple cleaning and disinfection procedures. Another argument for rigid lenses has been their reduced cost compared to that of soft lenses. In the era of PMMA lenses, this was true; but with the introduction of newer, rigid, gas-permeable materials, the material and manufacturing costs of rigid lenses have become greater than those of good-quality soft lenses. Improved manufacturing of soft lenses has also made their durability comparable to that of rigid gas-permeable lenses, negating replacement cost of lenses as a factor in choosing either product. Soft disposable lenses that are worn for one or two weeks and then discarded have eliminated the need for lens care and costly solutions, these unique products have become very cost-effective.

Simplicity in fitting is another advantage of soft lenses. Most soft lenses can be fitted with one or two sets of base curve/diameter parameters, whereas rigid lenses must be fitted precisely to a particular corneal radius of curvature. Thus inventory stocking of replacement soft lenses is feasible, but it is impractical for rigid lenses. Because of the simple, limited parameters for soft lenses, the use of trial lenses to determine the feasibility of disposable-lens wear for an individual patient is a practical reality. This is certainly not true of fitting rigid lenses for the same individual.

Because of numerous factors, the incidence of soft-lens complications had been declining. The most serious problem, microbial keratitis, has been reduced by improved, simple, effective disinfection systems, improved patient and practitioner education, and safer lens products, such as disposable or frequently replaced lenses. Improved lenses such as the new molded, ultrathin, high-water lenses—available as reusable, disposable, or frequent-replacement products—have improved oxygen flow to the cornea, making daily wear physiologically feasible. For the majority of patients with these lenses, adaptation to limited extended wear has become a safe and effective alternative.

Other deposit-induced complications (i.e., G.P.C. and superior limbal keratitis) are found among wearers of both rigid and soft lenses but are truly more common among soft-lens wearers. The incidence of these complications has been reduced recently by improved lens care systems such as enzymes and hydrogen peroxide systems and by the use of disposable or frequent-replacement lens regimens.

Contact-lens technology has made great strides in supplying the needs of the ametropic population with unique and effective rigid- or soft-lens devices. In theory, rigid lenses have numerous physiological and visual advantages, but soft lenses are at present the better modality for the reasons previously discussed. As a result of the effectiveness of these soft lenses, patients and fitters choose soft lenses by more than 5 to 1 over rigid lenses.

# The Superiority of RGP Lenses

**James E. Key, MD**

Largely because of relatively simple fitting techniques and initial patient comfort, soft hydrogel contact lenses account for the great majority of new contact-lens fits in the United States. Rigid gas-permeable lenses (RGPs) present the patient and practitioner with another choice, particularly in terms of recent advances in RGP-lens technology that overcome the discomfort problem.

The overriding consideration for both patient and practitioner, in terms of lens choice, should be the nature of contact-lens–induced changes in corneal metabolism and on the ocular surface. Depending on the lens material chosen, as well as the lens design and fitting technique, these changes may manifest in the epithelium, endothelium, or the conjunctiva and its vascular supply. The newer RGP lenses induce less ocular stress, primarily because of their greater oxygen transmissibility and fitting relationship to the cornea. This assertion is best examined by looking at the effect of contact lenses on the various affected parts of the eye.

## EPITHELIUM

The reported effects of corneal epithelial stress from contact lens wear include decreased mitosis of the basal cells, decreased epithelial thickness, decreased epithelial oxygen uptake, and increase in epithelial microcysts. Most of these changes are due to oxygen deprivation underneath the contact lenses with the resulting build-up of lactate and the production of edema.[1] Clinical syndromes associated with these changes are seen as a varying combination of punctate keratitis with staining, sterile corneal infiltrates, or even severe corneal ulceration.

At present, no soft contact lens achieves the theoretically safe level of oxygen transmission in the closed eye or extended wear state. Even when worn on a daily-wear regimen, soft contact lenses are at a significant disadvantage because they transmit oxygen only as a function of their water content and lens thickness. Increasing water content has a positive effect on oxygen transmission, whereas increasing lens thickness has a negative effect. Not only does increasing the water content lead to a deterioration in other aspects of lens performance, such as fragility, but it also obviously increases the lens thickness so that a practical limit to oxygen transmission is soon reached.

RGP lenses, on the other hand, transmit oxygen primarily as a function of their polymer structure. The addition of both silicone and fluorine greatly increases oxygen transmission through an RGP lens, and these substances do so by independent mechanisms.

Other factors are also important in oxygen transmission to the epithelium. These include contact-lens movement, tear exchange beneath the contact lens, the fit of the lens, and surface contamination. RGP lenses are not only more independent of tear evaporation rates than soft contact lenses but actively aid the tear-pump mechanism to exchange 20% of the tear volume per blink. RGP materials are likewise more resistant to protein and lipid deposits and more easily cleaned of such deposits.

Superficial corneal staining is frequently seen by the practitioner as a sign of epithelial stress. The pattern of central punctate staining, often associated with epithelial microcyst, is seen much less frequently with RGP lenses than with soft contact lenses because of the greater oxygen transmission of the RGP lenses. A more diffuse staining reaction, which can be seen from hypersensitivity to lens care products, is more typical of soft contact lenses as well, because more products containing preservatives are used in conjunction with those lenses.

More serious and attention-getting complications that affect the corneal epithelium include corneal abrasion, neovascularization, ulceration, and scarring. Soft contact lenses are implicated in the vast majority of cases of microbial keratitis reported in the literature. Several risk factors identified in recent studies as being responsible for microbial keratitis are poor compliance with the lens care regimen, the occasional overnight use of daily-wear lenses, and lens case contamination.[2] It is obvious why the users of soft contact lenses run a higher risk of microbial keratitis than users of RGP lenses if we consider these factors. To begin with, soft contact-lens disinfection is both more complicated than disinfection of RGPs and more likely to be misunderstood or simply skipped altogether. The lens cases tend to be contaminated more often due both to the complicated care regimen and to occasional confusion about lens care products. Last, if a patient wears a soft contact lens overnight, that lens will almost always provide less oxygen transmission and therefore less margin of safety to the cornea than any of the widely used RGP lenses available at present.

Another factor in the increased incidence of microbial keratitis with soft lenses is related to the greater growth of pathogenic bacteria on the surface of soft lenses. This is part due to the tendency of soft lenses to attract protein and lipid deposits on which the bacteria thrive. In addition, the soft lenses are more difficult to clean; and the comfort, or even bandage effect, of soft lenses may mask the symptoms of corneal ulceration until irreversible damage has occurred.

## ENDOTHELIUM

Endothelial polymegathism and pleomorphism occur naturally with aging, but they are more pronounced and occur earlier in contact-lens wearers. The underlying mechanism in polymegathism may be lens-induced corneal hypoxia with subsequent changes in the concentrations of lactic acid, endothelial cell hydrogen ions, cellular pH or cellular $pCO_2$. These physiologic changes cause osmotic swelling of the endothelial cells and thereby affect cell size and mosaic pattern. There is some evidence that higher degrees of polymegathism cause corneas to recover more slowly from stromal edema and swelling after periods of hypoxic stress or the stress induced by cataract surgery and lens implantation.[3] If polymegathism is irreversible and does indeed decrease the functional reserve of the endothelium, then its control is extremely important and must be considered in those people who wear contact lenses for many years.

Polymegathism is clearly associated with the duration of any type of contact-lens wear, but several studies suggest that RGP lenses induce less cell-size change than do soft contact lenses. Polymegathism is most advanced in patients who have used nongas-permeable hard (PMMA) lenses, is next most frequently seen in those wearing soft hydrogel lenses, and is the least evident in those who have worn or were switched to highly gas permeable RGP lenses.[4] An increase of 22% to 27% in polymegathism has been found in patients who have worn extended-wear soft contact lenses for five years, whereas no increase in polymegathism was found among patients wearing lenses similar to those that have the oxygen permeability of the present generation of RGP lenses.[5]

## CONJUNCTIVA AND OCULAR SURFACE

Superficial neovascularization, usually accompanied by corneal edema, is a more common finding with soft contact lenses than with RGP lenses. The cause, once again, is undoubtedly related to the lower oxygen transmission of soft contact lenses and to their larger diameter with its draping effect on the corneal limbal vessels.

A condition similar to classic superior limbic keratconjunctivitis has been reported in soft-contact-lens wearers but not in RGP-lens wearers. Mechanical factors and hypersensitivity, primarily to thimerisal, have been implicated; cessation of lens wear usually reverses the condition, but permanent scarring may result.

Of greater clinical significance, the direct mechanical irritation of the upper tarsal conjunctiva contributes to the development of giant papillary conjunctivitis (GPC). The sensitization of the conjunctival surface is most likely due to allergy to the mucoproteinaceous lens deposits on contact lenses. GPC is much more common in soft-contact-lens wearers, owing to the larger diameter of soft contact lenses and their greater tendency toward deposit adherence. Indeed, the only way patients with GPC can continue to wear contact lenses is usually to switch to RGP lenses.

## CONCLUSION

RGP lenses should be the lenses of choice for most contact lens wearers. This brief review has touched mainly upon the physiologic and clinical considerations in contact-lens wear that the ophthalmologist must consider. Other obvious advantages of RGP lenses include better visual acuity because of the ability to correct corneal astigmatism, the greater durability of RGP lenses, and the simplicity of lens care. The oxygen transmissibility of the newer materials leads me to the conclusion that only RGP lenses should be used for those patients who desire extended wear. The greater association of soft contact lenses with polymegathism, increased corneal edema, and increased corneal deswelling time renders such lenses, including disposable soft contact lenses, particularly unsuitable in the extended-wear patient.

The major difficulties and drawbacks to RGP lenses are those of superficial limbal staining and initial lens comfort. These problems will be solved by better quality lenses from the laboratories as well as new design factors such as aspheric peripheral curves with the proper edge lift to promote greater comfort and fitting stability. In conclusion, RGP lenses have clear advantages over soft lenses in providing the ideal lens characteristics desired both by contact lens practitioners and by their patients.

## References

1. Holden BA. Corneal requirements for extended wear: an update. CLAO J 1988; 14:3220-3222.
2. Schein OD, Glynn RJ, Poggio EG, et al. The relative risk of ulcerative keratitis among users of daily wear and extended wear soft contact lenses. N Engl J Med 1989; 321:773-778.
3. Rao GN, Aquavella JV, Goldberg SH, et al. Pseudophakic bullous keratopathy: relationship to preoperative corneal endothelial status. Ophthalmol 1984; 91:1135-1140.
4. Holden BA, Williams L, Sweeny DF, et al. The endothelial response to contact lens wear. CLAO J 1986; 12:150-152.
5. MacRae SM, Matsuda M, Shellans S. Corneal endothelial changes associated with contact lens wear. CLAO J 1989; 15:82-87.

# 29

# Wavelength Selection: Its Importance for Laser Treatment of Retinal and Choroidal Disease

## *Pro*

**Lawrence J. Singerman, MD**

Is laser wavelength important in the laser treatment of retinal and choroidal disease? Yes, at least sometimes. Is it the *most* important factor? No, never.

Randomized, controlled clinical trials have made invaluable contributions to improving the management of patients with macular and retinal vascular diseases. There are, however, higher truths than those created by clinical trials, and these include the principles of physics. Whether confirmed by a clinical trial or not, it remains a fact that yellow has a specific wavelength and that it is better absorbed in hemoglobin than is green and far better absorbed than is red. The wavelengths of other colors in the spectrum and their absorption in various media are also governed by physical laws.

Although it is easy—though often expensive—to buy the equipment used in laser treatment of macular and retinal vascular disease, the actual use of that equipment to provide the best possible treatment is complex. I believe that several factors, all managed optimally, are required for successful treatment both of choroidal neovascularization and of many other difficult lesions encountered in a retinal practice (Figure 29-1). Lack of thoroughness in taking any of these steps may lead to a poor result. Among these steps, the most important is proper patient selection and proper explanation to the patient of what can be expected from treatment.[1] In the management of choroidal neovascularization, excellent fluorescein angiography is important at several stages, both preoperatively and at frequent followup visits. Meticulous followup is particularly critical—in view of the high incidence of recurrences—in patients with choroidal neovascular membranes, especially in association with age-related macular degeneration, in which 59% of neovascular membranes recur within three years.[2] However, assuming all other factors are managed optimally, I believe that there are still certain cases in which the laser wavelength used may be a decisive factor in determining outcome. The relative value of different wavelengths may have been overemphasized by some laser manufacturers. Nevertheless, it is useful to have various wavelengths available as options in the management of many macular and retinal vascular diseases.[3]

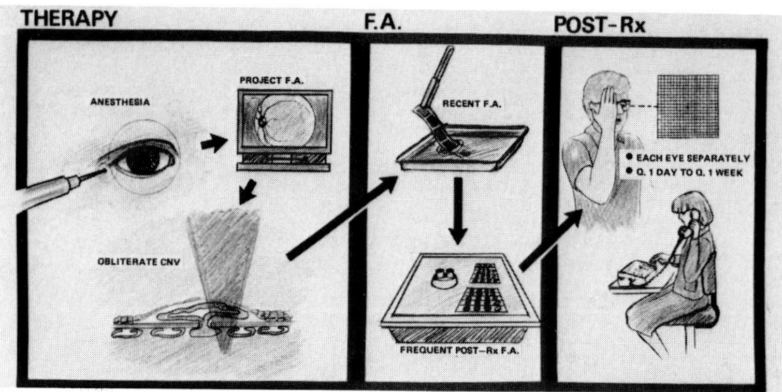


**FIGURE 29-1**     Adherence to the principles of management is more important than is the wavelength used. *(Reprinted with permission from JB Lippincott.)*

## PROLIFERATIVE RETINOPATHIES

A purist would treat proliferative diabetic retinopathy with the argon blue-green wavelength, because the efficacy of this treatment was proven by the Diabetic Retinopathy Study (DRS).[4] However, although the wavelength proved beneficial by the DRS was argon blue-green, subsequent research has demonstrated that the blue wavelength of the argon laser has several drawbacks. These are most evident in the management of choroidal neovascularization, in which the high absorption of blue by foveal xanthophyll pigment precludes safe treatment with blue-green in the juxtafoveal region. Other factors make blue undesirable in the management of proliferative retinopathies. It is highly absorbed by the xanthochrome in the nuclear sclerotic lens, which greatly increases the energy required and the difficulty of precisely placing burns of optimal quality (Figure 29-2). Furthermore, scatter treatment with the blue wavelength was found to induce a general retinal phototoxic effect.[5] Accordingly, we replaced blue-green with green argon laser in the treatment of proliferative retinopathies.

In proliferative retinopathies, there are several advantages, in selected cases, to the red wavelength of either krypton or the tunable dye laser (Figures 29-2 and 29-3).[6] These include the following:

- Better penetration of mild to moderate vitreous hemorrhage
- Better penetration of moderate nuclear sclerosis
- Less damage to normal retinal vasculature
- Less risk of epiretinal membrane formation and of increased vitreoretinal traction

In addition, the use of krypton or dye red is advantageous in patients with iris neovascularization, who usually also have corneal and lens opacities; red penetrates both of these better than blue, green, or yellow does.

However, the red krypton or dye laser wavelength also carries an increased risk of several complications. These include the following:

- Choroidal hemorrhage
- Choroidal detachment with possible angle-closure glaucoma
- Greater pain

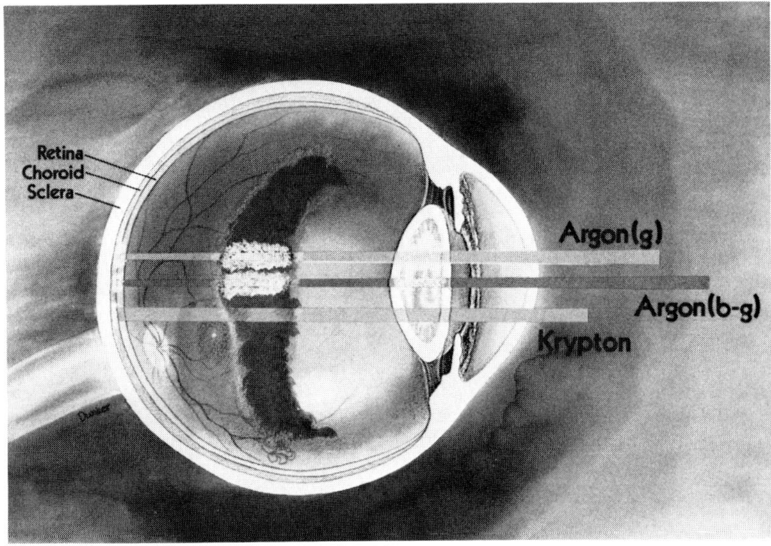



**FIGURE 29-2**   The blue and green wavelengths are absorbed in nuclear sclerotic lens and in vitreous hemorrhage, but the red wavelength penetrates these. *(Reprinted with permission from WB Saunders.)*

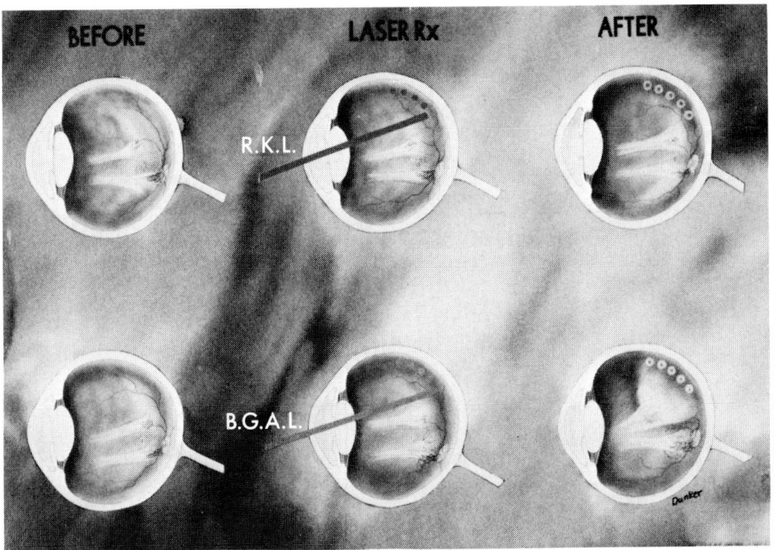



**FIGURE 29-3**   The blue wavelength may increase traction retinal detachment; the red wavelength may decrease the risk of this. RKL = red krypton laser, BGAL = blue-green argon laser. *(Reprinted with permission from WB Saunders.)*

- Breaks in Bruch's membrane with consequent choroidovitreal neovascularization (Figure 29-4).
- Inability to close surface neovascularization focally or stop a source of bleeding

The value of krypton or dye-red laser, compared with that of argon, in the management of proliferative diabetic retinopathy will be determined by the results

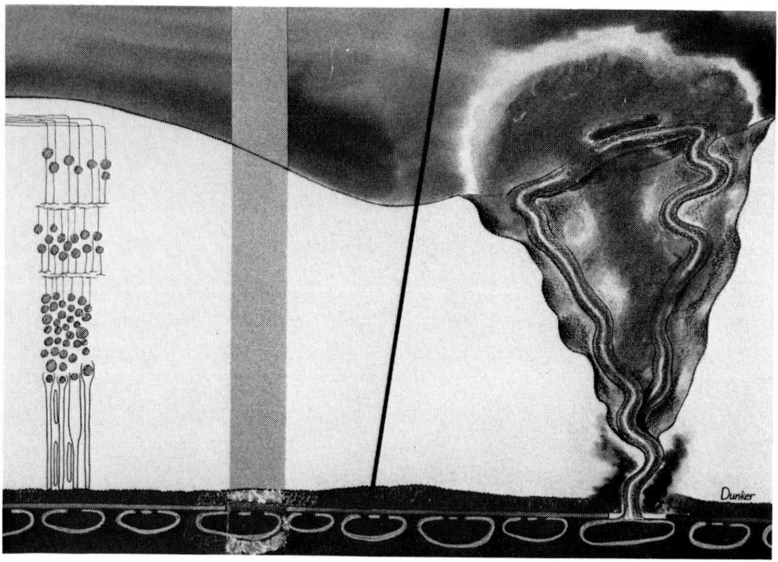

**FIGURE 29-4**     Choroidal-vitreal neovascularization may result from a break in Bruch's membrane, which occurs more frequently with red wavelengths, especially if used with short duration, high intensity burns.

of the Krypton Argon Regression of Neovascularization Study (KARNS), a multi-center, randomized, controlled clinical trial of more than 1000 patients, for which recruitment has recently been completed.[7] The protocol requires that patients in each treatment group receive identical treatment, except for exposure time: with argon, exposure time is 0.05 to 0.2 seconds; with krypton, 0.1 to 0.5 seconds. The aim of treatment is to place 1600 to 2000 burns, of 500-micron spot-size, on the retina.[8] Blankenship has shown that, in eyes with proliferative diabetic retinopathy, the histopathological and clinical effects of argon laser photocoagulation are similar to those of krypton laser photocoagulation.[9] However, significant differences could exist that his small sample size might not detect. The final KARNS data are being analyzed, and the results should be available soon.

The potential value of the diode laser in scatter laser therapy requires clarification. This modality is currently used in some practices because the small size of the laser allows portability and thus permits its use in offices that do not have other lasers. However, convincing data demonstrating the efficacy of the diode laser have not yet been evinced.

Recently, for scatter laser therapy we have often turned to the yellow wavelength because it is absorbed even less than green in the xanthochrome of the nuclear sclerotic lens. It is my clinical impression that treatment with yellow may be more comfortable than is treatment with other wavelengths, but this is not proven. Furthermore, one often wishes to pretreat diabetic maculopathy with focal therapy to microaneurysms at the same session as, but prior to, initiating scatter laser, and yellow may have an advantage in this setting. Focal treatment of microaneurysms should not be done with red laser, which is poorly absorbed in the hemoglobin of the microaneurysm.

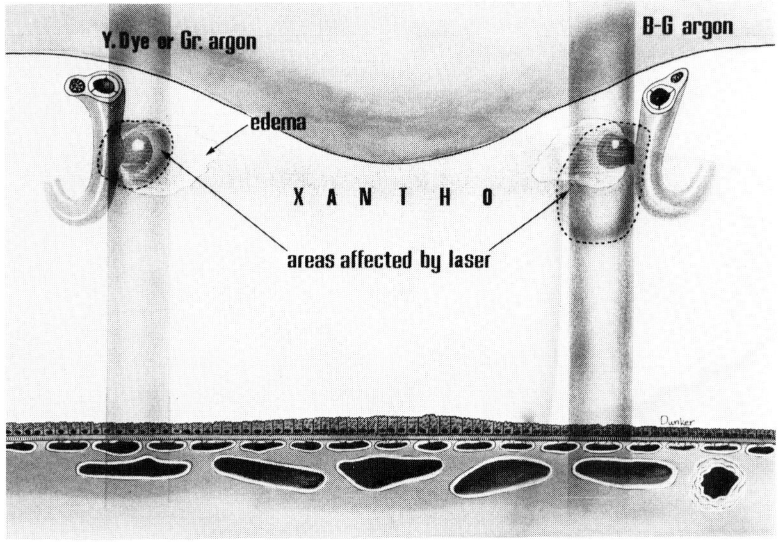



**FIGURE 29-5**    Yellow dye is optimally absorbed in the hemoglobin in microaneurysms and is now our wavelength of choice for diabetic maculopathy. Green argon is also acceptable, but blue-green argon is not because of high absorption in foveal xanthophyll pigment, resulting in more retinal

## DIABETIC MACULOPATHY

My distinct clinical impression is that the yellow wavelength is optimal for focal treatment of microaneurysms (Figure 29-5). While it is true that we often fail to occlude microaneurysms focally or change the color of the microaneurysm, as was one of the goals in the protocol for the Early Treatment Diabetic Retinopathy Study, I find it much easier to occlude these microaneurysms with yellow (577 nm) than with green. Certainly, we can close microaneurysms with green, but yellow requires less laser energy to do so. I avoid the use of argon blue-green because some microaneurysms requiring treatment might be near foveal xanthophyll pigment, in which the blue wavelength would be highly absorbed.

## CHOROIDAL NEOVASCULARIZATION

There are several reports of histopathologic results of dye laser. Smiddy et al found that in the primate retina intense treatment with the orange wavelength (595-600 nm) caused full-thickness burns in the retina, whereas the wavelengths on either side of it in the color spectrum, at similar powers, did not cause similar full-thickness burns.[10] Takahashi et al also reported that, of yellow (577 nm), orange (590 nm and 600 nm), and red (630 nm), orange had the most marked coagulative effects in the choriocapillaris.[11] A scanning electron microscopic study by the same authors showed that three months after photocoagulation burn areas caused by the orange wavelength showed less evidence of tissue repair than did those caused by red or yellow.[12] Smiddy et al found no difference among orange, red, and yellow in the effect of moderate-intensity burns but thought that the appearance of the lesion so achieved did not simulate a therapeutic one. One explanation for these findings is that the absorption in hemoglobin, melanin, and xanthophyll could be additive. Another possible explanation is that the neurosensory retina, retinal pigment epithelium, or choroid may contain a chromophore with substantial absorption around 600 nm.[13] I discontinued the use of orange wavelengths for treatment of choroidal neovascularization after treatment failure in four of my first six cases.[14]

My treatment of choice in most cases of choroidal neovascular membrane (NVM) is sequential red-yellow dye laser.[14] First the red wavelength is applied lightly, using a 200-micron spot size lesion. It is applied near the edges of the NVM and allowed to spread just beyond the margins of the NVM with 0.2 second burns. The faint whitening that occurs often enhances the visualization of the extent of the NVM. Next, the yellow wavelength is applied to the treated area, using 200 to 500 micron lesions at durations between 0.2 and 1.0 second, at power settings sufficient to create an intense white lesion. In cases with extensive subretinal hemorrhage adjacent to the NVM or large retinal vessels over the NVM, I often use mostly or only the red wavelength of the tunable dye or krypton laser. In cases with extensive atrophy of the retinal pigment epithelium, I may use only the yellow wavelength of the dye laser.

I use the red wavelength of the dye or krypton laser to penetrate nuclear sclerotic lens, turbid subretinal fluid, and peripapillary retinal blood vessels. The red wavelength is superior to other wavelengths in penetrating xanthochrome pigment in the nuclear sclerotic lens, which is very common in patients with AMD. In theory, red would best penetrate blood while causing the least nerve-fiber damage.[15] I use the red wavelength to try to treat through thin subretinal hemorrhage overlying a portion of the NVM because the absorption characteristics of red are more advantageous in that setting than are those of other wavelengths. I can place the red wavelength just over the edge of the NVM with more precision than I can obtain with any other wavelength. This is largely due to lower intraocular scatter and better lens penetration with red than with other conventional wavelengths. The red wavelength can be used to outline the NVM precisely; it penetrates the choroid deeply, often providing a faint whitening that enhances visualization of the NVM.

The yellow wavelength is absorbed directly in hemoglobin, with minimal absorption in the xanthophyll pigment. Closure of NVMs may be enhanced with yellow laser because of the increased absorption in the oxyhemoglobin in the NVM. I also prefer yellow for recurrent NVM after treatment with another wavelength, assuming it has a chance to enhance success, compared with another wavelength that failed to induce closure. It is also useful in attempts to eliminate feeder vessels, which we rarely identify in untreated eyes but do see, occasionally, in recurrences after treatment.

## OTHER RETINAL VASCULAR DISEASES

Yellow laser may also prove to be the treatment of choice in other, less common retinal vascular diseases. Because of its greater absorption in hemoglobin and the consequent reduction in laser energy required to achieve closure of vessel walls, there may be less risk of exudation or hemorrhage following treatment of intraretinal vascular lesions such as those associated with Von Hippel's disease,

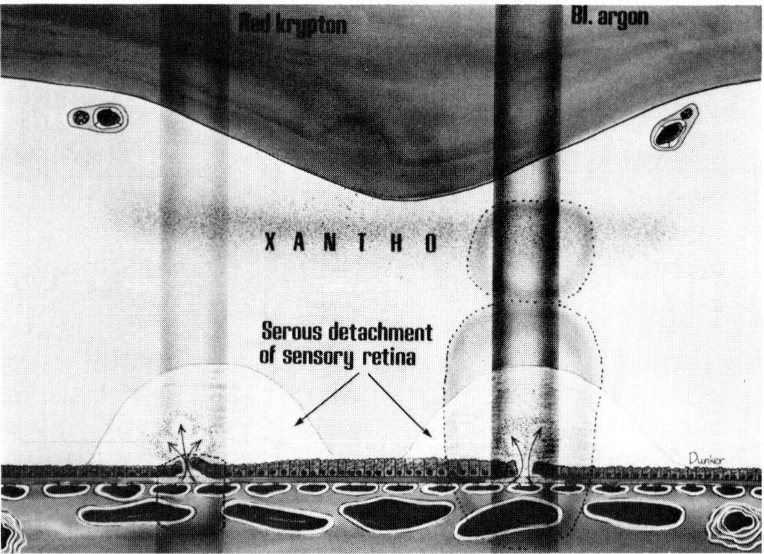


**FIGURE 29-6**  The red wavelength is absorbed only by melanin in the retinal pigment epithelium and choroid, whereas the blue-green wavelength is absorbed by foveal xanthophyll, hemoglobin, and melanin. *(Reprinted with permission from JB Lippincott.)*

Coats' disease, and retinal macroaneurysms.[16,17,18] Because these lesions are far from the retinal pigment epithelium, especially if there is associated exudative retinal detachment, there is less chance of thrombosis secondary to absorption of laser energy by melanin, and the absorption of laser energy by intravascular hemoglobin is more important in closing the vessel.

The krypton or dye-red laser wavelength may be advantageous in eyes with central serous chorioretinopathy.[19] The defect in this disorder is thought to be at the retinal pigment epithelium,[20] and recurrences occur most often near the initial leakage.[21,22] The absorption of the red wavelength by the melanin in the retinal pigment epithelium may make photocoagulation more effective and thus minimize recurrences, while causing less retinal damage than do other wavelengths (Figure 29-6).

In addition to the potential value of the dye laser, practitioners must also consider its potential drawbacks. Other lasers are more readily available and far less expensive to buy and maintain. In a large retinal referral practice or large ophthalmology program, the number of cases that might benefit from the availability of alternative wavelengths, especially yellow, is sufficient to justify the considerable expense of the dye laser. In practices with less retinal work, the expense might not be justifiable. Furthermore, it has been our experience that dye lasers malfunction much more frequently than do either argon or krypton lasers, and therefore a dye laser is probably not a good choice in a setting in which there is only one laser.

## CONCLUSION

It is indisputable that a number of steps, all managed optimally, are required for the successful management of patients with retinal and choroidal diseases. Wavelength selection can make a difference in selected cases. The flexibility of the dye laser offers the laser surgeon options in the different clinical settings encountered in the management of retinal and choroidal diseases. A randomized clinical trial using various wavelengths is required to prove the relative efficacy of one wavelength in comparison with another in any given disease. Such studies would be difficult to perform because of the multiple wavelengths and combinations thereof that are possible with the dye laser—precisely the features that make it valuable in our treatment armamentarium.

## References

1. Singerman LJ. Important points in the management of patients with choroidal neovascularization. Ophthalmol 1985; 92:610-614.
2. Macular Photocoagulation Study Group. Recurrent choroidal neovascularization after argon laser photocoagulation for neovascular maculopathy. Arch Ophthalmol 1986; 104:503-512.
3. L'Esperance FA Jr. Clinical photocoagulation with the organic dye laser. Ophthalmol 1985; 92:1592-1600.
4. Diabetic Retinopathy Study Research Group. Preliminary report on effects of photocoagulation therapy. Am J Ophthalmol 1976; 81:1-14.
5. Mainster MA, Ham WT, Delori FC. Potential retinal hazards: instrument and environmental light sources. Ophthalmol 1983; 90:927-932.
6. Singerman LJ. Red krypton laser therapy of macular and retinal vascular diseases. Retina 1982; 2:15-28.
7. Singerman LJ, Ferris FL, Mowery RP, et al. Krypton laser for proliferative diabetic retinopathy: the Krypton Argon Regression of Neovascularization Study. J Diabetic Complications 1988; 4:189-96.
8. Krypton Argon Regression of Neovascularization Study Group. Manual of Operations, Bethesda, Maryland, 1984 Office of Biometry and Epidemiology, National Eye Institute.
9. Blankenship GW. Red krypton and blue-green argon panretinal laser photocoagulation for proliferative diabetic retinopathy: a laboratory and clinical comparison. Trans Am Ophthalmol Soc 1986; 84:967-1003.
10. Smiddy WE, Patz A, Quigley HA, Dunkelberger GR. Histopathology of the effects of tuneable dye laser on monkey retina. Ophthalmol 1988; 95:956-963.
11. Takahashi K, Ohkuma H, Itagaki T, Uyama M. Histopathological study of the effects of photocoagulation on the retina and choroid with various wavelengths of dye laser. Acta Soc Ophthalmol Japan 1988; 92:1797-1808.
12. Takahashi K, Ohkuma H, Itagaki T, Uyama M. A scanning electron microscopic study of the retinochoroidal vascular casts following photocoagulation with various wavelengths of dye laser. Acta Soc Ophthalmol Japan 1988; 92:1809-1817.
13. Mainster MA. Wavelength selection in macular photocoagulation: tissue optics, thermal effects, and laser systems. Ophthalmol 1986; 93:952-958.
14. Singerman LJ, Kalski RS. Tunable dye laser photocoagulation for choroidal neovascularization complicating age-related macular degeneration. Retina 1989; 9:247-257.
15. Singerman LJ, Rice TA, Passloff RW. Krypton laser scatter photocoagulation treatment of proliferative diabetic retinopathy. In Ryan SJ, Dawson AK, Little HL, eds, Retinal diseases, Orlando; 1985, Grune & Stratton, pp. 43-48.
16. Blodi CF, Russell SR, Pulido JS, Folk JC. Direct and feeder vessel photocoagulation of retinal angiomas with dye yellow laser. Ophthalmol 1990; 97:791-795.
17. Singerman LJ, Saggau DD. Discussion; Blodi CF, Russell SR, Pulido JS, Folk JC. Direct and feeder vessel photocoagulation of retinal angiomas with dye yellow laser. Ophthalmol 1990; 97:796-797.
18. Joondeph BC, Joondeph HC, Blair NP. Retinal macroaneurysms treated with yellow dye laser. Retina 1989; 9:187-192.
19. Novak MA, Singerman LJ, Rice TA. Krypton and argon laser photocoagulation for central serous chorioretinopathy. Retina 1987; 7:162-169.
20. Gass JDM. Pathogenesis of disciform detachment of the neuroepithelium. II. Idiopathic central serous choroidopathy. Am J Ophthalmol 1967; 63:587.
21. Robertson D, Ilstrup D. Direct, indirect, and sham laser photocoagulation in the management of central serous chorioretinopathy. Am J Ophthalmol 1983; 95:457-466.
22. Gilbert CM, Owens SL, Smith PD, Fine SL. Long-term follow-up of central serous chorioretinopathy. Br J Ophthalmol 1984; 68:815-820.

## *Con*

**Stuart L. Fine, MD**

The issue is not whether wavelength selection is important but whether its importance has been overemphasized and overmarketed. For about 90% of the patients I treat, argon green, krypton red, dye red, or almost any other wavelength or color, would be acceptable. There is not more than an occasional situation where wavelength selection appears to be an important determinant of treatment outcome, particularly in comparison to the many other considerations involved in the management of patients with the retinal vascular and macular conditions amenable to treatment with laser photocoagulation.

In my practice, the approximate frequency of laser treatment for various conditions is as follows:

- Scatter treatment for proliferative retinopathy of varying etiologies (primarily diabetes and venous occlusion): 20%
- Focal treatment for diabetic macular edema: 30%
- Focal treatment for choroidal neovascularization of varying etiologies (primarily age-related macular degeneration and ocular histoplasmosis): 40%
- All others, including central serous chorioretinopathy, retinal tears, retinal telangiectasis, hemangiomas, etc.: 10%

Let us consider the potential role of laser wavelength in the management of these conditions.

## PROLIFERATIVE RETINOPATHY

Argon blue-green, or its variation argon green, is the wavelength which was employed in the three major collaborative clinical trials* assessing scatter laser treatment (formerly called panretinal photocoagulation or PRP) for retinal neovascularization.[1-3] Consequently, it is the wavelength whose treatment efficacy has been established unequivocally. While I suspect that krypton red can be employed just as effectively, argon green is more comfortable because the choroidal penetration is not as deep, so the laser energy is less likely to affect the sensory nerve fibers in the choroid. Clinicopathologic correlations comparing krypton red versus argon green lesions in human and primate eyes have shown no important differences in uptake when scatter-type lesions were delivered in a way that simulated the application of PRP in patients with proliferative retinopathy.[4] There are some situations, however, in which I do prefer krypton red, but these account for no more than 5% to 10% of the patients who require PRP. My indications for using krypton red are threefold: (1) media opacification by mild cataract, either lenticular or nuclear; (2) mild vitreous hemorrhage; and (3) presence of a condensed

---

*Diabetic Retinopathy Study (DRS), Early Treatment Diabetic Retinopathy Study (ETDRS), Branch Vein Occlusion Study (BVOS).

posterior vitreous detachment that behaves like a cataract (rare). In these situations, the penetration of red may be far superior to that of green, and in those instances I am pleased that the longer wavelength is available. But again, these situations account for no more than 5% to 10% of the patients who require PRP.

## DIABETIC MACULAR EDEMA

Since the Early Treatment Diabetic Retinopathy Study (ETDRS) has documented the value of focal treatment for diabetic macular edema, many patients with macular edema are being treated with laser photocoagulation.[5] So-called focal treatment actually encompasses three components: (1) efforts to occlude microaneurysms using repeated application of a small spot to whiten or darken the microaneurysm; (2) grid treatment to areas of diffuse leakage; and (3), grid treatment to areas of retinal capillary nonperfusion.

While any wavelength can be used to apply grid treatment, green is best for focal occlusion of microaneurysms. For focal treatment, red is not nearly as effective because the hemoglobin does not absorb in the red range. Although yellow is probably comparable to green, its efficacy has not been assessed in any clinical studies with long-term followup. Consequently, for most patients with diabetic macular edema, I use argon green. However, for a patient with macular edema and a substantial cataract, one might need to use krypton red or dye red for grid treatment to areas of diffuse leakage and areas of nonperfusion. Similarly, to apply focal treatment to microaneurysms in a patient with a cataract would be difficult with green, impossible with red, and possible with yellow. The relative role of focal occlusion in comparison to grid treatment in the successful outcome of treatment is not clear.

At the 1990 ARVO meeting in Sarasota, Rutledge and Wallow from the University of Wisconsin at Madison reported the histopathologic features in more than 125 laser lesions of five eyes treated for macular edema, more or less in accordance with the ETDRS protocol.[6] For most treated lesions, most of the damage was confined to the RPE/choriocapillaris layer, the photoreceptor layer, and the outer nuclear layer, with practically no damage to the inner nuclear, ganglion cell, or nerve fiber layers. Since all wavelengths are absorbed by the RPE and spread to involve adjacent choriocapillaris and photoreceptors, it may be that wavelength selection is irrelevant in the laser management of diabetic macular edema.

In a relevant experiment performed in rabbits, Marshall at the University of London showed that after laser treatment to the macula, radioactive tritium uptake was greater in retinal capillary endothelial cells of krypton-treated eyes than it was in argon-treated eyes.[7] The tritium uptake as an indication of protein synthesis in capillaries undergoing mitosis and repair suggests a mechanism of action for laser treatment for macular edema not previously considered.

In any event, the value of treatment, in comparison to no treatment, is firmly established. The mechanism of improvement after laser treatment and the role of wavelength is arguable and certainly not settled.

## CHOROIDAL NEOVASCULARIZATION

When treating new vessel membranes (NVMs) 200 microns or greater from the center of the foveal avascular zone (FAZ), I generally employ argon green because

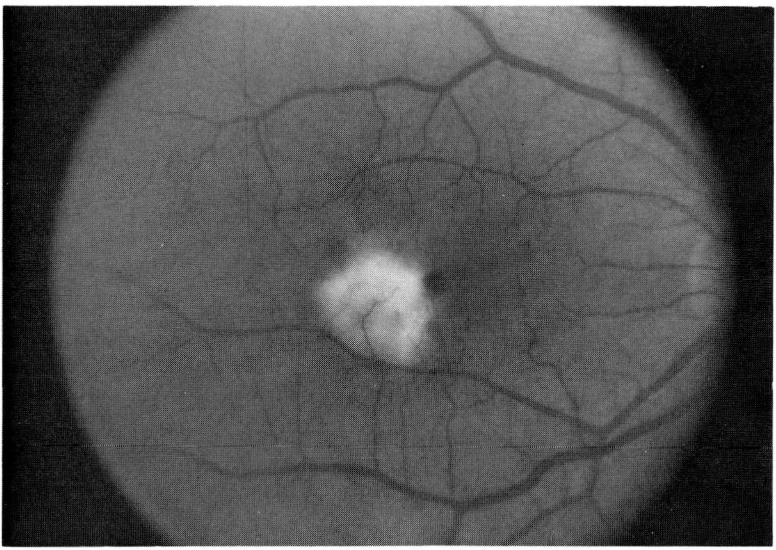

**FIGURE 29-7**  Photograph taken 12 hours after treatment of extrafoveal new vessel membrane with krypton red laser. Note intense "whitening" of pigment epithelium and retina.

the Macular Photocoagulation Study (MPS) has documented that argon laser treatment was preferable to observation in reducing the risk of severe vision loss in MPS-eligible eyes.[8] On the other hand, it seems likely that comparable results could be achieved using krypton red or dye red if all the other components of treatment, most particularly intense coagulations that cover the NVM adequately, are in place (Figure 29-7).

For the juxtafoveolar neovascular lesions in ocular histoplasmosis, I prefer krypton red or dye red for two reasons: (1) The MPS employed krypton red and documented the benefit of krypton red laser photocoagulation in comparison to no treatment;[9] and (2) histopathologic correlation shows that in the juxtafoveolar and peripapillary regions, krypton red tends to spare the inner retina from damage, in comparison to blue or blue-green (Figure 29-8).[4,10] Specifically, when human eyes to be enucleated for melanoma or primate eyes were used to assess laser damage of red versus green lesions delivered in a manner that simulated the treatment for choroidal neovascularization, there was full-thickness retinal destruction using blue-green, partial retinal destruction using green, and sparing of the inner retina using krypton red. All three wavelengths showed comparable destruction of choriocapillaris, RPE, and photoreceptors.

Should it become necessary to treat persistent or recurrent neovascular leakage and to extend the treatment into the laser scar, then one should anticipate full-thickness retinal destruction no matter which wavelength is used for the first or the subsequent treatment session. Because the retina is substantially thinned by the initial treatment, a second laser application several weeks or months later caused full-thickness retinal destruction in virtually every case in experimental primate eyes.[11]

Recent reports from MPS have emphasized the importance of covering the entire area of angiographically visible choroidal neovascularization with overlapping laser lesions of sufficient intensity to produce an endpoint of whiteness. The goal is to obliterate the NVM at the first treatment session. Following the MPS

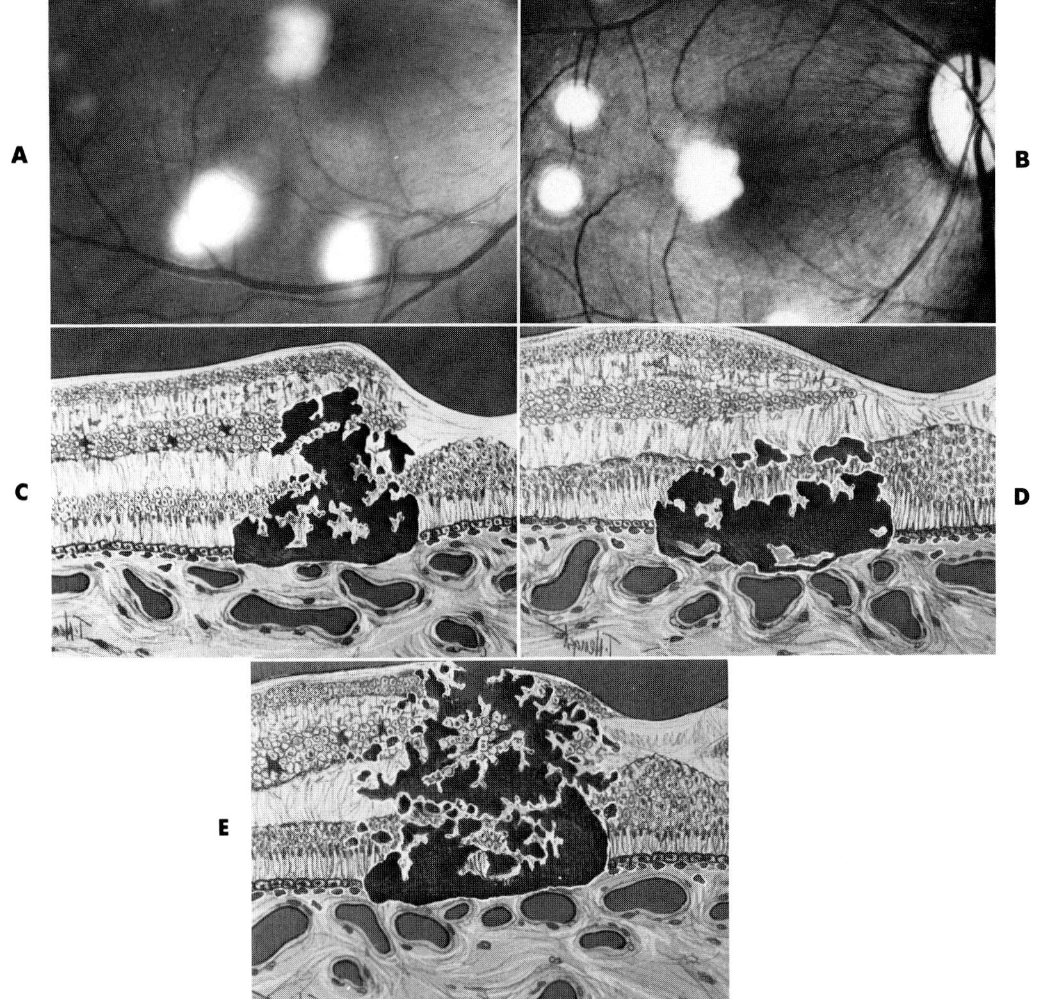

**FIGURE 29-8**  Clinicopathologic correlation of argon green and krypton red laser treatment in experimental primate eyes. **A,** Simulated treatment of juxtafoveal membrane with krypton red. **B,** Simulated treatment of juxtafoveal membrane with argon green. **C,** Sketch of histopathologic changes two weeks following krypton red treatment. Note loss of choriocapillaris, pigment epithelium, and outer two-thirds of retina with sparing of ganglion cell layer and nerve fiber layer. **D,** Sketch of histopathologic changes two weeks following krypton red treatment. Note loss of choriocapillaris, pigment epithelium, and outer half of retina. Note sparing of inner nuclear layer, ganglion cell layer, and nerve fiber layer. **E,** Sketch of histopathologic changes of simulated juxtafoveal lesion treated with argon blue-green laser. Note full-thickness retinal destruction.

treatment protocol to achieve this endpoint without treating an excessively large area of retina is associated with the best reported visual outcomes in treated eyes. It is not likely that achieving this goal has very much to do with wavelength selection, although that question is currently being addressed in three separate clinical trials for which data have not yet been reported.*

---

*(1) MPS trial of laser treatment for eyes with AMD and new subfoveal membranes; (2) MPS trial of laser treatment for eyes with AMD and recurrent subfoveal membranes; and (3) Canadian Study comparing argon with krypton laser treatment for eyes with neovascular membranes not involving the fovea.

## PIGMENT EPITHELIOPATHIES

For central serous chorioretinopathy and related conditions where laser applications of mild to moderate intensity are directed to focal leaks through the retinal pigment epithelium (RPE), any wavelength is satisfactory since all visible wavelengths are absorbed by melanin granules in the RPE. I generally choose green or red because those are the wavelengths with which I have had the most experience. I almost never treat serous detachments of the RPE that are not associated with choroidal neovascularization because there is no evidence that such treatment is preferable to observation, and there is at least one report indicating that laser treatment actually accelerates vision loss.[12]

However, if one were to treat serous RPE detachments, I think that any wavelength would be acceptable. In treating pigment epithelial detachments (PEDs) associated with choroidal NVMs, I would apply the same reasoning as that used in treating NVMs not associated with PEDs (i.e., green for extrafoveal membranes and red for juxtafoveal membranes or membranes in the papillomacular bundle).

## TUMORS

Vascular tumors, including retinal and choroidal hemangiomas, are uncommon. I treat retinal angiomas using two techniques of laser application. First, I treat the feeder vessel with repeated application of lesions lasting 0.5 to 1.0 second, applied repeatedly to the feeder vessel, while I apply pressure on the globe with a Goldmann contact lens in order to reduce flow in the central retinal artery. Second, I apply mild-intensity lesions in a scatter pattern over the surface of the tumor. I most often use green because of its absorption by hemoglobin. Undoubtedly, yellow would be acceptable because it has an absorption spectrum similar to that of green.

For the treatment of choroidal hemangioma, the use of green also has proven quite satisfactory. I can recall two occasions, however, when the availability of yellow has been important in the treatment of recurrent leakage from angiomas. One patient with a Von Hippel retinal angioma that apparently was closed five years earlier with argon green photocoagulation presented with recurrent tumor and localized preretinal hemorrhage. There were elevated feeder vessels in the mid-vitreous cavity. Yellow proved to be the most effective wavelength to close those feeder vessels.

Another patient treated successfully for choroidal hemangioma returned five years later with an accumulation of lipid around the base of an otherwise flat choroidal hemangioma laser-treatment scar. Apparently the lipid was leaking from viable vascular channels within the flat, atrophic, yellowish scar. Again, the yellow wavelength proved most advantageous in treating that lesion again.

## SUMMARY

A number of important points might influence the outcome in patients treated with photocoagulation. Perhaps nowhere are these more important than in the management of patients with choroidal neovascularization. I list the following considerations in order of importance in determining visual outcome:

1. Proper patient selection using criteria to identify eyes with discrete new vessel membranes not involving the center of the foveal avascular zone (FAZ).
2. Fluorescein angiograms with good resolution to identify the FAZ, the NVM, and their relationship to each other.
3. Use of posttreatment polaroid photographs to assess whether laser treatment has covered angiographically visible neovascularization.[13]
4. Informed consent that includes establishing the appropriate level of expectation on the part of the patient, the family, and the treating physician concerning a realistic outcome. Most patients with age-related macular degeneration and a NVM do not have good visual acuity with or without successful treatment.
5. Careful followup, including proper interpretation of the posttreatment angiogram and proper interpretation of the fundus findings, which might indicate the need for additional treatment or no additional treatment.
6. Wavelength. I believe that our ability to treat fundus diseases has been improved by the availability of a range of wavelengths, but I believe that wavelength plays a relatively minor role in comparison to the other considerations enumerated above.

## References


1. Diabetic Retinopathy Study Research Group. Preliminary report on effects of photocoagulation therapy. Am J Ophthalmol 1976; 81:1-14.
2. The Branch Vein Occlusion Study Group. Argon laser scatter photocoagulation for prevention of neovascularization and vitreous hemorrhage in branch vein occlusion. Arch Ophthalmol 1986; 104:34-41.
3. The Early Treatment Diabetic Retinopathy Study Research Group. Techniques for scatter and local photocoagulation treatment of diabetic retinopathy: Early Treatment Diabetic Retinopathy Study report no. 3. Int Ophthalmol Clin 1987; 27:254-264.
4. Smiddy WE, Fine SL, Green WR, Glaser BM. Clinicopathologic correlation of krypton red, argon blue-green, and argon green laser photocoagulation in the human fundus. Retina 1984; 4:15-21.
5. Early Treatment Diabetic Retinopathy Study Research Group. Photocoagulation for diabetic macular edema. Arch Ophthalmol 1985; 103:1796-1806.
6. Rutledge BK, Wallow IHL, Poulsen GL. Clinicopathologic correlation (CPC) of argon laser photocoagulation for diabetic macular edema. Invest Ophthalmol Vis Science 1990; 31:343.
7. Marshall J, Clover G, Rothery S. Some new findings on retinal irradiation by krypton and argon lasers. Doc Ophthalmol 1984; 36:21-37.
8. Macular Photocoagulation Study Group. Argon laser photocoagulation for senile macular degeneration: results of a randomized clinical trial. Arch Ophthalmol 1982; 100:912-918.
9. Macular Photocoagulation Study Group. Krypton laser photocoagulation for neovascular lesions of ocular histoplasmosis: results of a randomized clinical trial. Arch Ophthalmol 1987; 105:1499-1507.
10. Smiddy WE, Fine SL, Quigley HA, Hohman RM, Addicks EM. Comparison of krypton and argon laser photocoagulation in simulated clinical treatment of primate retina. Arch Ophthalmol 1984; 102:1086-1093.
11. Smiddy WE, Fine SL, Quigley HA, Hohman R, Dunkelberger G. Simulated treatment of recurrent choroidal neovascularization in primate retina. Arch Ophthalmol 1985; 103:428-433.
12. Moorfields Macular Study Group. Retinal pigment epithelial detachments in the elderly: a controlled clinical trial of laser. Brit J Ophthalmol 1982; 66:1-16.
13. Chamberlin JA, Bressler NM, Bressler SB, Elman MJ, Murphy RP, Fine SL, Macular Photocoagulation Study Group. Macular Photocoagulation Study Reading Center techniques to evaluate choroidal neovascularization and laser treatment. Ophthalmol 1988; 95(suppl):178.

# GRAND ROUNDS

# 30 Glaucoma and a Melanocytic Iris Lesion in an 18-Year-Old

**Presented by: Tamara R. Fountain**
**Discussed by: Morton F. Goldberg**
**Pathology Presented by: W. Richard Green**

**Dr. Goldberg:** Good afternoon. Who is presenting today's case?

**Dr. Fountain:** I am. Today's patient is an eighteen-year-old black male with unilateral glaucoma and a melanocytic iris lesion.

Report of case:

History: The patient was referred for evaluation of an increased cup-to-disc ratio noted at a routine examination. Past ocular history was negative except for wearing glasses for several years. A paternal uncle has glaucoma.

Examination:

**Manifest refraction:** OD $-0.25 + 0.50 \times 90 = 20/20$.
OS $-1.75 + 1.25 \times 97 = 20/40$.

**External examination:** The pupils were equal with a definite left afferent defect. The left pupil was round, though very sluggishly reactive, especially in the inferior temporal quadrant. The external exam was normal.

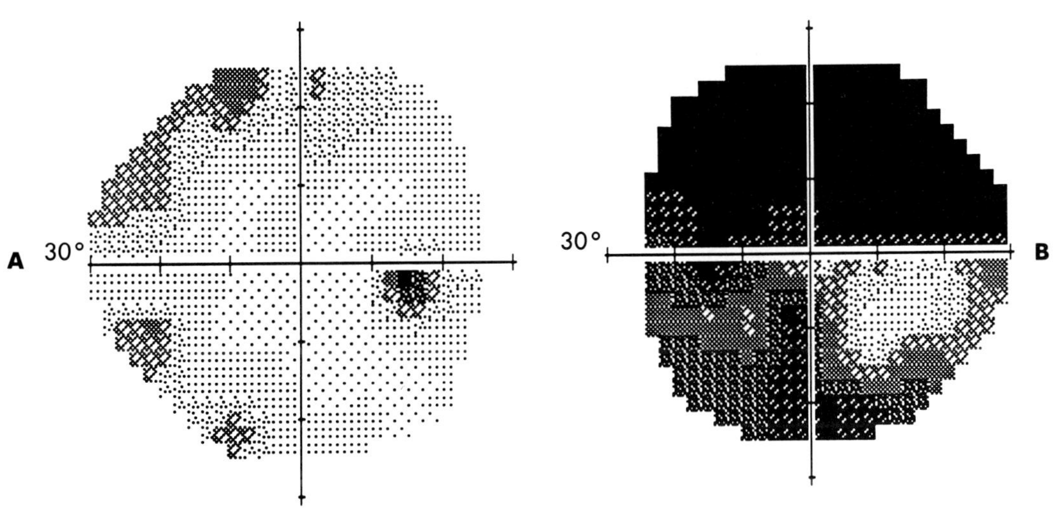

**FIGURE 30-1** Automated perimeter fields. **A,** Normal visual field, right eye. **B,** Dense superior defect, left eye, with residual nasal island.

"

**Visual fields and motility:** Automated perimeter fields showed a dense superior defect with generalized constriction OS (Figure 30-1). Extraocular motions were intact.

**Slit lamp examination:** Normal OD. The left eye was remarkable for multiple small slate-gray pigmentary episcleral patches with adjacent prominence of blood vessels. The cornea was clear. The iris was notable for a heavily pigmented, raised lesion measuring 6 × 2.5 × 1 mm extending from three-thirty to eight thirty o'clock (Figure 30-2). There was pigment speckled on the anterior lens capsule. The lens was clear. Gonioscopy demonstrated an elevated pigmented lesion extending from 3:30 to 8:00 with heavy pigment deposition of the trabecular meshwork for 360 degrees (Figure 30-3). The vitreous was free of cells.

**Tensions by applanation:** OD 12 mm Hg.

OS  35 mm Hg.

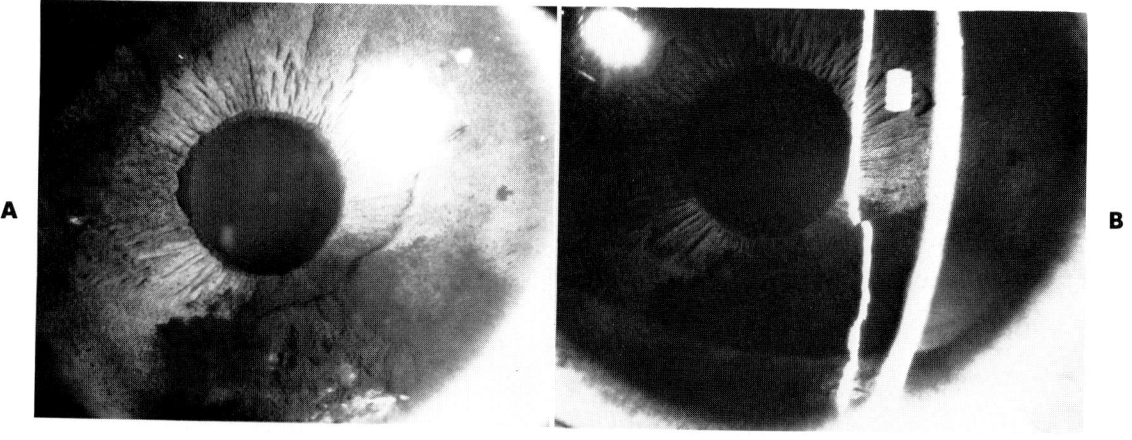

**FIGURE 30-2**    **A,** Iris lesion, relatively flat from 3:30 to 5:00, but then more elevated, extending to 8:30. **B,** Slit-beam photograph illustrating elevation of lesion.

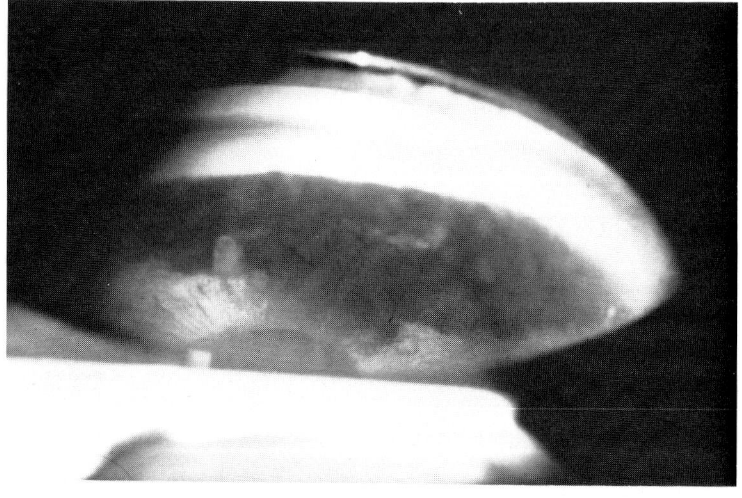

**FIGURE 30-3**    Gonioscopic view of the iris tumor.

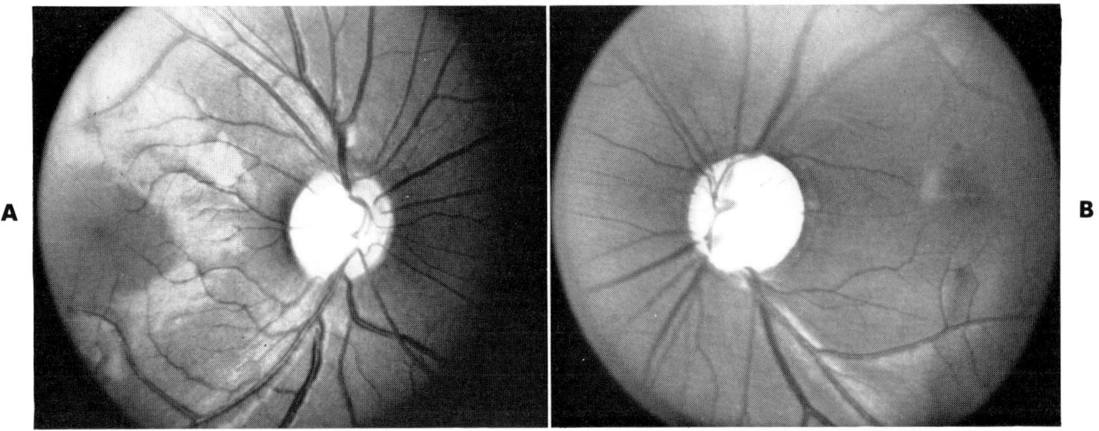

**FIGURE 30-4**    **A,** 0.5 cup-to-disc ratio, right eye. **B,** 1.0 cup-to-disc ratio, left eye.

**Fundus examination:** Showed a cup to disc ratio of 0.5 OD compared with a 1.0 ratio with a deeply excavated cup OS (Figure 30-4). The macula, vessels, and periphery were otherwise normal in both eyes.

**Laboratory:** A CT scan and bone-free plane films were negative for intraocular foreign body. Iris angiography showed no leak, even in the late frames. B-scan ultrasonography demonstrated the thickened inferior iris leaflet and marked optic disc cupping (Figure 30-5).

**Dr. Goldberg:** Thank you. Are the parents and grandparents all black?

**Dr. Fountain:** Yes.

**Dr. Goldberg:** What are sentinel vessels?

**Dr. Fountain:** They are abnormal dilated vessels visible in the sclera overlying a subjacent tumor. Although we noted some prominent vessels, true sentinel vessels were not noted in this case. We did not think that there was a ciliary body tumor.

**Dr. Goldberg:** What is the best kind of X-ray to diagnose a foreign body?

**Dr. Fountain:** Bone-free window-type studies are probably best. We also did an orbital CT scan.

**Dr. Goldberg:** What do you think about the results of the iris angiogram?

**Dr. Fountain:** I think that granulomas and most neoplasms will usually show at least some leakage, but this was not seen in this case.

*All participants recessed briefly to examine the patient. Dr. Goldberg pointed out a physical finding that had not been noted. There was a relative loss of the normal iris crypts on the superior "uninvolved" iris. The marked pigmentation in the angle was attributed to release of pigment and/or pigment containing cells from the lesion. A similar mechanism, layering of pigment cells on the superior iris stroma leading to a loss of the iris crypts, was also hypothesized.*

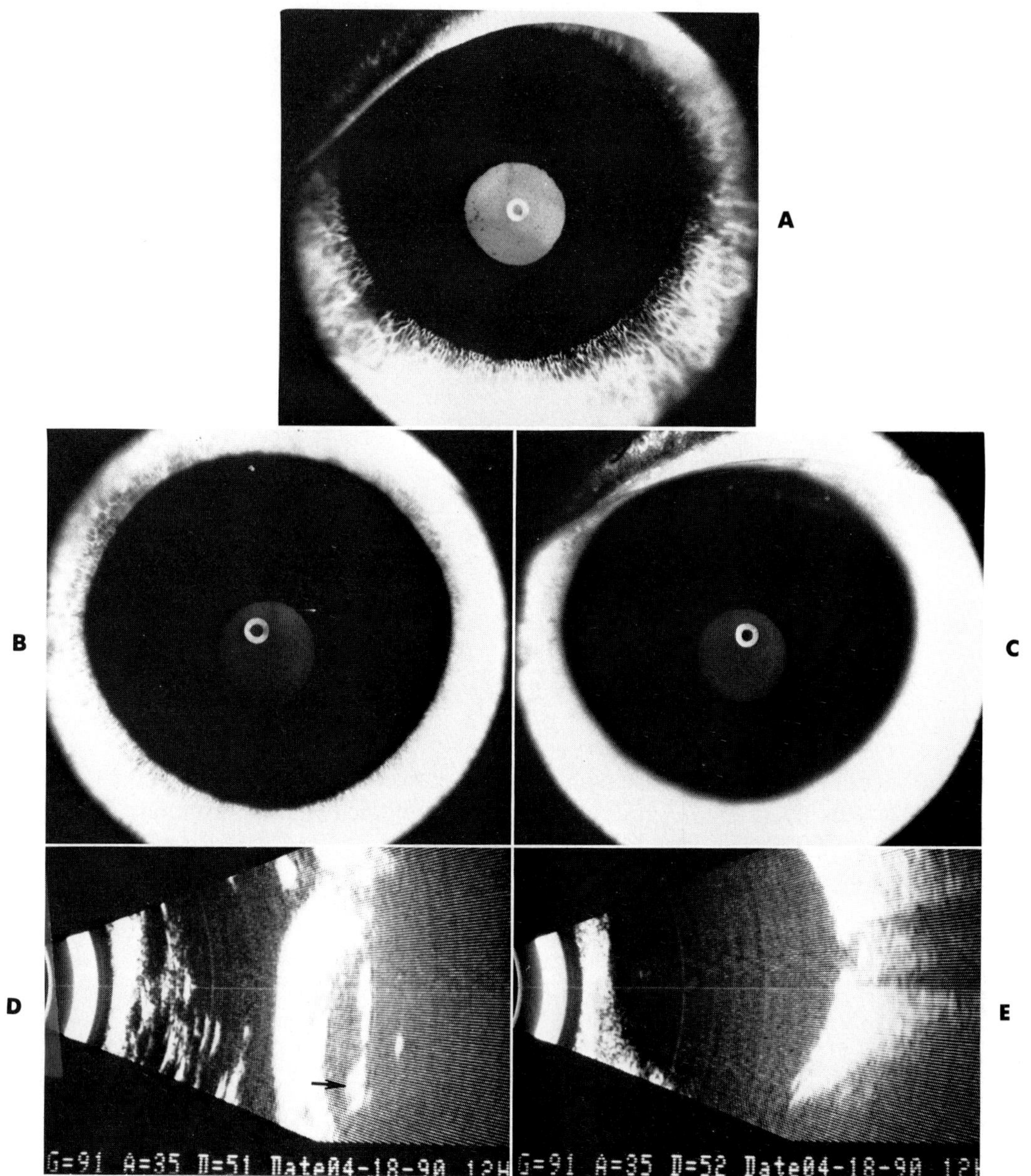

**FIGURE 30-5**     Iris angiography. **A,** Transit phase, 24 seconds. **B,** 123 seconds. **C,** 506 seconds. There is no late hyperfluorescence whatsoever. **D,** B-scan ultrasonography demonstrates thickening (arrow) of inferior iris leaflet and **E,** marked cupping of the optic disc.

**Dr. Goldberg:** Well, this is a fascinating patient. What are some of the diagnostic possibilities?

**Dr. Fountain:** The most likely lesions are nevus, melanoma, and melanocytoma. Alternative diagnoses include a long list of possibilities. (They are shown in the box on p. 375.)

## Dr. Fountain's Differential Diagnosis

Nevus
Melanoma
Melanocytoma
Foreign body
Irus nevus syndrome
Iridocorneal endothelial syndromes
Juvenile xanthogranuloma
Sarcoid and other granulomas
Primary iris cyst
Other iris cysts
Leiomyoma
Iris metastasis
Iris pigment epithelial hyperplasia
Rhabdomyosarcoma

**Dr. Goldberg:** Excellent. Which diagnosis do you favor? Let's go down the list and see which one is the most likely.

**Dr. Fountain:** Nevi, melanomas, and melanocytomas would be near the top of the list.

**Dr. Goldberg:** This is an eighteen-year-old black. Is melanoma likely?

**Dr. Fountain:** Well, melanomas are rare in blacks and, I suppose, rarer still in teenagers. But it is certainly possible.

**Dr. Goldberg:** In the past, certain clinical findings were felt to be clues that a lesion was more likely to be a melanoma than a nevus. Can you mention any?

**Dr. Fountain:** Features that previously have been felt to be clues that a lesion was malignant included growth across the angle, ectropion of the pupillary margin, and prominent vascularity. However, angle involvement and pupillary distortion are now known to be common features of nevi also, and I think prominent vascularity can be as well.

**Dr. Goldberg:** Good. Well, what are clinical features or clues that something is a melanoma and not a nevus?

**Dr. Fountain:** Evidence of growth and size are the most important factors. Melanomas are almost always 3 mm or more at the base and at least 1 mm thick, although so-called diffuse melanomas can be flatter. This lesion is big enough to be a melanoma. It is inferior, and iris melanomas are almost always inferiorly located. That may be related to light exposure. Secondary glaucoma, present in this case, is rarely seen with nevi. This is another reason melanoma is more likely than nevus.

**Dr. Goldberg:** What about melanocytoma?

**Dr. Fountain:** Unlike melanomas, which are uncommon in blacks, melanocytomas are more common in black patients than in white patients. This patient could easily have a necrotic melanocytoma. The marked pigment dispersion is typical, the dark color blocking a view of any vessels, and the host all make this a reasonable diagnosis. Melanocytomas are a subcategory of nevi, and this would be my number-one diagnosis.

**Dr. Goldberg:** Good. Let's quickly run down your other diagnoses.

**Dr. Fountain:** Foreign body should always be considered, especially in a young patient. The X-rays were negative, there is no previous history of significant trauma, and we looked carefully for a defect in Descemet's membrane but we could not identify a possible entry site. The secondary glaucoma would also be less likely, unless there was an inferior angle recession which has now closed up with PAS. The angle structures, where they can be seen, do not show recession.

**Dr. Goldberg:** OK. Let's continue down your list.

**Dr. Fountain:** Some of the iridocorneal endothelial syndromes are characterized by thinning, not thickening, of the stroma, so they can be ruled out. The iris nevus (Cogan-Reese) syndrome is possible, but we do not see multiple iris nodules and the PAS might be more prominent. Juvenile xanthogranuloma is not likely. The race of this patient makes sarcoidosis likely, but we have not seen prominent inflammation or keratic precipitates, and the chest X-ray was normal, as was the serum angiotensin–converting enzyme. Regarding a possible cyst, the lesion does not transilluminate and does not appear to be cystic. It is solid both clinically and on the ultrasound. Leiomyoma is rare, and I think that it is not usually so pigmented but I am not sure. The patient is healthy, and a metastasis in a eighteen year old must be very unlikely. The disc changes imply that the glaucoma has been present for some time, also making metastasis unlikely. One would have predicted that by this time the primary tumor would have caused symptoms. Rhabdomyosarcoma is vanishingly rare. Most likely, the tumor would be fast growing, making the chronic disc change less likely.

**Dr. Goldberg:** Good! It sounds like you favor melanocytoma or iris nevus. I think it is a partially necrotic melanocytoma, so I agree with you. How should we treat this, and how should we confirm the diagnosis?

**Dr. Fountain:** The patient has already been started on betagan and propine, and the pressure has come down to 30. I doubt that he would tolerate pilocarpine long term, or carbonic anhydrase medications for that matter. Argon laser trabeculoplasty might work, but only the superior half of the angle is visible, and I worry about scarring if one were to treat such a heavily pigmented angle. One option, if you are afraid he has a melanoma, is to treat the pressure topically and follow him. If the tumor grows or he gradually loses vision (he is 20/30 now) then one could do an enucleation.

**Dr. Goldberg:** What else?

**Dr. Fountain:** Iridocyclectomy is possible, but it would be rather extensive. The lesion involves the inferior six clock hours.

**Dr. Goldberg:** Are there other ways to diagnose this?

**Dr. Fountain:** There are no visible aqueous cells, so a paracentesis would probably be negative. At the time of an anterior chamber tap, you could rub the needle on the lesion or even put the needle into the lesion; but I suspect it would be hard for the cytopathologist to differentiate melanocytoma and melanoma reliably. Of course, you could do a diagnostic iridectomy or even a potential curative glaucoma-filtering procedure and do the inferior iridectomy at the same time.
**Dr. Goldberg:** What if it is a melanoma?

**Dr. Fountain:** Iris melanoma has very low metastasis rate. There is a tremendous amount of liberated pigment in this case; and if this is a melanoma, I suspect that there are tumor cells all over the angle and probably already outside the eye. Anyway, melanocytoma seems to be more likely.

**Dr. Goldberg:** I agree. How often do glaucoma-filtering procedures work, long term, in teenage blacks?

**Dr. Fountain:** We would probably use 5-FU in a young black patient. I need to ask Dr. Quigley or Dr. Jampel if they can estimate the success rate. I am not sure.*

*The patient was presented to W. R. Green, M.D., director of the Eye Pathology Laboratory. Dr. Green felt that the patient had a melanocytic lesion of the iris—a melanoma or nevus or possibly a melanocytoma. He suggested that an aspiration of aqueous with the bevel of the needle adjacent to the tumor could determine what type of cells were on the surface of the tumor and in the angle. Dr. Green also suggested a biopsy would be required to make a more definitive diagnosis. The patient was presented to A. E. Maumenee, M.D., director emeritus of the institute. Dr. Maumenee felt that the patient's medical regimen should be maximized by the addition of a carbonic anhydrase inhibitor. He agreed with trabeculectomy if medical therapy failed.*

**Dr. Goldberg's recommendation:** I think that you want a diagnosis. The patient can still see 20/30. You don't want to lose a very good eye. The risk of spreading the possible tumor is low. The situation should be discussed in detail with the patient and his parents. I recommend either of two approaches: (1) an incisional biopsy (through clear cornea to minimize conjunctival scarring) or an incisional biopsy followed by a filtering procedure superiorly if the lesion is not shown to be a melanoma; or (2) a simultaneous biopsy and filtering procedure performed either at the site of the biopsy inferiorly or at a separate site superiorly. In view of the widespread iris involvement, large tumor size, and advanced state of the glaucomatous optic nerve damage, I would not wait for further growth or attempts at topical pharmacotherapy of the glaucoma.

---

*Dr. Quigley, estimated that with 5-FU, the success rate for filtering surgery was near 0 in patients less than 8 years of age and rose to 80% in patients older than 21 but that the success rate has not been specifically studied in this patient's age group.

## SUMMARY

**Dr. Goldberg's diagnosis and recommendation:** Iris melanocytoma. A diagnostic iridectomy with or without a filtering procedure was recommended.

**Dr. Green's diagnosis and recommendation:** Melanocytoma rather than melanoma. A needle biopsy or diagnostic biopsy was recommended.

**Dr. Maumenee's diagnosis and recommendation:** Melanocytoma rather than nevus or melanoma. Medical management of the glaucoma but no diagnostic procedure was recommended. Biopsy was not recommended unless it was planned as part of a glaucoma-filtering procedure.

**Dr. Fountain's decision:** The issues were discussed in detail with the patient and his family. A course of medical management of the glaucoma was planned.

## CONCLUSION

The patient was started on a topical beta-blocker, epinephrine, and pilocarpine. The pressure dropped to 20 mm Hg but then promptly rose to 30 mm Hg. Acetazolamide was not well tolerated, and methazolamide was substituted, but the pressure was 32. Prior to a planned filtering procedure, an inferior partial iridectomy was performed.

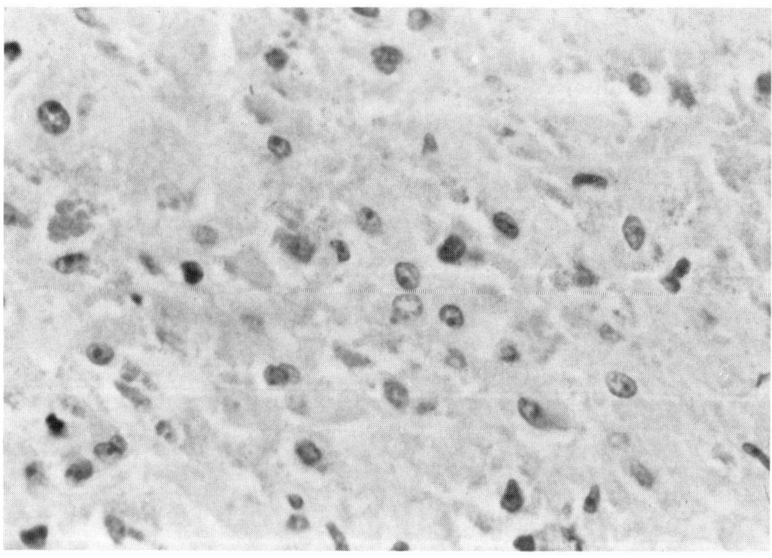

**FIGURE 30-6**     Melanocytoma composed of large, fairly uniform, plump round or oval cells with abundant, densely pigmented cytoplasm and small nuclei with a small nucleolus.

**Dr. Green's Pathology Report:**

**Microscopic:** Exam reveals a densely pigmented iris tumor composed of large, fairly uniform, plump round or oval cells with abundant, densely pigmented cytoplasm and small nuclei with a small nucleolus. A more prominent nucleolus is present in some cells. Other large round cells with similar features but having clumped pigment (macrophages) were scattered throughout the lesion. A few interspersed spindle-shaped cells are present. No mitoses are present per 40 HPF (Figure 30-6).

**Transmission electron microscopy:** Examination of 1-micron-thick section of epon-embedded sections shows a densely pigmented iris tumor composed of large, plump, round or oval cells with a distended cytoplasm containing uniform spherical pigment granules and small, fairly uniform nuclei, some of which have a prominent nucleolus. Similar cells contain nonuniform pigment with some aggregates of pigment granules. There are two populations of cells—one of which is uniformly packed with round or oval-shaped pigment granules 230 to 650 microns in diameter. These pigment granules do not appear to be enclosed by a membrane (Figure 30-7).

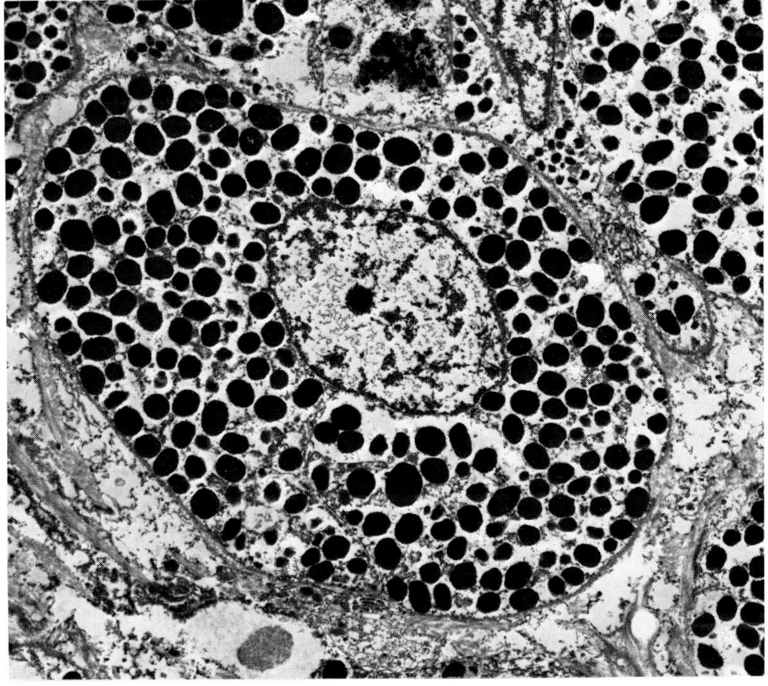

**FIGURE 30-7**     Transmission electron micrograph of melanocytoma cells. EP86044, × 5,000.

A second population of cells consists of macrophages, which contain aggregates of similar pigment granules in a background of finely granular material (Figure 30-8). No distinct membrane is seen around most of these phagosomes. No basement membrane or junctional complexes are seen on either cell type. Large collagen, 50 to 75 microns in diameter, is interspersed between the cells.

**Dr. Green's diagnosis:** Iris melanocytoma.

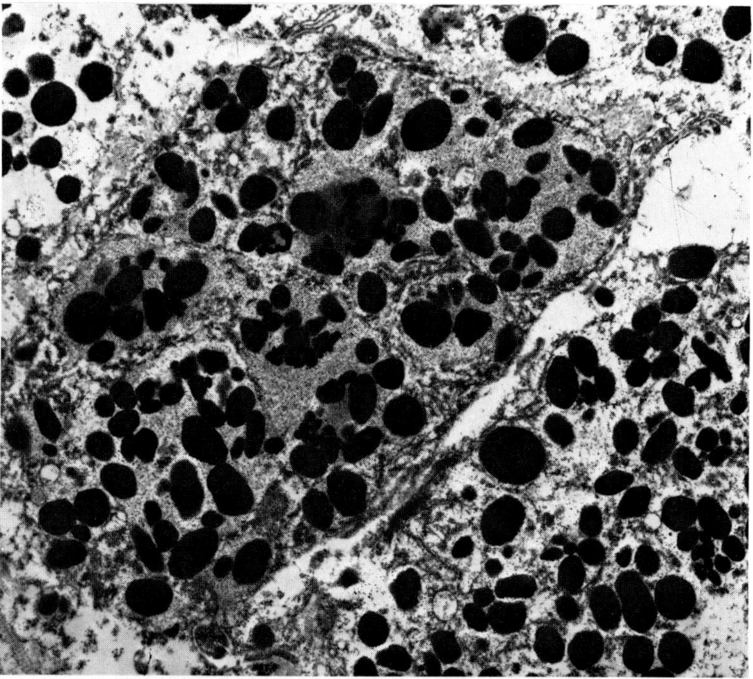

**FIGURE 30-8**     Transmission electron micrograph of macrophages. EP86044, × 10,500.

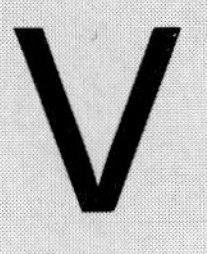



# PART V

# LITERATURE COMMENTARY

# 31

# A Comparison of the Radiation Dose to the Lens of the Eye from Four Modern C T Scanners

**Lawrence W. Hirst, MD**
Professor of Ophthalmology
University of Queensland Lions
Brisbane, Australia

This study examined the radiation dose to which the crystalline lens is exposed during computerized tomography scanning using a phantom model on five current-generation computerized tomography scanners. Using 3-mm slices in a fashion similar to what would normally be part of a routine scanning plan for the head, the five scanners delivered from 25-milli Gray (mGy) to 49-mGy doses. Slice thickness, interslice gap, and half value layer (HVL) are important parameters determining the final dose for the crystalline lens. It is suggested that it would be conceivable that a dose of 1400 mGy could be given with a single scan.

Sim LH, Case CC. *Australasian Physical and Engineering Sciences in Medicine* 1988; 11(2):76-80.

## COMMENT

Although it would appear that 10 Gy units are needed in a single dose invariably to lead to delayed cataract formation, the doses achieved with single, maximal scanning of an eye would be at least one order of magnitude less than this. Nonetheless, it becomes clear that a consequential dose of radiation is delivered to the eye if the phantom model was appropriately constituted. The effect of repeated scans and the resultant cumulative radiation dose and its influence on cataractogenesis remains unclear. However, the knowledge that a dose of up to 1400 mGy can be delivered to the lens by a lengthy examination with and without contrast, with parameters set that raise radiation exposure, should lead radiologists to evaluate carefully the parameters they use in routine scanning and minimize radiation exposure to the lens.

# 32

# Perifoveal Photocoagulation for Subfoveal Subretinal New Vessels with Monochromatic Laser and Dye Laser

**Gisèle Soubrane, MD**
University of Créteil France


Subfoveal new vessels are not at present considered amenable to laser treatment. The goal of the perifoveal technique is to treat large, subfoveal new vessels in which the peripheral neovascular network extends more than 200 microns from the fovea, in order to obtain an atrophic, flat scar allowing visual rehabilitation.

The treatment approach is to occlude the entire membrane with overlapping, intense burns but spare the foveal avascular zone. A randomized controlled trial is under way to evaluate the benefit of this treatment.

To evaluate the effect of the different wavelengths of the dye laser in a clinical setting, the perifoveal technic was applied. The area to be photocoagulated was divided into 4 quadrants in which the following wavelengths were used: 578 nm (yellow), 590 nm (orange) or 514 nm (green), 600 nm (orange), and 640 nm (red).

Use of the green wavelength (514 nm) resulted in occlusion of the retinal capillaries overlying the photocoagulation site. The choriocapillaris was no longer visible. The red wavelength (640 nm) caused an early exudative response in the treated area, with a sparing of the retinal capillaries. With the yellow wavelength (578 nm), the exudation was moderate. The capillary bed of the retina and of the choriocapillaris was disturbed. There was no clinical or angiographic difference between 590 nm and 600 nm (orange). Both wavelengths resulted in an atrophic scar. Two months after treatment, all parts of the scars were comparable.

In the perifoveal photocoagulation, all wavelengths studied demonstrated a similar efficacy in occluding the large subfoveal membranes.

Coscas G, Ramahefasolo C, Soubrane G. *Bull Soc Ophthalmol Fr* 1989; 8-9:1017-1022.

## COMMENT

This inventive approach was selected to compare the effect of different wavelengths in the same neovascular lesion in a diseased eye. However, due to the high level of energy required by the treatment of subretinal new vessels, it is not surprising that no major difference could be observed. One of the areas where the absorption of the different wavelengths varies theoretically is the xanthophill pigment, in which no burns were applied according to the perifoveal technic. Differences might have been observed if subfoveal treatment techniques had been employed.

# 33

# Clinical Results of Multifocal Lens Implantation

**Francesco Bandello, MD**
Department of Ophthalmology
University of Milan, Italy

The authors report on their clinical experience with a new multifocal anterior-chamber IOL manufactured by 3M Vision Care (St. Paul, Minn.). They report the results obtained in a group of ten patients with their IOLs implanted in the sulcus after cataract extracapsular extraction. The cases were observed within the context of a multicenter clinical trial supervised by FDA.

One month after intervention, corrected mean visual acuity was 6.9 (median 0.7, range 0.6-0.9). The near visual acuity with distance correction in place was at least Jaeger 2 in all cases and Jaeger 1 in four.

A glare test (Brightness Acuity Tester) demonstrated a reduction from 0.12 to 0.37 lines from the lowest to the highest brightness level.

Brancato R, Menchini U, Scialdone A, et al. First Clinical Results of a New Multifocal IOL with Diffractive Optics, *Italian Journal of Ophthalmology* 1989; 3:35-39.

The authors report their clinical experience with a multifocal posterior-chamber IOL. The optic diameter of this polypropylene lens, manufactured by IOLAB, is 7 mm. The lens is provided with two C-flex loops for capsular bag and sulcus fixation. Its major advantage is good visual acuity for either distance or near vision with no need for further correction.

A group of ten patients within an international protocol supervised by FDA underwent extracapsular cataract extraction with IOL implantation in the bag (nine cases) and in the sulcus (one case).

Corrected distance visual acuity was 0.8 and more in nine cases (near vision: Jaeger 1). In these patients, Brightness Acuity Test demonstrated a reduction of visual acuity equal to 10% in presence of high light.

No relevant intraoperative or postoperative complications occurred. The mean followup lasted eight months for all patients.

Frezzotti R, Caporossi A, Simi C. Clinical Results of Multifocal Lens Implantation, *Italian Journal of Ophthalmology* 1989; 3:31-34.

## COMMENT

At present, extracapsular cataract extraction with posterior-chamber IOL implantation is the standard cataract surgical technique in Italy. Multifocal intraocular

IOLs are technically innovative and provide a correction for near visual acuity with no need for optical correction, and consequent greater comfort for the operated patients.

The absence of remarkable side-effects evidenced in these two studies, despite the small number of cases, leads to the conclusion that this new type of intraocular lenses may improve the quality of life for pseudophakic patients.

# 34 Retinoscopy at Two Meters
## A Test to Detect Amblyogenic Factors in Preverbal Children

**Carlos A. Moreira, Jr., MD**
Prof de Oftalmologia da Fac Evangelica de Medicina
Curitiba, Brasil

To detect amblyogenic factors in the preverbal population, mainly aniso-metropia, the authors conducted a prospective study on 100 children. Eighty percent were less than 2 years old. Retinoscopy at two meters was performed by a nonmedical technician. The results were expressed as symmetrical or asymmetrical and compared to refractions made by an ophthalmologist in a double-blind mode. The number of positive and negative findings were highly concordant ($p = 0.005$). The high sensitivity (77%) and specificity (90%) of this simple test lead the authors to recommend it for amblyopia screening programs. Only one of the children did not cooperate for the testing.

Brik M, Brik D. *Arquivos Brasileiros de Oftalmologia* 1989; 52:108-109.

## COMMENT

Of all amblyogenic factors, anisometropia may be the most difficult to diagnose at an early stage. The present work describes retinoscopy at two meters as a simple method to detect anisometropia, media opacities, and strabismus in preverbal children. Advantages of this test are that it can be performed by a technician; there is little contact with the infants to be examined; and there is no need for pupil dilation. Results were recorded, with regard to the intensity of fundus reflex, as symmetrical or asymmetrical. Later they were compared to the results of conventional refraction made by an ophthalmologist. Results proved highly concordant by statistical analysis. The simplicity and reliability of this test indicate that it may be useful as a component of some amblyopia screening programs.

# Index



---

Tables are indicated by *t*. Figures are indicated by *f*.